CRC
Handbook
of the
Laboratory Diagnosis
and
Treatment of Infertility

Editors

Brooks A. Keel

Associate Professor
Department of Obstetrics and Gynecology
Director, Reproductive Medicine Laboratories
Scientific Director
Women's Research Institute
University of Kansas School of Medicine
Wichita, Kansas

Bobby W. Webster

Associate Professor
Director, Division of Reproductive Endocrinology
Department of Obstetrics and Gynecology
University of Kansas School of Medicine
Wichita, Kansas

CRC Press
Boca Raton   Ann Arbor   Boston

Library of Congress Cataloging-in-Publication Data

Handbook of the laboratory diagnosis and treatment of infertility/
    editors. Brooks A. Keel, Bobby W. Webster.
        p.   cm.
    Includes bibliographical references.
    ISBN 0-8493-3549-3
    1. Infertility—Diagnosis—Handbooks, manuals, etc. 2. Diagnosis,
    Laboratory—Handbooks, manuals, etc. I. Keel, Brooks, A.
    II. Webster, Bobby W.
        [DNLM: 1. Diagnosis, Laboratory—methods—handbooks.
    2. Infertility—diagnosis—handbooks. WP 39 H236]
    RC889.H258   1990
    616.6'92—dc20
    DNLM/DLC
    for Library of Congress   90-1661
                                                                                      CIP

Direct all inquiries to CRC Press, Inc., 2000 Corporate Blvd., N.W., Boca Raton, Florida 33431.

© 1990 by CRC Press, Inc.

International Standard Book Number 0-8493-3549-3

Library of Congress Card Number 90-1661
Printed in the United States

FOREWORD

Those who work in the field of reproductive medicine can no longer isolate themselves as clinicians vs. basic scientists vs. technicians. We must all speak the same language and speak it knowledgeably. Each of us must actively enhance our understanding of the methodology and application of the increasingly numerous tests becoming available, and interact with one another. Doctors Keel and Webster have taken the initiative in this book. Their leadership will ensure that IVF, GIFT, ZIFT, PROST, and TET have meaning other than as letters of the alphabet, and that the term 'sperm micro-injection' will not be taken lightly.

This book presents for technician and physician alike a single source of expert and practical advice on laboratory testing of infertility. The editors have very successfully convinced some of the most expert individuals in the field to participate in its production. With these resources, they have put together a handbook that not only tells you what tests should be done, but when they should be done. The text takes you from the drawing of the blood or collection of the specimen, to the finished product, and covers every step in between. It discusses the choosing of the appropriate solution, how to mix it, and how to use it. It suggests appropriate containers, glassware, and pipettes necessary for each test, and at what temperature the test should be performed. It speaks to the pitfalls that can be encountered, and discusses normal, abnormal, and erroneous results that could be received. It elucidates the newest equipment and identified sources for materials. It also lists laboratories with special facilities and individuals with special expertise available for reference.

This book encompasses the entire field of reproductive laboratory technique and its interpretation. Its authoritative, concrete, ''hands-on'' approach will be of invaluable assistance to me as a gynecologist, pathologist, and reproductive laboratory director. It will serve as an excellent guide for my technicians as well.

The two editors are themselves well-known experts in this field, and run one of the outstanding reproductive centers in the country. Their center is unique in its synthesis of basic science, clinical laboratory, and patient management principles. I praise Doctors Keel and Webster for having taken of their time and talent to put this book together and to have assembled such an astute group of authors. They have provided an important service to us all.

Daniel K. Roberts, M.D., Ph.D.
Professor and Chairman
Department of Obstetrics
  and Gynecology
University of Kansas School
  of Medicine-Wichita
HCA/Wesley Medical Center
Wichita, Kansas

PREFACE

It has been estimated that 1 in 6 couples suffers from infertility. With the advent of *in vitro* fertilization and its related technologies a virtual knowledge explosion has occurred concerning the laboratory diagnosis and treatment of infertility. As a consequence of this new and rapidly progressing field, laboratory and clinic personnel are performing a variety of novel and highly sophisticated procedures often without benefit of a detailed laboratory handbook or procedure manual. The objective of this publication is to provide both the clinician and technician with a comprehensive, detailed, and step-by-step handbook describing the various procedures frequently utilized in the infertility clinic. The resulting product represents a materials and methods ''notebook'' which can be used at the bench by a technician or clinician who has a basic knowledge of general laboratory procedures. The information contained is detailed enough to allow accurate performance of the procedure, specific enough to ensure accurate interpretation of results, and general enough to enable an individual not familiar with infertility testing to comprehend the scope and importance of the procedure. It was our hope that each chapter would provide enough background to interest and assist the clinician who may not wish to perform the tests himself but who desires sufficient information to become knowledgeable about when to order the procedure, how to interpret the results, and how to fit the results into the scheme of the infertility workup. Emphasis has been placed on detailed methodology, buffer recipes, equipment, and supplies required, and quality control procedures. An appendix was constructed to provide details on the various buffer and reagents used, addresses of suppliers, and forms referenced throughout the book. In short, this handbook provides the necessary information to allow the clinician and/or technician to accurately perform and interpret the described procedures.

This handbook has been generally organized such that the techniques involved in the routine laboratory evaluation and treatment of the male and female partner are presented. These topics include (1) the analysis of sperm and seminal plasma, including sperm motility and kinematics as well as *in vitro* sperm concentration techniques, (2) cryopreservation of sperm, (3) the evaluation of cervical mucus and sperm-mucus interaction, (4) antisperm antibody detection, (5) sperm penetration assays, and (6) serum hormone assays. In addition, the general infertility evaluation and other clinical diagnostic procedures, such as the microbiological examination of the couple, and the endometrial biopsy are discussed. Finally, the laboratory techniques involved in the evaluation and cryopreservation of human oocytes and pre-embryos and in the set up and quality control monitoring of the *in vitro* fertilization/ embryo transfer laboratory are provided in detail.

The book was designed by inviting a group of internationally recognized experts in the field of infertility diagnosis and treatment to describe in detail the various clinicial tests currently utilized in their respective laboratories and clinics. We have allowed these experts freedom in terms of the organization and presentation of their information which has resulted in a most interesting blend of presentation style and scientific interpretation of the various procedures. Clearly, although the clinical usefulness and interpretation of the information derived from some of these techniques may be debated, we believe that this single text represents a comprehensive coverage of the state-of-the-art techniques and procedures currently used in the practice of the laboratory diagnosis and treatment of infertility. It is our hope that this text may serve as a guide for current investigation and as a stimulus for future developments in the field.

Brooks A. Keel, Ph.D.
Bobby W. Webster, M.D.

THE EDITORS

Brooks A. Keel, Ph.D., is Associate Professor of Obstetrics and Gynecology and Pathology at the University of Kansas School of Medicine-Wichita, and Adjunct Professor of Clinical Sciences at The Wichita State University. Dr. Keel serves as Scientific Director of The Women's Research Institute, the Director of the Reproductive Medicine Laboratories, and is an Andrologist for the Center for Reproductive Medicine in Wichita, Kansas.

Dr. Keel received his B.S. degree in biology from Augusta College in 1978 and his Ph.D. in endocrinology from the Medical College of Georgia in 1982. Dr. Keel completed 3 years of postdoctoral training in reproductive endocrinology at the University of Texas Health Science Center in Houston and the University of South Dakota School of Medicine in Vermillion. He accepted his current position in 1985. Dr. Keel has been certified as a Clinical Laboratory Director by the American Board of Bioanalysis since 1987.

Dr. Keel is a member of the Endocrine Society, the Society for the Study of Reproduction, the American Society of Andrology and the American Fertility Society. He also serves on the editorial board for *Archives of Andrology* and *Biology of Reproduction*. Dr. Keel has published more than forty publications in national and international journals and has served as editor on several books in the area of reproductive endocrinology.

Dr. Keel's research interests include the study of physiological role and biochemical basis for glycoprotein heterogeneity, and the mechanisms controlling pituitary-testicular function. His grant support is from the Wesley Medical Research Institutes, The Wesley Foundation, the Women's Research Institute, and the National Institutes of Health.

Bobby W. Webster, M.D., is an Associate Professor of Obstetrics and Gynecology at the University of Kansas School of Medicine-Wichita, and Adjunct Professor of Clinical Sciences at The Wichita State University. Dr. Webster is Director, Division of Reproductive Endocrinology and Fertility, Department of Obstetrics and Gynecology and Director of the Center for Reproductive Medicine, and President and CEO of the Women's Research Institute, Wichita, Kansas.

Dr. Webster did his undergraduate work in Pharmacy at Southwestern Oklahoma State University. He attended Medical School at the University of Texas in Galveston and completed a residency in Obstetrics and Gynecology at the University of Kansas School of Medicine-Wichita.

Dr. Webster had a General Obstetrics and Gynecology practice in Wichita before completing a Fellowship in Reproductive Endocrinology at Vanderbilt University in Nashville, Tennessee. He is Board-certified in General Obstetrics and Gynecology as well as in the sub-speciality of Reproductive Endocrinology and Infertility.

Dr. Webster is a member of The Society of Reproductive Endocrinologists, The American Fertility Society, Society for the Study of Reproduction and The Society of Reproductive Surgeons.

EDITORIAL ADVISORY BOARD

To facilitate this undertaking, an Advisory Board of recognized authorities was organized. This board assisted the editors in evaluating the data and information for accuracy and made suggestions concerning the organization and presentation of the information. The editors wish to express their appreciation to these individuals for their participation. Their input and support have been invaluable.

CONTRIBUTORS

Anibal A. Acosta
Professor
Department of Obstetrics and
  Gynecology
The Jones Institute for Reproductive
  Medicine
Eastern Virginia Medical School
Norfolk, Virginia

Nancy J. Alexander
Professor
Department of Obstetrics and
  Gynecology
Eastern Virginia Medical School
Norfolk, Virginia

Brenda Bassham
Senior Research Assistant
Laboratory for Male Reproductive
  Research and Testing
Scott Department of Urology
Baylor College of Medicine
Houston, Texas

Lani Johnson Burkman
Assistant Professor
Department of Obstetrics and
  Gynecology
The Jones Institute Research
  Laboratories
Eastern Virginia Medical School
Norfolk, Virginia

Gary N. Clarke
Senior Scientist
Department of Pathology
Royal Women's Hospital
Carlton, Victoria, Canada

Charles C. Coddington, III
Assistant Professor
Department of Obstetrics and
  Gynecology
The Jones Institute for Reproductive
  Medicine
Eastern Virginia Medical School
Norfolk, Virginia

Andrew S. Cook
Chief Resident
Department of Obstetrics and
  Gynecology
School of Medicine
University of Kansas
Wichita, Kansas

William E. Findley
Assistant Professor
Director of Research and Quality
  Assurance
Division of Reproductive Endocrinology
Department of Obstetrics and
  Gynecology
Baylor College of Medicine
Houston, Texas

Daniel Franken
Head
Infertility Laboratory
University of Stellenbosch
Tygerberg Hospital
Tygerberg, South Africa

David L. Fulgham
Senior Research Associate and Project
  Officer
Department of Obstetrics and
  Gynecology
Eastern Virginia Medical School
Norfolk, Virginia

Catherine Garner
Administrative Director
Reproductive Resource Center
Overland Park, Kansas

William E. Gibbons
Associate Professor
Director, Division of Reproductive
  Endocrinology
Department of Obstetrics and
  Gynecology
Baylor College of Medicine
Houston, Texas

Ruth Greenblatt
Assistant Professor
Department of Medicine
University of California
San Francisco, California

Kelly K. Hanshew
Laboratory Manager
IVF Laboratory
Department of Obstetrics and
 Gynecology
H.C.A. Wesley Medical Center
Wichita, Kansas

Gary D. Hodgen
Professor and Scientific Director
Department of Obstetrics and
 Gynecology
The Jones Institute for Reproductive
 Medicine
Eastern Virginia Medical School
Norfolk, Virginia

Brooks A. Keel
Associate Professor
Department of Obstetrics and
 Gynecology
University of Kansas School of
 Medicine-Wichita
Scientific Director
Women's Research Institute
Wichita, Kansas

Mary K. Korte
Laboratory Technologist
Department of Obstetrics and
 Gynecology
Immunoinfertility Laboratory
University of Michigan Hospitals
Ann Arbor, Michigan

Rajasingam S. Jeyendran
Associate Professor
Department of Obstetrics and
 Gynecology
Northwestern University Medical School
Chicago, Illinois

Aron Johnson
Research Associate
Scott Department of Urology
Baylor College of Medicine
Houston, Texas

Thinus Kruger
Professor
University of Stellenbosch
Tygerberg Hospital
Tygerberg, South Africa

Dolores J. Lamb
Director of Laboratory for Male
 Reproductive Research and Testing
Assistant Professor of Urology, and
Assistant Professor of Cell Biology
Scott Department of Urology and Cell
 Biology
Baylor College of Medicine
Houston, Texas

Larry I. Lipschultz
Professor
Scott Department of Urology
Laboratory for Male Reproductive
 Research and Testing
Baylor College of Medicine
Houston, Texas

Richard P. Marrs
Director
Institute for Reproductive Research
Hospital of the Good Samaritan
Los Angeles, California

Jeffrey V. May
Assistant Professor
Department of Obstetrics and
 Gynecology
Director of IVF/ET Laboratory
University of Kansas School of
 Medicine-Wichita
Wichita, Kansas

Alan C. Menge
Professor
Department of Obstetrics and
 Gynecology
University of Michigan
Ann Arbor, Michigan

Kamran S. Moghissi
Professor and Chairman
Department of Obstetrics and
 Gynecology
Wayne State University
Detroit, Michigan

David Mortimer
Associate Professor
Department of Obstetrics and
 Gynaecology
University of Calgary
Calgary, Alberta, Canada

Sergio Oehninger
Assistant Professor
Department of Obstetrics and
 Gynecology
The Jones Institute for Reproductive
 Medicine
Eastern Virginia Medical School
Norfolk, Virginia

Michael P. O'Leary
Assistant Professor of Urology
Tufts University School of Medicine
Director of Andrology
New England Medical Centers Hospitals
Boston, Massachusetts

Tim H. Parmley
Professor
Department of Obstetrics, Gynecology
 and Pathology
University of Arkansas for Medical
 Sciences
Little Rock, Arkansas

Patrick Quinn
Director of Gamete Laboratories
Institute for Reproductive Research
Hospital of the Good Samaritan
Los Angeles, California

Jerome K. Sherman
Professor
Department of Anatomy
University of Arkansas for Medical
 Sciences
Little Rock, Arkansas

Ajit K. Thakur
Principal Scientist and Biostatistician
Department of Biostatistics
Hazleton Laboratories America, Inc.
Vienna, Virginia

Lucinda L. Veeck
Director of Embryology
Department of Obstetrics and
 Gynecology
Eastern Virginia Medical School
Norfolk, Virginia

Bobby W. Webster
Associate Professor and Director
Division of Reproductive Endocrinology
Department of Obstetrics and
 Gynecology
University of Kansas School of
 Medicine-Wichita
Wichita, Kansas

Lourens J. D. Zaneveld
Professor
Department of Obstetrics and
 Gynecology, and Department of
 Biochemistry
Rush University
Rush-Presbyterian-St. Luke's Medical
 Center
Chicago, Illinois

TABLE OF CONTENTS

Chapter 1

THE INFERTILITY EVALUATION

Bobby W. Webster, Andrews S. Cook, and Catherine H. Garner

TABLE OF CONTENTS

I. INTRODUCTION

Infertility, generally defined as the inability to conceive after 1 year of unprotected intercourse, is a medical tragedy to most affected couples and deserves the same diagnostic consideration and expertise as any other complicated medical problem. With the rising incidence of infertility has come greater demands upon clinicians and scientists interested in both the diagnosis and management of problems in this increasingly complex area of medicine.

Contributing factors to this rising incidence and subsequent increasing patient demands for services include:

1. Increasing tendency to postpone childbearing until after age 30 because of education and/or career goals
2. Widespread availability and use of various contraception methods decreasing the number of unplanned conceptions
3. Liberalization of abortion laws with the subsequent decrease in the numbers of babies available for adoption
4. Increasing incidence of the numbers of single women choosing to raise children as a single parent
5. Rising incidence of multiple sexual partners and its attendant risk of contracting a sexually transmitted disease resulting in damage to the reproductive organs

The infertility evaluation is unique in that one deals with a biologic unit consisting of two adults. This biologic unit is failing to function as expected and potentially may stress the very foundation of the relationship. The problem of infertility must be addressed with honesty and meticulous attention to detail both on the part of the physician and the couple. The evaluation should proceed rapidly and efficiently in an attempt to make a diagnosis and provide answers, explanations, and a prognosis. Once a diagnosis is made, efforts should then be directed at correcting the problem(s) in the most efficient manner available which offers the greatest potential for achieving a conception.

An explosion of knowledge and technology development in the subspecialty of reproductive endocrinology makes demands on the clinician working with the infertile couple and subsequently on the laboratory providing services and diagnostic testing for the reproductive endocrinologist.

II. INCIDENCE OF INFERTILITY

It is estimated that one of every six married couples find themselves involuntarily infertile which translates to between two and four million couples in the U.S. alone. At the end of 1 year of unprotected intercourse, 88% of fertile couples will have achieved pregnancy. (Figure 1). Each year between 300,000 and 1 million couples seek medical treatment for infertility spending an estimated $1 billion in pursuit of pregnancy.[1]

III. ETIOLOGY OF INFERTILITY

The causes of infertility vary among patient populations studied. In general, however, it is estimated that in the routine infertility practice, compromised seminal quality is etiologic in approximately 40% of cases. Purely female factors are apparent in 40% of cases with an additional 20% having a combination of both male and female factors.

With respect to female factors, tubal pathology exists in 30 to 40% of cases including both endometriosis and pelvic inflammatory disease. Ovulatory dysfunction is found in

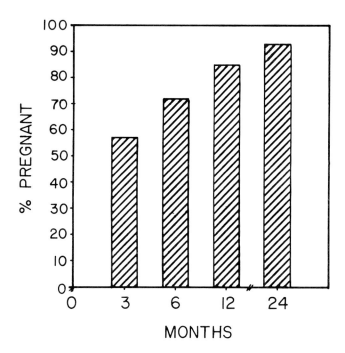

FIGURE 1.   Time required for conception to occur in the general population. Graph drawn from the data presented in Guttmacher, A. F., *JAMA*, 161, 855, 1956.

approximately 30% with cervical pathology accounting for 5 to 10% and uterine pathology for less than 10%. Medical diseases or problems such as hypothyroidism, metabolic disorders, and nutritional factors are present in less than 5% of cases.

IV. THE EVALUATION

A rapid, meticulous, and thorough evaluation can be accomplished in from two to three menstrual cycles and can do much to alleviate the anxiety associated with the problem of infertility as well as provide emotional support toward resolution of the problem.

A. INITIAL INTERVIEW

The initial assessment for the infertile couple should ideally begin with an interview which includes both partners and the clinician. If applicable, results of previous therapies and treatments are reviewed and interpreted. An evaluation plan is then developed, discussed, and outlined with its purposes being to establish a firm diagnosis and ultimately a prognosis for successful therapy.

B. HISTORY AND PHYSICAL EXAMINATION

The history and physical examination of both members of the infertile couple are directed toward detecting an etiology of the infertility. Previous pregnancies related to either partner and their outcomes, sexual frequency, coital practices, previous contraceptive practices, associated past or present medical problems, and current medications should be thoroughly explored in each partner. A detailed menstrual history is obtained seeking information to establish the potential for ovulatory capacity as well as the possible presence of endometriosis.

If history or initial screening semen analysis leads to suspicion of male factor, serum gonadotropins and testosterone determinations are obtained as well as early urologic consultation.

Physical examination of the female is conducted with special emphasis on signs of possible androgen excess, abnormal breast secretion, as well as evidence of vaginal, cervical, or uterine abnormalities. Physical findings may dictate inclusion of additional testing.

The basic diagnostic studies to be performed in the routine infertility evaluation include the following:

1. Semen analysis
2. Basal body temperature charting in conjunction with urinary LH testing
3. Hysterosalpingography
4. Postcoital testing
5. Endometrial biopsy
6. Laparoscopy $+/-$ hysteroscopy

C. SEMEN ANALYSIS

Semen analysis is performed ideally with an abstinence time equal to that of the couple's usual coital frequency around the predicted time of ovulation. This assay will provide the initial and most comprehensive evaluation of the fertility potential of the male and is the cornerstone in the evaluation of the male partner. The semen analysis provides detailed information relative to sperm concentration, motility, kinetics, and morphology (see Chapter 3). A semiquantitative and somewhat subjective clinical assessment of the various parameters has been traditionally used. Recent advances in automated systems has allowed for a more objective evaluation with less chance for technical error (see Chapter 6). Discussions of the definitions and terminology commonly used are found in Chapter 3.

As semen quality in an individual may vary, a minimum of two samples must be processed even if the results of the first analysis are satisfactory. Collection of the specimen should be by masturbation, if possible, with notation made as to duration of abstinence, method and time of collection, post collection handling of the specimen, time received at laboratory, and the loss of any part of the specimen.

Normal values of the various parameters will vary according to the laboratory's method of analysis. More advanced systems using undiluted specimen will generally show somewhat lower ranges of normal particularly with respect to sperm concentration and motility. Please refer to Chapter 3 for a more detailed explanation.

D. OVULATORY TIMING
1. Basal Body Temperature

Basal body temperature (BBT) evaluations require detailed instruction and compliance if they are to provide useful information with respect to the occurrence of probable ovulation. Their value is retrospective in allowing for estimation of time of ovulation, follicular phase length, luteal phase length, and appropriateness of coital timing.

2. Urinary LH Testing

Urinary LH testing allows for the detection of the preovulatory LH surge and thus allows for precise and accurate timing of other tests in the routine infertility evaluation including postcoital testing and the endometrial biopsy.

E. HYSTEROSALPINGOGRAPHY

The hysterosalpingogram (HSG) allows for the radiographic display of the uterine cavity contour and documentation of tubal patency. It is appropriately scheduled in the follicular phase of the cycle 2 to 3 d after cessation of normal menses.

One of the more serious potential complications of an HSG is infectious morbidity in the form of acute salpingitis. The incidence varies from 0.3 to 3.1%.[2,3] This complication

TABLE 1
Risk Factors for Post-HSG Infection

Risk factor	Score
Major	
Secondary infertility	2+
Prior pelvic infection	2+
Prior pelvic surgery for infection	2+
Prior adnexal tenderness	2+
Prior adnexal mass	2+
Minor	
Primary infertility	1+
Undocumented history of salpingitis	1+

From Stumpf, P. G. and March, M. M., *Fertil. Steril.*, 33, 487, 1980. With permission.

of a dignostic test in the infertility evalution can result in tubal occlusion and thus have a devastating effect on fertility potential. Ideally one would like to screen and identify prospective high risk patients. This group could then be excluded from testing altogether, or treated prophylactically with antibiotics both before and after the procedure. Stumpf and March identified major and minor risk factors for development of infection following HSG.[4] The major risk factors are assigned a score of 2 + and the minor risk factors are assigned a score of 1 + (Table 1). In this retrospective study, 8 of 15 (53%) patients with a score of 6 or greater became infected while only 6 of 449 (1.3%) patients with a score of 5 or less became infected.

It is our practice to pre-screen all patients with a complete blood count (CBC) and erythrocyte sedimentation rate (ESR). If either is elevated, the procedure is canceled and a course of broad spectrum antibiotics is prescribed. The CBC and ESR are repeated in the next cycle and if normal and the patient is not at high risk, the study is completed. If abnormal again and the patient is not at high risk, the procedure is completed with prophylactic broad spectrum antibiotic coverage both before and after the procedure. If the patient is at high risk for infectious morbidity, the procedure is eliminated with tubal patency and uterine cavity contour assessed by combination laparoscopy/hysteroscopy in conjunction with intraoperative chromoperturbation as well as prophylactic antibiotic coverage.

If the patient is inadvertently discovered to have hydrosalpinges in spite of a negative history and normal CBC and ESR, she is begun immediately on oral broad spectrum antibiotics and observed on an out-patient basis.[5]

Increased pregnancy rates during the first 4 months following HSG has been well documented.[6,7] The therapeutic benefit of HSG may be greater with the use of oil-based dye as compared to a water-based dye, however controversy exists over which type of dye should be used because of potential complications. Historically, a high-viscosity oil-base contrast media (Lipiodol; iodized poppy seed oil with 40% iodine) was used. Complications included embolization and granuloma formation.[8,9] Pulmonary embolism has resulted in four deaths, three with oil-based contrast medium and the most recent in 1959 with a water-based contrast medium. No serious embolism complications have been reported with the use of low-viscosity oil-base contrast medium (Ethiodol; ethiodized poppy seed oil with 37% iodine). Granuloma formation seems to be associated with prolonged absorption of the dye which can occur with diseased fallopian tubes. The presence of Lipiodol has been documented in the peritoneal cavity years after instillation, however, Ethiodol is absorbed within a month.

Post-HSG pregnancy rates using oil-base contrast medium (29%) have been reported as higher than with water-base contrast medium (13%).[10] DeCherney has proposed that the

HSG be performed initially with water-base contrast medium, and if tubal patency is documented, oil-base contrast medium be used to enhance fertility.

F. POSTCOITAL TESTING

Historically, the postcoital test (PCT) has been a poor predictor of fertility.[11,12] It does however provide the means to eliminate the possibility of sexual dysfunction and provide for a crude examination of sperm-cervical mucus interaction which may lead to the performance of more elaborate and expensive testing.

The cervical mucus is receptive to sperm for only a "window" of time throughout the cycle around the time of ovulation. As the "window" of receptivity varies from patient to patient, proper timing of the test is important to eliminate a false interpretation. The use of urinary LH monitoring allows for the prospective estimation of the time of ovulation thus decreasing the likelihood of poor timing being a factor should poor results be obtained.

If menstrual history is compatible with ovulatory cycles, patients are instructed to begin urinary LH testing on morning samples 2 to 3 d before the anticipated time of ovulation. Upon detection of the LH surge, the patient calls to schedule an appointment for the next morning and is instructed to have intercourse that night. On the morning of the appointment, an intracervical specimen is obtained with a 16 gauge blunt needle attached to a tuberculin syringe. The sample is then evaluated with respect to the quality and quantity of cervical mucous (see Chapter 8) as well as the quantity and motility characteristics of sperm present.

Controversy exists with respect to what constitutes a normal number of progressively motile sperm in cervical mucous. Studies have shown that pregnancy rates of couples with 1 to 5 motile sperm per high power field did not differ significantly from couples with 11 to 20 motile sperm per high power field, and that 20% of couples with proven fertility had less than one sperm per high power field.[11,12] Likewise, sperm have been recovered from peritoneal fluid of patients with repeated poor postcoital tests undergoing insemination just prior to laparoscopy performed at midcycle.

Accepted definitions of normal include 1, 5, 10, and 20 progressively motile sperm per hpf.[13,15-17] Our laboratory uses five or greater progressively motile sperm per high power field as adequate. In the presence of a documented well-timed test with good cervical mucus showing unacceptable numbers of progressively motile sperm, both parties are routinely treated with doxycycline for 10 d with onset of the next menses and the test is repeated in the following cycle. This therapy should eliminate low grade infection in either partner as being contributory to the poor test result. A repeated poor test is subsequently followed by *in vitro* testing (see Chapter 8).

If the cervical mucous is consistently of poor quality, treatment of the female with low doses of supplemental estrogens in the follicular phase may prove helpful. The requirement of higher doses, however, may suppress ovulation and lead to consideration of techniques such as intrauterine insemination.

Significantly, some immunologic causes of infertility may be detected by the presence of "shaking" or nonmotile sperm in the cervical mucus and thus be an indicator for the early evaluation of the couple for antisperm antibodies (see Chapters 9 and 10).

Although subject to wide variation in performance and interpretation, the properly timed postcoital test should be a prerequisite of more invasive and expensive laboratory testing procedures.

G. ENDOMETRIAL BIOPSY

Although the uterus itself is rarely a cause of the inability to conceive, it may be etiologic for early pregnancy wastage and reproductive failure. Since the first description of luteal phase deficiency (LPD) in 1949,[18] many methods of diagnosis have been proposed including luteal phase length, evaluation of basal body temperature, ultrasonographic evaluation of follicular development, and endometrial biopsy.

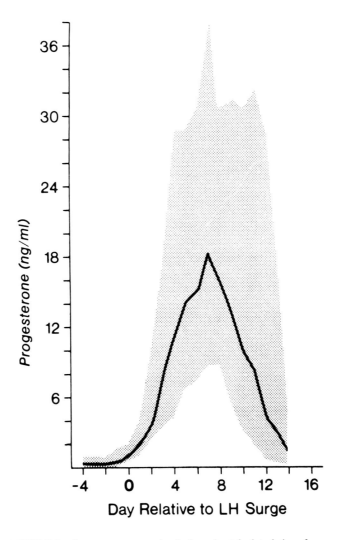

FIGURE 2. Serum progesterone levels throughout the luteal phase from a group of 14 normal women are illustrated. The daily mean (geometric) P level with two standard deviations (calculated after logarithmic conversion) is indicated. A P level in a blood sample from a patient would need to be outside the 2 SD margin on a given cycle day to be abnormal. (From McNeely, M. J. and Soules, M. R., *Fertil. Steril.*, 50, 1, 1988. With permission.)

LPD implies either an inadequate amount of progesterone being secreted by the corpus luteum or inability of the endometrium to respond to what would otherwise be considered adequate progesterone concentrations. The measurement of serum progesterone levels in the luteal phase to diagnosis LPD is subject to inherent sampling variability due to the pulsatile nature of progesterone secretion (Figure 2). Individual patient variation and difficulty in timing may dramatically affect the single progesterone level and to a lesser extent serial progesterone levels thus making interpretation subject to wide variability.[19,22]

Compromised follicular development as an etiology of LPD was investigated sonographically in a group of patients with histologically confirmed LPD. Only 40% of patients were found to have dominant follicles less than 17 mm in size.[23]

Use of the endometrial biopsy for the diagnosis of LPD has the advantage of evaluation of the status of the target organ independent of daily hormone fluctuation. BBT and urinary

LH testing are used to time the endometrial sampling within 1 to 2 days of the predicted onset of menses. The histologic dating is based on the classic work of Noyes et al.[24] with the most advanced area in the specimen evaluated to enhance the sensitivity of the interpretation as recommended later by Noyes[25] (see Appendix VIII). The diagnosis of LPD is made with two biopsies greater than 48 h out of phase with the onset of menses being considered ideal cycle day 28 or postovulatory day 14. The reader is referred to Chapter 2 for further details. Although accepted treatments of LPD vary, a repeat biopsy is mandatory to confirm therapeutic correction of the LPD.

H. LAPAROSCOPY/HYSTEROSCOPY

Evaluation of the peritoneal factor is accomplished by laparoscopy as indicated by symptomatology, failure to conceive after correction of previously discovered factors, or a failure to detect an etiology after completion of the routine evaluation.

Laparoscopic visualization of the peritoneal cavity allows for the diagnosis of mechanical or physical abnormalities which can contribute to infertility such as endometriosis and/or pelvic adhesions. The increasing utilization of treatment modalities administered via laparoscopy allows the procedure to be therapeutic as well as diagnostic in many patients.

Hysteroscopy is performed simultaneously in those patients in whom the screening HSG has demonstrated abnormalities or in those patients in whom direct visualization of the uterine cavity and tubal ostia will be useful in either diagnosis or formation of a treatment plan.

The accurate documentation and treatment of detected disease states allows for the couple and the physician to intelligently develop the remainder of the treatment plan with emphasis on the greater probabilities of achieving pregnancy.

I. ADDITIONAL TESTING

In those couples in whom no etiology of infertility is detected, further evaluation is indicated. It should be noted that these evaluations are rarely positive but are necessary before labeling the couple as "unexplained infertility".

A few of the more common tests (covered elsewhere in this text) include immunologic testing, sperm functional capability evaluation and, occasionally, genetic evaluation.

CONCLUSION

Appropriate, meticulous, and thorough evaluation of the infertile couple should result in a diagnosis in 90 to 95% of cases. An individualized treatment plan based on diagnostic findings should result in either a successful pregnancy or assist in bringing to resolution the problem of infertility.

Each stage of the infertility evaluation evokes particular psychological stresses for the couple. Attention to the emotional well being of the individuals may necessitate referral to a mental health professional or, in rare cases, discontinuation of the medical evaluation and treatment.

REFERENCES

1. U.S. Congress, Office of Technology Assessment, Infertility: Medical and Social Choices. OTA-BA 358, U.S. Government Printing Office, Washington, D.C., May 1988.
2. **Marshak, R. H., Roole, C. S., and Goldberger, M. A.,** Hysterography and hysterosalpingography, *Surg. Gynecol. Obstet.,* 91, 182, 1950.

3. **Measday, B.,** An analysis of the complications of hysterosalpingography, *J. Obstet. Gynecol. Br. Emp.,* 67, 663, 1960.

4. **Stumpf, P. G. and March, M. M.,** Febrile morbidity following hysterosalpingography: Identification of risk factors and recommendations for prophylaxis, *Fertil. Steril.,* 33, 487, 1980.

5. **Pittaway, D. E., Winfield, A. C., Maxson, W., Daniell, J., Herbert, C., and Wentz, A. C.,** Prevention of acute pelvic inflammatory disease after hysterosalpingography: Efficacy of doxycycline prophylaxis, *Am. J. Obstet. Gynecol.,* 147, 623, 1983.

6. **Wahby, O., Sobrero, A. J., and Epstein, J. A.,** Hysterosalpingography in relation to pregnancy and its outcome in infertile women, *Fertil. Steril.,* 17, 520, 1966.

7. **Palmer, A.,** Ethiodol hysterosalpingography for the treatment of infertility, *Fertil. Steril.,* 11, 311, 1960.

8. **Levinson, J. M.,** Pulmonary oil embolism following hysterosalpingography, *Fertil. Steril.,* 14, 21, 1963.

9. **Bateman, B. G., Nunley, W. G., Jr., and Kitchin, J. D., III,** Intravasation during hysterosalpingography using oil-base contrast media, *Fertil. Steril.,* 34, 439, 1980.

10. **DeCherney, A. H., Kort, H., Barney, J. B., and DeVore, F. R.,** Increased pregnancy rate with oil-soluble hysterosalpingography dye, *Fertil. Steril.,* 33, 407, 1980.

11. **Jette, N. T. and Glass, R. H.,** Prognostic value of the postcoital test, *Fertil. Steril.,* 23, 29, 1972.

12. **Kovacs, G. T., Newman, G. B., and Henson, G. L.,** The postcoital test. What is normal?, *Br. Med. J.,* 1, 818, 1978.

13. **Asch, R. H.,** Laparoscopic recovery of sperm from peritoneal fluid, in patients with negative or poor Sims-Huhner test, *Fertil. Steril.,* 27, 1111, 1976.

14. **Templeton, A. A. and Mortimer, D. M.,** The development of a clinical test of sperm migration to the site of fertilization, *Fertil. Steril.,* 37, 410, 1982.

15. **Danezis, J., Sujan, S., and Sobrero, A. J.,** Evaluation of the postcoital test, *Fertil. Steril.,* 13, 559, 1962.

16. **Davajan, V. and Kunitake, G. M.,** Fraction in vitro and vitro examination of postcoital and cervical mucus in the human, *Fertil. Steril.,* 20, 197, 1969.

17. **Glass, H. G. and Mroueh, A.,** The postcoital test and semen analysis, *Fertil. Steril.,* 28, 1289, 1977.

18. **Jones, G. E. S.,** Some newer aspects of the management of infertility, *JAMA,* 141, 1123, 1949.

19. **Israel, R., Mishell, D. R., Jr., Stone, S. C., Thorneycroft, I. H., and Moyer, D. L.,** Single luteal phase serum progesterone assay as an indicator of ovulation, *Am. J. Obstet. Gynecol.,* 112, 1043, 1972.

20. **Ross, G. T., Cargille, C. M., Lipsett, M. B., Rayford, P. L., Marshall, Jr., Strott, C. A., and Rodbard, D.,** Pituitary and gonadal hormones in women during spontaneous and induced ovulatory cycles, *Rec. Prog. Hormone Res.,* 26, 1, 1970.

21. **Johansson, E. D. B.,** Progesterone levels in peripheral plasma during the luteal phase of the normal human menstrual cycle measured by a rapid competitive protein binding technique, *Acta Endocrinol.(Copenhagen),* 61, 592, 1969.

22. **Radwanska, E. and Sawyer, G. I. M.,** Plasma progesterone estimation in infertile women and in women under treatment with clomiphene and chorionic gonadotropin, *J. Obstet. Gynecol. Br. Commun.,* 81, 107, 1974.

23. **Check, J. H., Goldberg, B. B., Kurtz, A., Adelson, H. G., and Rankin, A.,** Pelvic sonography to help determine the appropriate therapy for luteal phase defects, *Int. J. Fertil.,* 29, 156, 1984.

24. **Noyes, R. W., Hertig, A. T., and Rock, J.,** Dating the endometrial biopsy, *Fertil. Steril.,* 1, 3, 1950.

25. **Noyes, R. W. and Haman, J. O.,** Accuracy of endometrial dating. Correlation of endometrial dating with basal body temperature and menses, *Fertil. Steril.,* 4, 504, 1953.

Chapter 2

THE ENDOMETRIAL BIOPSY

Tim H. Parmley

TABLE OF CONTENTS

I. HISTORY

The histopathologic description of the normally cycling endometrium has a history that stretches back into the 19th century, primarily in Germany. Many of these very early observations culminate in the description by Hitschmann and Adler in 1908.[1] This eighty three page tome was typical of the thorough German literary style of the time. The medical history of 58 women from which the endometria were removed at a known time in their cycle were cataloged. As the histologic material encompassed the cycle the authors were able to describe the sequential changes in the endometrium as the cycle progressed. They divided their description into postmenstrual, interval, premenstrual, and menstrual phases. Although their description has since been amplified and also correlated with the corpus luteum in man and other primates, it has never been superseded. The history of these additional developments has been recently reviewed by Bardawil.[2] It was Rock and Bartlett, however, who first described the use of endometrial biopsies to ''date'' the endometrium in the sense discussed in this chapter.[3] They made a series of valuable observations that remain pertinent. One was that the location from which the biopsy is taken matters and that high on the anterior or posterior wall is the appropriate site. Another was that the biopsy should be evaluated in order to determine if it has been taken from an appropriate site before being interpreted. They pointed out that proliferative phase endometrium could not be assigned to any given day and they described the day by day changes that may be observed in the secretory phase endometrium. They then discussed the limits of accuracy inherent in the method. A detailed discussion of this topic concludes this chapter, but from the historical point of view it is appropriate to note that they made no excessive claims and they anticipated most of the issues. Subsequently, Rock collaborated with Noyes and Hertig in the publication of one of the most widely quoted papers in gynecology.[4] Beginning on page 3 of the new journal, *Fertility and Sterility,* this offering added an emphasis on using the most advanced date ascertainable from any given biopsy as well as a set of beautiful pictures. It also contained a discussion of the limits of accuracy and made the point that when it is possible to do so, the method correlates better with the known time of ovulation than with the next menstrual period. This point recurs in subsequent literature as will be detailed below. This was based on their use of the basal body temperature chart to achieve better correlation than they achieved with the next menstrual period.

II. TECHNICAL PRINCIPLES

The pathologic evaluation of endometrial biopsies is highly sensitive to the technical quality of the biopsy. It is difficult to over emphasize this point and I will return to it. Of almost equal importance is the site from which the biopsy is taken. Maximal physiologic development of the endometrium takes place over the middle of the anterior or posterior walls so that biopsies must be taken from these sites in order to yield the most useful information. The lower uterine segment, the sides, the cornua, and the top of the fundus may possess endometrial surfaces which are less well developed (Figure 1).

It is equally important that the biopsy be taken with sufficient confidence that a large orientable piece of endometrium be obtained and not fragments too small to place into context. That this is a feature of operator performance is suggested by the fact that a pathologist may learn to recognize that good biopsies are consistently sent to the pathology laboratory by some individuals and not by others.

III. TRANSFER AND FIXATION

Once obtained a biopsy should be transferred to fixative as promptly as possible and as atraumatically as possible. Any instrument which grasps, pokes or pushes the tissue com-

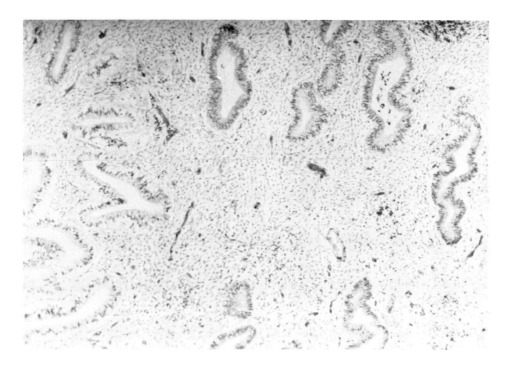

FIGURE 1. To the left, all the glandular epithelium contains well developed subnuclear vacuolization. To the right as one approaches the lateral wall of the uterine cavity the glandular epithelium has not responded to rising postovulatory progesterone.

promises the interpretation. The endometrium is very soft, and almost any force will crush it.

The fixative used is important. Details of cellular morphology are important in interpreting the epithelial changes that accompany the early secretory phase as well as in interpreting the stromal changes that characterize the late secretory phase. Both are made more difficult by fixatives such as formalin which produce cytoplasmic shrinkage of decidual cells, condensation of mitoses, or clumping of secretory products. Bouin's is a very good fixative for the endometrium but most rely on buffered formalin for economic reasons. Routine hematoxylin and eosin sections are prepared from paraffin blocks and the tissue should be sectioned thinly enough to allow for the interpretation of individual cells. Biopsies should be thoroughly sampled.

IV. INTERPRETATION

It is the basics that are most commonly omitted. Is the biopsy sufficiently large and intact and free of artifact to be interpretable? Is it from a reactive portion of the endometrium? Is it possible to tell whether or not there is both a zona compacta and a zona spongiosa present? And does the tissue lack obvious abnormality such as inflammation or focal areas of nonresponse? If the answer is not yes to these questions, then the biopsy cannot be satisfactorily interpreted and attempts to do so result in errors of interpretation. When the uninterpretable nature of the biopsy is communicated to the clinician, the frequent result is a request for "the best estimate you can give me." This is a clinical error. It may lead a pathologist who is cynical, insecure, or too eager to help, to offer an estimate based on inadequate data.

In the immediate postmenstrual phase, the endometrium is low. The basalis will reveal

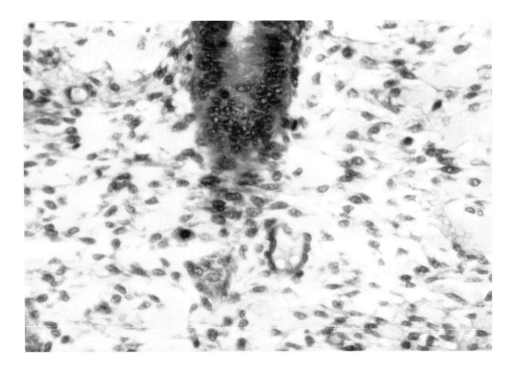

FIGURE 2.   High nuclear cytoplasmic ratios characterize both stromal and epithelial cells in this proliferative endometrium. Two stromal mitosis are seen.

simple glands that are lined by columnar, pseudostratified epithelium. These are embedded in a cellular stroma consisting of mononuclear type and fibroblastic cells. At the surface the stroma will continue to contain a few fragments of clumped necrotic stroma and there is some associated inflammatory infiltrate. The epithelium lining the remaining glands will be clear and filled with secretion. That on the surface may still be relatively flattened with a lot of eosinophilic cytoplasm. This is the repairing state. It is quickly replaced by a truly proliferating endometrium. The necrotic fragments of stroma, the secretory and repairing epithelia are all removed. The secretory epithelium may reveal dramatic apoptosis as the inflammatory infiltrate clears.

The proliferating endometrium is characterized by mitotically active epithelium and stroma (Figure 2). Most of the mitoses occur above the basal level in the developing upper portion of the glands and stroma. Straight tubular glands embedded in a loose matrix are the result (Figure 3). The glandular epithelium is composed of columnar cells arranged in a pseudostratified epithelium. The stroma is composed of fibroblasts and mononuclear cells. This tissue is fundamentally undifferentiated with high nuclear cytoplasmic ratios in epithelium and stroma, mitoses, and little evidence of function. Occasionally small subnuclear vacuoles do appear in the epithelial cells of a proliferative endometrium stimulated only by estrogen, but they are invariably small and sharply angulated in the light microscope. There is some increase in stromal edema in the mid-proliferative phase, but this has not proven to be a reliable microscopic feature of biopsy material.

With ovulation and rising progesterone levels the epithelial cells in the most reactive portion of the endometrium begin to accumulate subnuclear glycogen (Figure 4). The most reactive portion of the endometrium is the middle portion of the tubular glands in the middle of the anterior and posterior walls of the uterine cavity. The basal portion of the glands does not respond and the most superficial portion tends to respond in a laggard manner.

On approximately the second postovulatory day, day 16 of a 28-d cycle, subnuclear

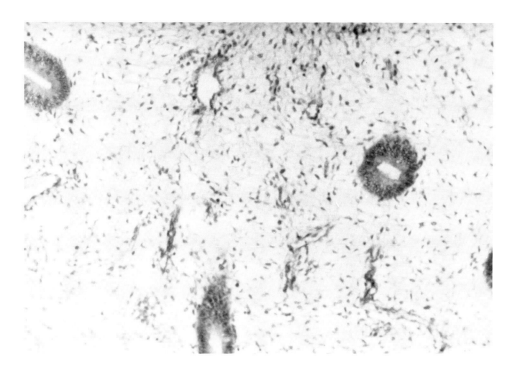

FIGURE 3. Straight tubular glands cut across produce small ''donuts'' in a loose matrix which dominates the field in this proliferative endometrium.

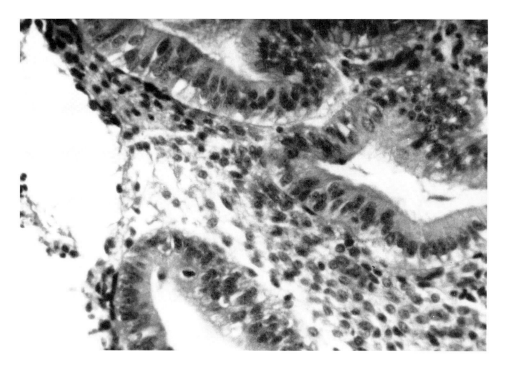

FIGURE 4. Irregular subnuclear vacuoles are seen in this epithelium which is still pseudostratified and still contains mitosis.

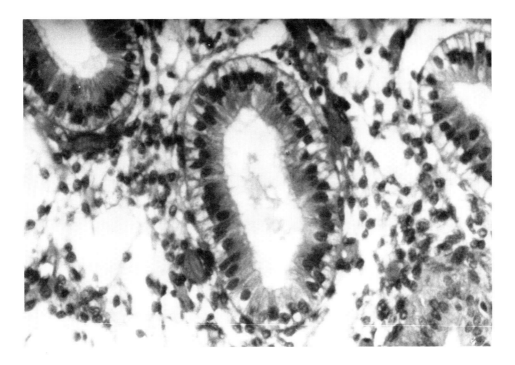

FIGURE 5.   Subnuclear vacuoles uniformly elevate the epithelial cell nuclei to the center of the cell.

vacuoles are widespread in the epithelium of the mid-portion of the glands. By the 17th d, a consistent subnuclear layer uniformly elevates the nuclei to the mid-portion of the cell (Figure 5). On the 18th d, these vacuoles slip past the nuclei. By the 19th d, they have reached the luminal pole of the cell. Here on the 19th, 20th, and 21st d they are secreted by an apocrine mechanism into the lumen of the gland (Figure 6). This apocrine mechanism produces intact, secretory vacuoles above the cell surface in the lumen of the gland. On the 21st d the secretion begins to form a dense inspissated core within the lumen of the gland (Figure 7).

The importance of technical factors cannot be over emphasized. These glandular events take place in the middle or spongiosa layer of the endometrium. The epithelium of the more superficial portions of the glands lags behind, and even late in the secretory phase of the cycle, vacuoles will be subnuclear in these sites. Therefore, in order to appropriately "date" an endometrial biopsy one must have a piece of tissue sufficiently large and intact to insure that one is evaluating glands located some distance from the endometrial surface.

It is also in the mid- to late secretory phase that the reactive middle portion of the glands becomes quite tortuous and converts the middle zone of the endometrium into the so called zona spongiosa (Figure 8). The development of the zona compacta, the third and most superficial layer in the classic description, is a feature of the last week of the cycle.

Normally, implantation takes place on the 20th or 21st d of the 28-d cycle. Coincident with this potential occurrence, there is a relatively acute increase in intercellular fluid or stromal edema in the functional portion of the endometrium (Figure 9). This specifically stromal event heralds a shift in emphasis from the epithelium of the glands which have been used to date the endometrium to this point. Subsequent datable events will occur in the stroma and will result in the production of the most superficial of the classic three layers, the zona compacta. On about the 23rd d, the spiral arterioles high in the interglandular spaces begin to exhibit perivascular cuffs composed of stromal cells that are accumulating cytoplasm and thus becoming decidual cells (Figure 10). The term pseudodecidual is mis-

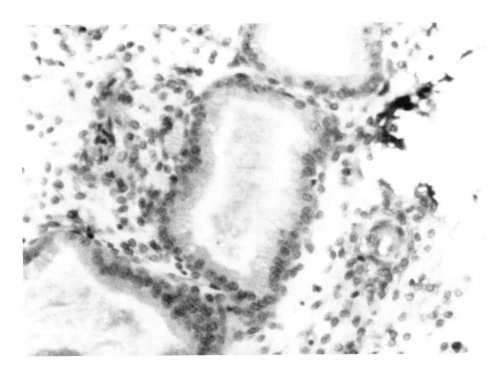

FIGURE 6.   Peak secretory activity is indicated by the abundant fluffy secretion in the gland lumen and multiple secretory vacuoles above the epithelial surface.

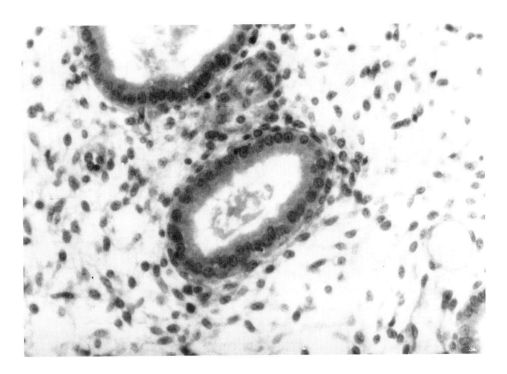

FIGURE 7.   Inspissated secretion is suggested by the dense core of secretory material in this gland. The gland epithelium is becoming cuboidal and less vacuolated.

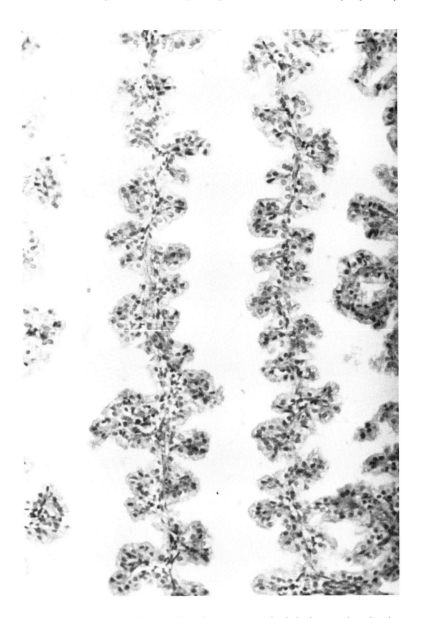

FIGURE 8.   So tortuous and crowded are these secretory glands in the spongiosa that they have been mistaken for malignancy.

leading, however, it refers to the progesterone induced changes in endometrial stromal cells which are less pronounced than those produced by pregnancy.

Decidualization of the stromal cell, a cellular differentiation induced by progesterone, consists of the circumnuclear accumulation of cytoplasm. The spindle-shaped stromal cells are converted into polyhedral cells. The general increase in cellular cytoplasm and relative 'isappearance of intercellular space gives the stroma a dense look. This appearance can be simulated and such simulation may lead to diagnostic error. Dense stromal proliferation associated only with estrogen may result in apparent decidualization due to increased cellularity and thus increased cytoplasm. In this case, however, the cells remain spindle cells. Similarly, intracellular matrix, such as the scarring that may occur in polyps, has been misinterpreted as decidual. It is important, therefore, in determining whether or not 23 d

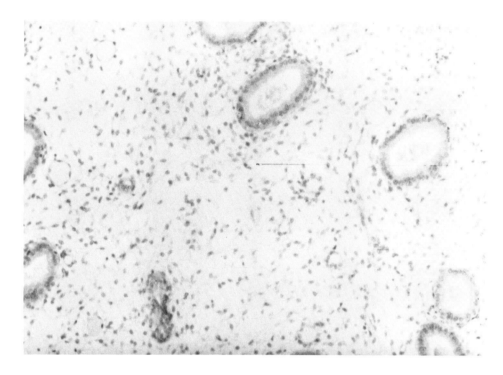

FIGURE 9. Stromal edema is a prominent accompaniment of mid secretory activity.

are indicated by the biopsy that the perivascular cuff is composed of decidual type cells. Occasionally stromal edema that leaves only structural cells around a vessel will create a picture that simulates a cuff. Again in this case the stromal cells are spindle shaped.

On the 24th d of the cycle spiral arterioles possess cuffs composed of clearly decidualized cells and by the 25th d foci of such decidualized cells are appearing underneath the surface epithelium (Figure 11). By the 26th d, many spiral arterials are contained within columns of decidualized stroma that extend from the spongiosa to the surface where they spread laterally to produce the so called zona compacta. This process is generalized on the 27th d and in association with it, the endometrial granulocytes which are not decidualized become more prominent (Figure 12). Small round cells with oval, often indented nuclei, possess eosinophilic cytoplasmic granules visible in the light microscope. They have been present throughout the cycle but are more visible when their neighbors become decidualized. The glandular epithelium in the gland necks in the zona compacta still resembles early secretory epithelium with intracellular vacuoles.

It is seen, therefore, that the most superficial portion of the endometrium is required for evaluating the last week of the cycle. A biopsy so cut that only the spongiosa is visualized will not demonstrate extensive decidualization. Further, the zona compacta does not develop well in nonreactive portions of the endometrial cavity. Also the glandular epithelium in the gland necks in the zona compacta still resembles early secretory epithelium with intracellular vacuoles, and in order not to be mislead by this phenomenon, one must have a biopsy that allows one to determine that the gland epithelium is superficial.

The first signs of endometrial breakdown also occur superficially. They consist initially of small foci of stromal cells which have clumped and become much more basophilic. These may be associated with slight hemorrhage or a fibrin thrombus in an adjacent capillary. These foci tend to be subepithelial which leads to the overlying epithelium becoming separated. Both the stromal and epithelial process become generalized and involve much of the zona compacta and spongiosa of the reactive portion of the endometrium. Epithelial repair

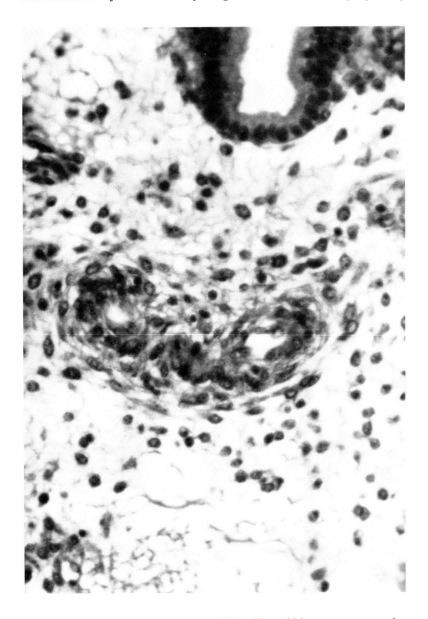

FIGURE 10. More cells are present around this capillary which possess more cytoplasm than those more distant from it.

begins immediately and frequently being simultaneously with slough. The repairing epithelial cells with abundant eosinophilic cytoplasm have led to their being misinterpreted as squamous in character.

In a conception cycle, the sequence described above is somewhat altered beginning as early as the 24th d. It may be noted that as described above, the cycling endometrium demonstrates peak secretion on day 20 to 21, peak edema on day 21 to 22, and peak decidualization in the immediate premenstrual phase. When conception occurs, the edema persists and secretion begins again on about day 24. This resumption of function produces enlargement of the glands that now contain light and fluffy new secretion around a more dense eosinophilic core of old secretion (Figure 13). The epithelium becomes newly vacuolated and the enlarged clear cells are termed hypersecretory. The combination of marked

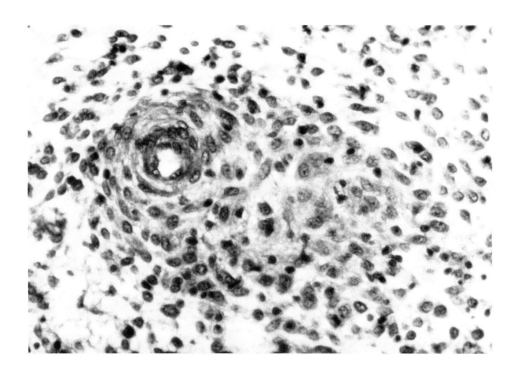

FIGURE 11.   Cells surrounding this capillary have acquired much more cytoplasm than those more distant from it giving it an investment of decidual cells.

decidualization, persistent edema, and hypersecretory glands has been termed gestational hyperplasia by Hertig. It preceeds more complete decidualization as pregnancy progresses.

V. ACCURACY

From its inception the practice of endometrial dating has been criticizied as inaccurate and defended as accurate. Careful study of this literature not only reveals the degree to which accuracy has been achieved but other insights as well. In the original publication, Rock and Bartlett state, "we do not claim exact accuracy" and just prior to their detailed description of the secretory phase reiterated: " . . . we make no claim to exact accuracy".[3] Indeed they predicted the date of menstruation exactly only 16% of the time and were within ± 2 d 70% of the time. In the subsequent landmark article by Noyes et al., the methodology was discussed again.[4] Noyes, utilizing the most advanced area in 300 biopsies, was able to pick the day of menstruation only 20% of the time and he was within ± 1 d only 60% of the time. Multiple observers produced much wider variation and even a single observer had errors ranging from 6 d early to 10 d late. The importance of observer variation has been repeatedly shown. These initial publications were followed by the criticism of, among others, Emil Novak.[5] Although this author produced no data, his eminent stature provoked a response. Noyes and Haman published over a thousand cases, independently read by the two of them, in which the endometrial biopsy results were correlated with that predicted by the basal body temperature record and the date of the next menstrual period.[6] Haman used the initial criteria of Rock and Bartlett and Noyes used the modification of these published by himself, Hertig, and Rock. The modification was primarily to use the most advanced data observed in the tissue rather than an overall average. Noyes dates might therefore have been expected to be consistently advanced with respect to those of Haman. All their data suggests that this is true early in the cycle, but that the reverse is true after the 24th d. In any case,

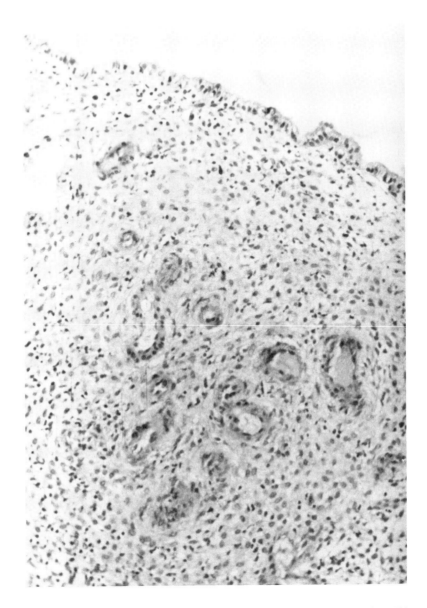

FIGURE 12.   Decidualization is becoming generalized beneath the surface epithelium. This produces a zone of decidualization, the zona compacta, in which the mononuclear endometrial granulocytes are much more apparent.

the two observers agreed exactly 29% of the time and within a day 62% of the time and within 2 d 81% of the time. However, in individual cases they disagreed as much as twelve days in either direction with the greatest deviation occurring early and late in the secretory phase. Obviously, if an endometrial biopsy is dated in the middle of the secretory phase there is only room for 7 d of deviation on either side of it. The length of the phase and the closeness of the chosen date to either cyclic end point limits possible deviation which they pointed out. In view of this individual variation, the authors' data also gives precious little support to the idea that the modified criteria do any better than the original ones. They were able to predict the date of menstruation exactly about 25% of the time, they were within a day about 60% of the time and within 2 d about 80% of the time.

Several subsequent attempts to improve or to document the accuracy or inaccuracy of

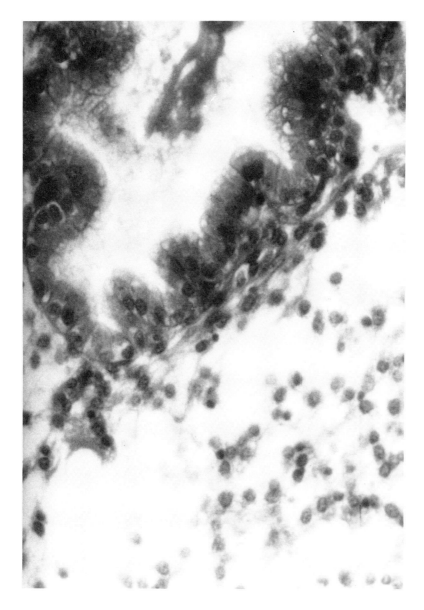

FIGURE 13.   Inspissated secretion occupies the lumen of this gland but the epithelial cells are large and contain secretory vacuoles.

endometrial dating have occurred. Treadway et al. biopsied 11 patients in cycles being monitored with daily LH determination.[7] The correlation between the day of ovulation (LH peak + 1) and the day of the endometrial biopsy was 0.79. Only one pathologist was involved in this study. Five of eleven patients had endometrial biopsy dates 2 d behind the date predicted by the LH peak and three had dates 2 or 3 d beyond the date predicted by the LH peak. These cases are of interest, but the numbers are too small for comparison with the previous studies. It is of interest that one standard deviation around the mean of luteal phase cycle length was 1.9 d in this study.

Lundy et al. have published the best correlations between the endometrial histologic date and the LH peak (r = 0.97). This was the result of having two pathologists review the material using the most advanced date given.[8] This does provide some support for the common dictum about endometrial dating being most accurate when based on the most advanced endometrium. The two pathologists in this study correlated with each other, r = 0.85.

Koninckx et al. also correlated biopsies with LH peaks and demonstrated accuracy similar to that achieved by others.[9] The standard deviation of their correlations was 1.2 and 1.3 d in two groups of women.

Johannisson et al. quantitated several histologic criteria and correlated them with the LH surge and with daily estradiol and progesterone levels.[10] Again they were able to agree within a day with the LH surge in 64% of cases and in 81% within 2 d. The spread in their data was similar to that of others. These authors also attempted to take biopsies from both lateral walls and from the anterior wall of the cavity and could demonstrate no differences in these biopsies. As complete sections of the endometrium have repeatedly demonstrated that the endometrium of the lateral walls, does not respond as consistently to progesterone as does the anterior and posterior walls, it must be assumed that biopsies presumably taken from the lateral walls are less accurate. While admonitions are here given to ensure the tissue is from the correct site, the histology should be assayed, not the operators intention.

Balasch et al. further documented variability of results by pointing out that subsequent biopsies tend to reverse the initial impression. However, of the 17 patients whose first two biopsies documented a luteal phase defect, only 1 demonstrated a normal biopsy at a third sampling.[11] In contrast, 83 of 172 patients whose initial biopsies suggested a deficiency were normal when a second biopsy was done. This is of interest as two successive biopsies demonstrating a deficiency is a common clinical criteria for a luteal phase defect.

In a most recent paper, Li et al. obtained a correlation of .70 between two observers and each of these observers got better results R = 0.65 and 0.75 with the LH surge than with the next menstural period, R = 0.28 and R = 0.41, respectively.[12] These authors also noticed a tendency to err toward the center of the cycle.

In summary, two observers are capable of agreeing on an endometrial date only around 75% of the time. Exact dating is achievable about 20% of the time. Sixty percent of the time one can get within ± 1 d and around 75% of the time within ± 2 d. These figures are of course generalizations from the above reviewed literature. If one chooses to see them as documenting accuracy one may do so and obviously the reverse is also true. Carefully interpreted endometrial biopsies may help clinicians who use them intelligently. Perhaps they demonstrate a more general truism which is that both clinicians and pathologists tend to have higher expectations than are reasonable when one tries to quantitate ever variable biology.

REFERENCES

1. **Hitschmann, F. and Adler, L.,** Der Bau der Uterusschleimhaut des geschlechtsreifen Weibes mit besonderer Berucksichtigung der Menstruation. in *Monatsschrif fur Geburtshulfe u. Gynakologie,* Bd. XXVII, Heft 1, 1908.
2. **Bardawil, W. A.,** Endometrium, in *Gynecologic Endocrinology,* 4th ed., Gold, J. J. and Josimovich, J. B., Eds., Plenum Medical Book Company, New York, 1988.
3. **Rick, J. and Bartlett, M. K.,** Biopsy studies of human endometrium, *JAMA,* June 12, 1937, 2022.
4. **Noyes, R. W., Hertig, A. T., and Rock, J.,** Dating the endometrial biopsy, *Fertil. Steril.,* 1, 3, 1950.
5. **Novak, E.,** Editorial, *Obstet. Gynecol. Surv.,* 5, 564, 1950.
6. **Noyes, R. W. and Haman, J. O.,** Accuracy of endometrial dating: correlation of endometrial dating with basal body temperature and menses, *Fertil. Steril.,* 4, 504, 1953.
7. **Tredway, D. R., Mishell, D. R., and Moyer, D. L.,** Correlation of endometrial dating with luteinizing hormone peak, *Am. J. Obstet. Gynecol.,* 8, 1030, 1975.

8. **Lundy, L. E., Lee, S. G., Levy, W., Woodruff, J. D., Wu, C. H., and Abdalla, M.,** The ovulatory cycle: a histologic, thermal, steroid and gonadotropin correlation, *Obstet. Gynecol.,* 44, 14, 1974.

9. **Koninckx, P. R., Goddeeris, P. G., Lauweryns, J. M., Hertogh, R. C., and Brosens, I. A.,** Accuracy of endometrial biopsy dating in relation to the midcycle luteinizing hormone peak, *Fertil. Steril.,* 28, 443, 1977.

10. **Johannisson, E., Parker, R. A., Landgren, B. M., and Dieczfalusy, E.,** Morphometric analysis of the human endometrium in relation to peripheral hormone levels, *Fertil. Steril.,* 38, 564, 1982.

11. **Balasch, J., Vanrell, J. A., Creus, M., Marquez, M., and Gonzalez-Merlo, J.,** The endometrial biopsy for diagnosis of luteal phase deficiency, *Fertil. Steril.,* 44, 699, 1985.

12. **Li, T. C., Rogers, A. W., Lenton, E. A., Dockery, P., and Cooke, I.,** A comparison between two methods of chronological dating of human endometrial biopsies during the luteal phase, and their correlation with histologic dating, *Fertil. Steril.,* 48, 928, 1987.

Chapter 3

THE SEMEN ANALYSIS

Brooks A. Keel

TABLE OF CONTENTS

I. INTRODUCTION

Infertility is generally defined as an inability to conceive after 12 months of unprotected intercourse. Infertility is a serious problem affecting an estimated 2.4 million married couples today.[1] It has been suggested that 40% of diagnosed infertility can be related to a problem with the male partner, 40% to a problem with the female partner, and the remainder due to problems with both partners. Thus, infertility should be considered a couple problem and the evaluation of infertility must involve both male and female factors.

Perhaps the most important aspect of the laboratory diagnosis of male factor infertility involves a careful evaluation of the semen. Theoretically, the semen analysis is an easy test to perform. One simply places a drop of semen on a slide and observes the relative number and mobility of sperm. However, if careful attention is not paid to this analysis, gross misinformation about the male partner results. For example, it has become increasingly clear that knowing subjectively how many sperm are present and moving may not provide enough information concerning the fertility potential of the male patient. Objective information on the qualitative and quantitative characteristics of sperm movement (kinematics) is often needed. It is because of the misconception that the semen analysis is "simple" or routine in nature that this test is often one of the most abused laboratory tests performed in the infertility evaluation.

Several excellent articles have reviewed the processes and methods involved in the semen analysis.[2-11] In this chapter I will attempt to provide the reader with step-by-step methodology for performing the semen analysis, point out some of the pitfalls associated with the test, provide some explanation for abnormal results, and review recent advances in the analysis of male factor infertility.

II. SPECIMEN COLLECTION

Several reports have shown significant variation of semen parameters within normal men.[11,12] These studies have indicated that a single semen specimen provides an unreliable assessment of the fertility potential of the male. Most investigators agree that at least two to three ejaculates spaced 2 weeks apart provide a reliable initial evaluation and baseline values. A repeat analysis is particularly important in the face of an abnormal result. In addition, significant annual variation in semen parameters has been reported.[13] Thus, multiple analyses are often required. The patient should be informed of the possibility of producing multiple specimens before he collects the first ejaculate.

Without a doubt, more erroneous semen analysis results have resulted from improper attention to specimen collection and handling than all other possibilities combined. Careful attention to several key points will eliminate these potential errors. The proper methods of specimen collection should be carefully discussed with the patient prior to collection of the specimen. Our laboratory provides an instruction sheet to each patient prior to collection (Appendix IV). This sheet provides the laboratory with important demographic data on the patient as well as information about the ejaculate including time of collection, whether any of the specimen was lost and the period of abstinence. Several key points should be remembered when discussing a semen analysis with the patient: the length of sexual abstinence, method used for collection, the container used for collection, and the method of specimen transport to the laboratory. These points will be discussed below.

A. ABSTINENCE
The period of sexual abstinence before collection of an ejaculate can have profound effects on the results of a semen analysis. In one study evaluating sperm count and semen volume after serial daily ejaculations, sperm concentration and semen volume was reduced

by 70% of control within the first 4 d.[14] Semen variables have been shown to increase linearly between 1 and 5 d of sexual rest.[12] Mean daily increments of approximately 15 million sperm/ml and 0.5 ml semen volume have been reported with abstinence.[11,12] On the other hand, extended periods of abstinence (weeks) can also have detrimental effects on ejaculate quality resulting in cell death and abnormal morphology. The optimal time appears to be 2 to 3 d, and this period of abstinence should be consistent from one analysis to another. The patient should be instructed that abstinence means refraining from any ejaculation, not just intercourse. The period of abstinence should be recorded on each analysis report form.

B. COLLECTION METHOD

Masturbation is the most widely used and in many cases the only acceptable technique for collecting a semen specimen. It has the advantage of most often resulting in the collection of a complete and uncontaminated specimen. Lubricants and lotions may be used in the collection of ejaculates. However, one study has shown that high concentrations (16.7% v/v) of glycerin may adversely affect sperm motility while similar concentrations of egg white showed no effect.[15] Therefore, before recommending lubricants to patients, the lubricants should be tested for sperm toxicity effects. We currently recommend Today℗ personal lubricant (Whitehall Laboratories, New York, NY) which is commercially available from most medical suppliers. These lubricants should be readily available for the patient in the collection room.

Some patients because of religious or moral convictions refuse masturbation. For these patients, a specially designed condom is available for collection of the specimen by intercourse (a silastic seminal collection device; see below). One study has, in fact, reported better quality ejaculates collected by this method.[16] However, spillage of the specimen upon removal of the condom from the penis is very possible as well as incomplete collection from the condom prior to analysis.

Coitus interruptus (or "withdrawal") should, however, be discouraged because of the difficulty of withdrawing the penis from the vagina at the time of ejaculation and collecting the entire specimen without loss of some of the ejaculate. Since the first portion of the ejaculate usually contains the greatest number of sperm, the resulting analysis may be erroneous.

In patients with an excessive semen volume, the collection of a "split ejaculate" may be beneficial. By this process, the patient collects the first portion of the ejaculate into one container and the remainder into another container. Since the first portion of the ejaculate contains the largest proportion of sperm, collecting this portion separate from the rest of the ejaculate can result in a higher concentration of sperm in a reduced volume of seminal plasma. Collection of the split ejaculate can be performed by providing the patient with two specimen jars taped together and labeled as #1 and #2. The patient is then instructed to collect the first fractions in jar #1 and the remainder in jar #2. An analysis is then performed on each container. Obviously, this technique is not an easy task for some patients and often requires more than one attempt to achieve accurate results. Furthermore, with the advent of sperm washing techniques and the sperm wash and rise procedure (see Chapter 11), the use of the split ejaculate is now less frequently indicated.

Regardless of the method used, the patient must be properly instructed prior to collection and then questioned afterwards for possible collection errors. Patients will seldom volunteer information concerning collection errors because of ignorance or embarrassment. Thus the importance of the patient questionnaire.

C. CONTAINER

The container used for the collection of semen should be provided by the laboratory or clinic. Bottles and jars obtained from the patients home often are contaminated with detergents and/or water and are unsuitable. The container should be wide-mouthed to allow ease of collection. Glass containers are perhaps the best. Several reports have indicated that some plastics may have spermicidal characteristics.[17,18] However, glass containers are easily broken and the plastic containers are less expensive and can be discarded after use. For this reason we use plastic 128 ml nonsterile disposable specimen containers (Fisherbrand, Fisher Scientific, Cat. No. 14-375-112A). A sterile disposable Seminal Fluid Collection Container (Apex Medical Technologies, Inc., San Diego, CA) is also available commercially. This device comes with a large collecting funnel attached to a 6 ml graduated plastic tube. It has the advantage of ease of collection, and the graduated tube allows accurate measurement of semen volume without having to transfer the specimen to another container.[19] The kit contains a collection container, graduated vial, vial cap, patient I.D. label, and directions for use. Other laboratories have also used household Zip Loc Storage Bags (Dow Chemical Company) for semen collection.[9] This storage bag has the advantage that is readily available, and can be tightly sealed, folded and placed in a brown lightproof bag or shirt pocket. The disadvantage is that it is sometimes difficult to remove all of the specimen from the bag prior to analysis.

Regardless of the container used, it should be checked for sperm toxicity before use. This can easily be checked by collecting a sperm specimen in a glass container, dividing the ejaculate equally between this container and the test container, incubating both containers at 37°C, and comparing sperm motility at 30 min, 1, 2, and 3 h. The percent motility of the test container should be comparable to that observed in the glass container.

If the patient refuses masturbation as a method of collection, condoms may be utilized. Because most readily available condoms contain spermicides, appropriate condoms must be provided by the laboratory or clinic and be specially designed for the purpose of collecting semen for analysis. Polyethylene sheaths made by Milex Corporation (Chicago, IL) have been used in the past, but are uncomfortable for most patients. This has led to the investigation of the use of silastic condoms which are more comfortable and aesthetic for patients.[20,21] More recently, a silastic Sperm Collection Device (SCD; HDC Corporation, Mountain View, CA) has become available. The use of this condom has been reported to increase the quality of ejaculates, particularly in individuals with low sperm counts.[16]

D. TRANSPORT

It is our opinion that it is advantageous to have the patient collect the specimen in close proximity to the laboratory, hospital, or clinic where the analysis is going to be performed. This allows the technician performing the analysis to evaluate the coagulation/liquefaction phenomenon (see below), reduces the chance of the specimen being exposed to extremes of temperature during transport, and keeps the time interval between collection and analysis minimal.

Consideration for patients privacy must be recognized. As one might imagine, it is difficult for some patients to be given a specimen container, directed to a small bathroom near the nurses station or gynecologist's waiting room, and be expected to masturbate. In our clinic, we have designated a room which is quiet, secluded, and away from patient traffic and is utilized for the collection of semen specimens only. We also encourage participation of the female partner during this process. Naturally, some patients are totally uncomfortable with collecting a semen specimen in a clinic or doctor's office. These individuals are carefully instructed on collection and transport of the specimen and are allowed to collect elsewhere.

Although visible light may have deleterious effects on animal sperm, it has minimal effects on human sperm motility.[22] Temperature can, however, markedly affect initial sperm motility and velocity as well as motility longevity.[23,24] We advise patients to protect the ejaculate from extremes of temperature while transporting the specimen to the laboratory.

During the winter months, we suggest that the specimen be carried in an inside coat pocket and during the summer months the specimen should be protected from direct sunlight.

The relative temperature and condition of the specimen should always be evaluated when the specimen arrives to the laboratory. If the specimen container (and hence the ejaculate) is excessively cool or warm to the touch, this fact should be noted on the semen analysis report form. If the specimen was not collected at the laboratory or the clinic, or if the container was not provided by the laboratory, this should also be noted.

III. MACROSCOPIC ANALYSIS

A. OVERVIEW OF PROCEDURES
1. Note and record condition of container (warm, cold, damaged, etc.), and time of specimen collection and arrival to laboratory.
2. Evaluate liquefaction. Record time required or "complete".
3. Evaluate viscosity. Record as normal or 1+ to 4+. If hyperviscous (3 to 4+), mechanically reduce viscosity.
4. Measure semen volume. Record to the nearest 0.1 ml.
5. Record unusual semen color or turbidity.
6. Measure and record pH.

B. SPECIMEN CONDITION
Note the general condition of the specimen. Make sure it is properly labeled with patient's name and, if necessary, the doctor's name as well. The patient information sheet or questionnaire should also accompany each specimen (Appendix IV). Check this information for completeness. Record the period of abstinence.

C. LIQUEFACTION
Semen is normally ejaculated as a coagulum. The specimen will usually liquify within 30 min. It is considered abnormal if liquefaction requires more than 1 h.[25] If the specimen has been collected in the laboratory, note the time of collection and evaluate liquefaction after 30 min. If the actual time required for this process can be noted, record this time on the report form. If the specimen has been collected elsewhere and transported to the laboratory, evaluate liquefaction upon arrival. If liquefaction has occurred, record "complete" for this process.

Liquefaction is usually evaluated visually. The coagulum is a thick, viscous gel-like mass. The specimen container is held up next to a light source and tilted sideways so that the specimen is "spread out". The liquified specimen should have a uniform fluid appearance. If the specimen has not liquified, reevaluate in 15 to 20 min. There have been more quantitative methods reported for analyzing liquefaction[25] but we have found this approach unnecessary on a routine basis.

Liquefaction and viscosity are two completely different phenomenan. A viscous sample (see below) should never be reported as "specimen did not liquify". This is a common error among laboratories performing semen analyses, and it is very important to differentiate between these two processes.

Failure of a specimen to coagulate immediately after ejaculation may be indicative of seminal vesicle dysfunction. In many cases, it is not possible to evaluate the semen specimen so soon after ejaculation. Therefore, noncoagulation is difficult to evaluate by the laboratory. On the other hand, failure of the clot to liquify may be indicative of prostatic dysfunctin. Although accurate evaluation of this process may provide important diagnostic information for the physician, infertility due to liquefaction abnormalities is rare. Several techniques are available for reducing the viscosity of semen and these are discussed below.

TABLE 1
Arbitrary Subjective Scale for Evaluating Semen Viscosity by the Pipette Method

Rating	Observation
Normal	Semen easily drawn and released in distinct drops.
1 +	Semen easily drawn and released with slight stringing.
2 +	Semen can be drawn but is released with moderate stringing. Mucoid strings "connect" drops.
3 +	Semen difficult to draw into pipette. Release requires moderate pressure. No distinct drops seen with significant mucoid stringing.
4 +	Semen cannot be drawn into a pipette. Semen pours as a solid mass.

D. VISCOSITY

Excessive viscosity (hyperviscosity) and nonliquefaction are two separate phenomenon. Viscosity is measured after complete liquefaction has occurred. Viscosity can be measured by pouring the specimen from the collection container into a graduated cylinder used for measuring volume. Normal viscosity is defined as that which will allow semen to be poured drop by drop from the container.[4] Alternatively, viscosity may be evaluated by the ability of semen to be drawn up into and released from a Pasteur pipette. Normal viscosity will allow the semen to be easily drawn into the pipette and will be released easily in distinct drops without excess mucoid stringing. Extremely viscous semen often cannot be drawn into the pipette, or will be expelled as a continuous string. We use an arbitrary subjective scale for evaluating viscosity by the pipette method (Table 1). Obviously, this scaling system is very subjective and requires practice before consistency is noted. More objective methods of viscosity have been reported (see References 3 and 4), but with experience the above method is quite satisfactory for routine use.

The role of hyperviscosity in infertility is currently poorly understood. This condition can be transient and can vary widely between and within patients. It is conceivable that extremely viscous samples may inhibit sperm from leaving the vagina and entering the cervical mucus. However, if the postcoital evaluation of the couple is normal than hyperviscosity as a cause for infertility can be ruled out.[2] Hyperviscosity can, however, cause technical problems with the semen analysis. An extremely viscous sample (3 to 4 +) can make accurate sperm counts and motility determinations very difficult to measure. Under these conditions, the viscosity can be markedly reduced by adding the specimen to a syringe fitted with an 18 gauge needle. The specimen is then forced through the needle. This process may have to be repeated several times to completely reduce the viscosity. For samples with moderate viscosity (2 to 3 +), repeated pipetting with a Pasteur pipette can often significantly reduce the viscous nature of the specimen and allow a more accurate analysis of sperm count and motility. The use of mucolytic agents to reduce semen viscosity has been reported[4,26] but generally are not required for routine analysis.

E. VOLUME
1. Methods

The volume of the semen can easily be measured by transferring the specimen to a graduated cylinder or centrifuge tube. Volume should be recorded to the nearest 0.1 ml. The use of glass graduated cylinders necessitates washing and reuse of the cylinder. If this method is used, extreme care must be used to ensure that the cylinder is completely free of contaminating water or detergents. Therefore, disposable graduated 15 ml conical centrifuge tubes are generally used.

2. Normal Values

Normal values for semen volume range from 1.5 to 5.5 ml (Table 2). The suffix "spermia" is used to refer to semen volume (Table 3). Reduced semen volume (<1.5 ml)

TABLE 2
Reference Values for a Normal Semen Analysis

Parameter	Normal range	Units
Count	20 to 250	$\times 10^6$/ml
Motility	>40	%
Velocity	>20	μm/sec
Motile density	>8	$\times 10^6$/ml
Motility index	>8	μm/sec
Morphology	>60	% normal forms
Volume	1.5—5.5	ml
Liquefaction	10—30	Minutes
Viscosity	0—1+	Subjective scale
Agglutination	Absent	Subjective scale

Note: Values represent the normal range of reference semen analysis values using an objective microcomputerized multiple exposure photography system. Motile density is defined as the product of the motility and the sperm count. Motility index is defined as the product of the motility and the velocity. Velocity is determined as straight line velocity.

TABLE 3
Nomenclature for Characterizing Semen Specimens Based on the Results of the Semen Analysis

Phrase	Definition
-spermia	Refers to abnormalities of semen
-zoospermia	Refers to abnormalities of spermatozoa
Hypospermia	Semen volume <1.5 ml
Hyperspermia	Semen volume >5.5 ml
Aspermia	No semen volume
Pyospermia	Leukocytes (WBCs) present in semen
Hematospermia	Red blood cells present in semen
Oligozoospermia	Sperm count <20 $\times 10^6$/ml
Polyzoospermia	Sperm count >250 $\times 10^6$/ml
Asthenozoospermia	Sperm motility <40%
Teratozoospermia	>40% abnormal morphological forms
Necrozoospermia	Nonviable sperm
Oligoasthenozoospermia	Motile density <8 $\times 10^6$ motile sperm/ml

is classified as hypospermia. Increased semen volumes (>5.5 ml) is classified as hyperspermia. Total absence of semen indicates aspermia.

3. Abnormal Results

a. Hypospermia

Abnormalities in semen volume can be diagnostically very important. Hypospermia can have several potential causes. Perhaps the most frequent cause of hypospermia is a collection error. This can be ascertained by questioning the patient. If the first part of the ejaculate was lost during collection, the analysis should reveal a reduced sperm count. Biochemically, the ejaculate will have reduced levels of prostate specific secretions such as acid phosphatase. If the last portion of the ejaculate was lost, the sperm count may be normal to high, and the secretions of the seminal vesicle, such as fructose, will be reduced. Reduced semen volume may also be related to the period of abstinence. Exceptionally short periods of abstinence (1 d or less) may reduce the volume of semen. Repeat analysis with longer periods of abstinence (3 d) should correct this problem.

Hypospermia is also caused by pathological conditions including retrograde ejaculation, congenital absence of the seminal vesicles and vas deferens, and ejaculatory duct blockage. Retrograde ejaculation, a backward ejaculation of semen into the bladder, can be easily ruled out by examining a postejaculation urine sample. The presence of many sperm in the urine, especially after centrifugation of the sample, is indicative of a retrograde ejaculation. Sperm can be harvested from this urine sample and prepared for insemination (see below). Congenital bilateral absence of the vas deferens is associated with a similar absence of the seminal vesicles, since both are embryonically derived from the same tissues. In this condition, the specimen will lack sperm and fructose, the marker for the seminal vesicles. Total ejaculatory duct obstruction gives similar findings.

b. Hyperspermia

Seminal volumes >5.5 ml are technically considered as hyperspermic. Unless the sperm concentration is severely reduced fertility is seldom compromised by this condition. An excess of seminal fluid may "dilute" sperm so that a reduced number of sperm come in contact with the cervical mucus. In cases of severe hyperspermia in the face of a reduced sperm count, collecting a split ejaculate may be indicated. However, as mentioned above, with the advent of sperm wash and rise procedures (see Chapter 11), motile sperm can be concentrated easily *in vitro* and artificial insemination with the concentrated specimen performed.

c. Aspermia

A total absence of semen is termed aspermia. If this condition is detected, a gross collection error must first be ruled out. Pathologically, this condition can result from retrograde ejaculation or ejaculatory duct obstruction. Examination of a post-ejaculation urine specimen should be performed to rule out retrograde ejaculation. In some instances patients who have undergone retroperitoneal lymph node dissection (RLND), or operations for vesicle neck obstruction, may have an aspermic ejaculation unrelated to retrograde flow as a result of interruption of the sympathetic nerve supply to the vas deferens.[27] These patients will have the sensation of orgasm without emission.

F. COLOR AND TURBIDITY

Semen is normally translucent or whitish-gray opalescent in color. The presence of blood in semen (termed hematospermia) can color the semen pink to bright red to brownish red. The presence of blood in semen is obviously abnormal and should be reported. Certain drugs such as antibiotics used in the treatment of cystitis may also stain the semen.[3] Report any unusual coloration observed. The presence of gross macroscopic particles, nonliquified streaks of mucus, or particulate debris should also be reported.

G. pH

The pH of semen is measured using litmus paper ranging from 6.6 to 9.0. The pH of normal semen is slightly alkaline ranging from 7.2 to 7.8. The secretions of the prostate are acidic while the secretions of the seminal vesicles are alkaline. Therefore, alterations in semen pH may be indicative of sex accessory gland dysfunction. However, we have not found this semen parameter to be particularly useful or reproducible in the diagnosis of male factor infertility.

IV. MICROSCOPIC ANALYSIS

A. OVERVIEW OF PROCEDURES
1.   Perform wet mount analysis. Analyze the following:
    a. Turbidity
    b. Agglutination
    c. Estimate of count and motility
2.   Determine percent motility and kinetics by:
    a. Subjective methods
    b. Objective methods
3.   Determine sperm count by:
    a. Hemocytometer
    b. Makler chamber
    c. Computer-assisted semen analysis (CASA)
4.   Prepare semen smear, stain the smear, perform morphology differential

B. WET MOUNT ANALYSIS
Regardless of the technique used for determination of sperm count and motility, a wet mount or "wet prep" analysis should be performed on each specimen. This analysis will give the technician a subjective overview of sperm count, motility and kinetics and will allow determination of turbidity and agglutination. The temperature at which sperm count and motility is assessed is important. Obviously, performing the analysis at 37°C is optimal. However, without the use of a temperature-regulated microscope stage, complete analysis at this temperature is not always possible. We routinely perform semen analysis at room temperature. As expected, large fluctuations in room temperature can occur, and changes in the temperature at the location where the semen analysis is performed must be carefully monitored.

1. Methods
After complete liquefaction, thoroughly mix the semen in the container. Place a drop of undiluted semen on a clean glass slide and cover with a coverslip. Reproducibility can be improved by using an automatic pipettor and placing 10 µl of semen on the slide. Observe 20 microscopic fields using a power of 200 to 400× (high power field; hpf). Estimate the approximate percentage of motile sperm, the relative speed and direction of travel, and the approximate numbers of sperm per hpf. Estimate turbidity and the presence or absence of agglutination. Determine the relative percentage of "round cells" (immature germ cells and white blood cells).

2. Turbidity
Mature sperm obviously make up the largest percentage of cells found in semen. However, other cells and debris may sometimes be found in semen. Epithelial cells which arise from the male genital tract may be seen in semen. Rare to occasional epithelial cells per hpf is probably not indicative of pathology. However, many epithelial cells may be present in men with urethritis. Epithelial cells of vaginal origin are sometimes seen and may indicate that the specimen was collected by coitus interruptus. If these cells are observed, this should be noted on the analysis report form.

Immature germ cells and white blood cells (WBCs) are often seen in semen. It can be difficult to differentiate between these two cell types from stained smears (see below) and almost impossible on wet prep analysis. We routinely perform a Papanicolaou (PAP) stain on specimens that demonstrate a large amount (10% or more relative to mature sperm) of these "round cells". Therefore, wet prep analysis can be helpful in determining which

TABLE 4
Arbitrary Subjective Scale Used to Evaluate
Sperm Agglutination by Wet Mount Analysis

Rating	Observation
Absent	No agglutination observed
1+	Occasional sperm agglutinated
2+	25% or less of sperm agglutinated
3+	25—50% sperm agglutinated
4+	Gross agglutination, few sperm free swimming

specimens need to be prepared in this manner. The actual number of WBCs and percentage of immature germ cells should be determined and recorded (see below).

Other particulate matter such as spermine crystals, talcum powder, and spermicidal powders can be seen in seminal plasma. If materials are observed in excess, it should be recorded. Obviously, gross bacteria, Trichomonas, and Candida should be reported.

3. Agglutination

In some, but not all, semen specimens which contain specific antisperm antibodies spontaneous agglutination of sperm will occur. If agglutination is observed, this should be noted along with a subjective determination of the degree and type of agglutination. We use a 1+ to 4+ scale to evaluate agglutination (Table 4). The type of sperm agglutination should also be noted: head-to-head, head-to-tail, tail-to-tail, or mixed. Sperm will occasionally adhere to debris and other particulate matter in semen. This should not be confused with true agglutination and not reported unless severe. The presence of sperm agglutination may indicate that specific antisperm antibody testing should be performed (see Chapters 9 and 10).

4. Estimate Sperm Count, Motility, and Kinetics

The approximate sperm count should be determined. This subjective measure (few, several, many, numerous sperm/hpf) need not be reported. However, if numerous sperm/hpf are observed but an objective sperm count reveals a reduced number of sperm, one should question the results and repeat the analysis. In much the same way, a subjective estimate of sperm motility (25, 50, 75, or >80%) and kinetics (sluggish random movement vs. rapid straight line movement) should also be made and compared with the more objective determinations. Clearly, this type of analysis is very subjective and prone to within and between technician error. However, with practice these ''mental notes'' can often indicate potential errors in the objective analysis.

C. MOTILITY
1. Subjective Determinations

Sperm motility can be estimated by placing a 10 μl drop of well-mixed semen on a slide, covered by a coverslip, and evaluating 10 to 20 fields at 200 to 400× power (wet mount analysis). The relative percentage of motile sperm is then estimated. The percent motility is then reported to the nearest 5%. Obviously, this technique is potentially fraught with reproducibility errors. With practice, this method can give reasonable estimates of motility. More accurate methods of sperm motility determination can be made by actually counting the motile and nonmotile sperm in at least five separate microscopic fields (count at least 200 total sperm) and calculating the percentage of motile sperm from these counts.

2. Objective Determinations

Several objective methods have recently been introduced allowing for more accurate

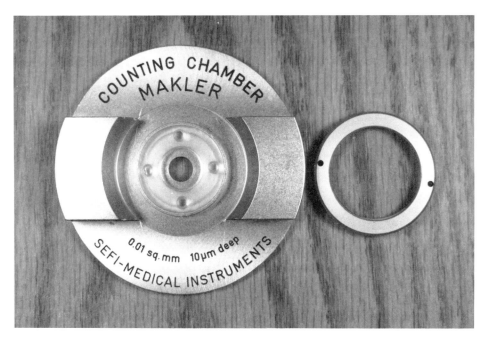

FIGURE 1.   The Makler Counting Chamber.

and reproducible determination of sperm motility. The use of the Makler Counting Chamber (Figure 1) and CASA have markedly improved our ability to measure the mobility of sperm. These methods will be discussed below.

a. Makler Counting Chamber

The Makler Counting Chamber (Sefi-Medical Instruments, Israel; available in the U.S. from Zygotek™ Systems, Inc., Springfield, MA) has been specially designed for the counting of sperm and estimating sperm motility.[28] This chamber is composed of two parts (Figure 2). The lower main part is made up of a circular metal base and two handles. The semen sample is placed on a flat glass disc in the center of the base. Four quartz-tipped posts are arranged along the periphery. Each post is 10 μm in height. The upper part of the chamber is a cover glass which contains a marked 1 mm² grid which is subdivided into 110 squares each 0.1×0.1 mm (Figure 3). When the cover glass is placed onto the base, the semen sample is spread out over a field 10 μm in depth. The space bounded by the two surfaces and ten of the small squares is 0.001 mm³ or one millionth of ml. Thus, the number of sperm counted in ten squares is equal to $\times 10^6$ sperm per 1.0 ml. The use of this chamber for sperm counts is detailed below. For motility determination:

1. Clean and dry the chamber completely.
2. Mix specimen well, place one drop (8 to 10 μl) onto the center of the lower disk.
3. Place the cover glass on the four posts. Semen should spread over the entire area of the lower glass disc. Avoid adding excess semen which will flood over the four posts and render the analysis inaccurate.
4. Lift the chamber by the handles, place on the microscope stage and view using a $\times 20$ objective and $\times 10$ eyepiece.
5. Count all of the nonmotile sperm within 9 or 16 squares.
6. Count all of the motile sperm within this same area.
7. Repeat this procedure in another area of the same grid.
8. Clean the chamber and repeat above three to four times. Calculate the average number.

39

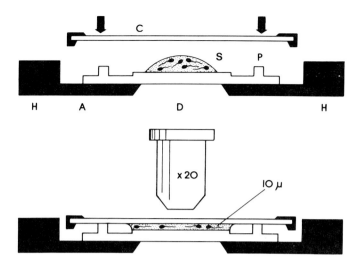

FIGURE 2. Diagrammatic representation of the Makler Counting Chamber. A, metal base, C, cover glass. D, flat disc on which the sperm sample (S) is placed. H, handles. Makler Counting Chamber Instructions for Use, Sefi-Medical Instruments, Haifa, Israel. With permission.

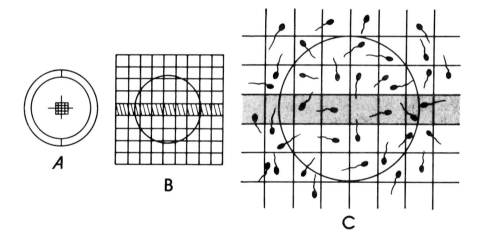

FIGURE 3. Diagrammatic representation of the Makler Counting Chamber cover glass showing a magnification of the counting grid incorporated into the cover glass. Makler Counting Chamber Instructions for Use, Sefi-Medical Instruments, Haifa, Israel. With permission.

Because of the difficulty of counting motile sperm, several alternatives are possible. These alternatives are based on counting all nonmotile sperm in a fresh specimen, immobilizing the sperm by heat or cold, and counting the total number of sperm. In the first alternative, load the chamber with fresh semen and count the nonmotile sperm as above. Place the chamber at −20°C for 10 min to immobilize the motile sperm. Count the total number of sperm. In the second alternative, perform the count of nonmotile sperm in the fresh specimen as above. Transfer a small part of the fresh specimen to test tube and heat at 50 to 60°C for 5 min to immobilize the sperm. Clean, re-load the chamber, and count the total number of sperm as above. In each case, the motility is calculated as:

$$\text{(total sperm — nonmotile sperm)/total sperm} \times 100$$

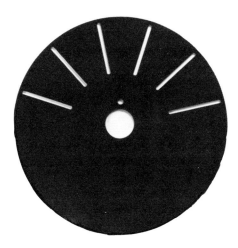

FIGURE 4. The six-slotted disk used in multiple-exposure photography (MEP) semen analysis.

b. *Photomicrography*

Development of the Makler Counting Chamber was an important advance in andrology. Because of its well-defined and constant depth, sperm could be visualized in a single plane. This allows sperm to be photographed on the microscope stage while swimming perpendicular to the film plane. Amnon Makler developed a multiple-exposure photography (MEP) technique for photographing sperm in motion.[29,30] In this technique, the Makler chamber is loaded and placed on the stage of a phase contrast microscope. The microscope is fitted with a still camera (recent versions utilize a Polaroid instant camera) and a stroboscope. The stroboscope consists of a motor which rotates a six-slotted disk (Figure 4). The disk is situated between the light source and the stage such that when initially placed, the light source is blackened by the darkened half of the disk. At the time the shutter of the camera is opened, the disk is rotated and the specimen in the chamber is illuminated by six bursts of light at $1/6$-s intervals as each slot passes by the light source, exposing the film. In the resulting photograph (Figure 5), nonmotile sperm show up as a single brightly lit sperm head and associated tail, while the motile sperm appear as six-ringed chains. The nonmotile and motile sperm can be readily differentiated. To obtain the percent motility, one simply counts the numbers of motile and nonmotile sperm and calculates the percent motile. Others have used videomicroscopy and analysis of individual video frames to assess sperm motility.[31]

c. *CASA*

The use of computer assisted semen analysis has advanced the field of male fertility testing. These systems not only have increased the accuracy and reproducibility of sperm count and motility determinations, but also have allowed the measurement of the speed and direction of sperm travel. Two basic methodologies are currently available. One utilizes computer assisted MEP[32-35] and the other videomicroscopy.[36] These methods are described in detail in Chapter 6. We have utilized the MEP system (available commercially from Zygotek™ Systems, Inc. Springfield, MA) in our laboratory for the last four years.[32-34] This system consists of an Olympus BH-2 microscope with a ×20 phase-contrast objective, 7000 Polaroid 4 × 5 camera using type 57 black and white film, stroboscope, IBM PC computer, and graphics tablet. The multiple exposed film is placed on the graphics tablet (Figure 6) and with the aid of the computer and the graphics tablet the motile and nonmotile sperm

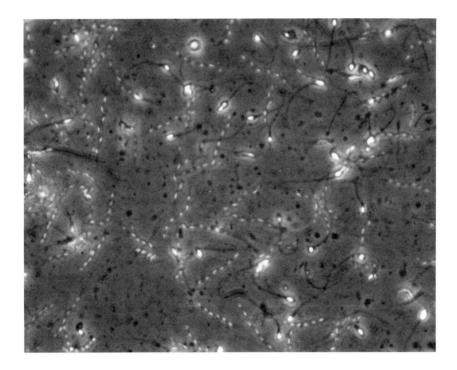

FIGURE 5. A multiple exposed photograph of human spermatozoa used in MEP semen analysis. The nonmotile sperm show up as a single brightly lit sperm head and associated tail, while the motile sperm appear as six-ringed chains. Film used was Polaroid type 57 black and white.

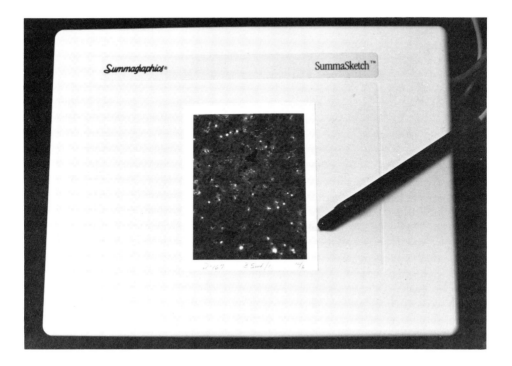

FIGURE 6. Illustration of the graphics tablet, multiple-exposed photograph of sperm, and graphics pen used in computerized MEP semen analysis. The graphics pen is used to touch the motile and nonmotile sperm seen in the photograph. This touch is registered by a computer which tallies the sperm numbers.

are counted. The computer automatically tallies sperm numbers (see below) and calculates motility.

The CASA systems have the advantage of providing objective semen analysis data. The disadvantages include price and potential errors induced by computer system parameter settings and extremes of sperm numbers.[37-40] The price for the system can range from $15,000 to well over $35,000. However, the objectiveness of the results, the information derived and the time-saving features of these systems often override the costs, especially if a large number of semen analyses are to be performed. The potential user-induced errors can be minimized by careful attention to the settings used.

d. Turbidimetric Method

Several investigators have reported on a turbidimetric method for objective evaluation of sperm motility.[41,42] This method is based on the fact that sperm will swim upward from a concentrated cell suspension at the bottom of an optical cuvette into a layer of clear medium.[41] This movement will result in a time-dependent increase in turbidity in the medium which can be measured as an increase in absorbance. Clinically, it has the advantages of providing a quantitative measure of sperm motility, does not rely on arbitrary ratings by individuals, and the sperm must perform work (i.e., they must swim upward) in order to be measured.[42] Although this technique has these advantages, it is currently not routinely used to measure sperm motility in most clinical laboratories.

3. Initial vs. Repeated Measures of Motility

Several investigators have suggested that sperm motility should be evaluated every hour for 4 or more hours and again at 24 h to determine motility longevity. It is well known that sperm motility is a temperature-dependent phenomenon.[24] Clearly, sperm longevity is important since coitus and ovulation rarely coincide and the sperm must therefore remain viable in the female reproductive tract for some time if fertilization is to take place.[3] Thus, analysis of sperm motility longevity in vitro may provide important information concerning the fertility potential of the male. However, we and others[8] do not routinely perform repeated measurements of sperm motility because (1) sperm survival is not optimal in seminal plasma and longevity studies in this media probably are totally unrelated to survival in the female tract, (2) sperm leave seminal plasma within minutes after ejaculation for the cervical mucus, which is a more compatible media for sperm survival, and (3) *in vitro* measurements in a defined media other than seminal plasma are time consuming and expensive to perform on a routine basis. Until more proven *in vitro* techniques for assessment of motility longevity are defined and related positively to fertility potential, we have opted to report only initial motility values.

4. Normal Values

In many laboratories using subjective methods of analysis, normal sperm motility in semen is defined as >60%. However, in one report subjective motility determinations tended to overestimate motility by approximately 20%.[29] In our laboratory, using the MEP methodology, we have set 40% as a lower limit for "normal" motility (Table 2). Samples having motilities less than 40% are classified as asthenozoospermia. Others have used 50% as the cutoff for normal semen quality, 40 to 50% as marginal (borderline) and <40% as abnormal.[5]

5. Vital Live-Dead Staining

The total lack of motility in the ejaculate is definitely cause for concern. One must initially determine whether the lack of motility is due to motility dysfunction in the sperm or sperm cell death. A simple vital staining procedure can help to differentiate between these two abnormalities.

Eosin Vital Live-Dead Stain Method 1

1.   Prepare a 0.5% solution of blue eosin (Eosin B, Certified, Kodak #C5322; 0.5 g/100 ml distilled H_2O). Solution should be prepared fresh each day of use.
2.   Mix one drop of well-mixed semen with one drop of the eosin solution on a slide.
3.   Cover with a coverslip and examine after 1 to 2 min.
4.   Viable spermatozoa remain unstained against a pink background. Dead sperm are stained red ("red = dead").
5.   Count at least 200 total sperm and calculate percent viable.

Eosin Vital Live-Dead Stain Method 2[45]

1.   Prepare 0.125 M sodium phosphate buffer, pH 7.4.
2.   Dissolve 0.25 g Eosin B in 100 ml buffer.
3.   Spread 20 μl of the stain over a 15 mm diameter area on a glass slide.
4.   Allow the slides to air dry. Prepared slides may be stored at room temperature for at least 2 years.
5.   To test semen, place one drop of well-mixed semen on the eosin spot.
6.   Dissolve the eosin by gentle stirring. Let stand 1 min.
7.   Cover with a coverslip and read as above.

Eosin penetrates damaged sperm membranes. Occasionally, only part of the spermatozoa may take up the stain. If any part of the sperm cell shows the red color of the stain the sperm should be considered nonviable.[3] The percent nonviable should always be equal to or less than the percentage of nonmotile sperm.

6. Abnormal Results

a. Asthenozoospermia

Decreased sperm motility may be due to several factors. The most obvious and easily correctable causes of asthenozoopsermia are related to specimen collection and transport errors. If containers other than those provided by the laboratory are used, these should be checked for sperm toxicity. Any condom used for semen collection other than those described above should automatically be suspected as being sperm toxic. If the patient provided his own container, he should be asked if he washed the container prior to collection. Contamination with detergents or water can severely reduce motility. If the specimen was not collected in the laboratory, question the patient on the method used.

Abstinence can also effect sperm motility. Extended periods of sexual rest (several weeks) is often associated with decreased motility. Re-collection after 3 d of abstinence should rule out this cause of asthenozoospermia. Interestingly, relatively short abstinence, while decreasing sperm numbers, does not usually cause reductions in motility.

Medical causes of asthenozoospermia are related to abnormal spermatogenesis, epididymal sperm maturation and transport dysfunction, abnormal secretions of the sex accessory glands and infection. Decreased sperm motility is also often associated with the presence of a varicocele. Unfortunately, treatment of asthenozoospermia, especially unexplained or "idiopathic" asthenozoospermia, is often difficult and frustrating. Treatment modalities which offer some promise include intrauterine insemination (IUI) and *in vitro* fertilization procedures.

b. Necrozoospermia

If a total absence of sperm motility is observed on semen analysis, it becomes important to distinguish between nonviable sperm and those sperm with motility apparatus abnormalities. The eosin vital staining methods described above are simple means of making this distinction. A significantly high number of nonviable sperm (true necrozoospermia) may indicate that a collection and/or transport error has occurred as described above. The presence

TABLE 5
Subjective Grading System Used to Evaluate Sperm Kinetics

Numerical value	Descriptive value	Observation
0	None	No forward progression
1	Poor	Weak, sluggish forward progression or random directional movement
2	Fair	Moderate, forward progression, primarily unidirectional
3	Good	Good forward unidirectional progression
4	Excellent	Rapid forward unidirectional progression

of viable nonmotile sperm may indicate severe motility apparatus abnormality. One such condition is the immotile cilia syndrome, or Kartagener's syndrome.[46] In this condition, ciliary immotility is due to the absence of dynein arms on the outer microtubules of the anexonemal complex, resulting in total nonmotility of sperm. Other forms of ciliary dyskinesis, resulting in severe asthenozoospermia (1% motile forms) have also been reported.[47] While these abnormalities lead to nonmotility, normal penetration of zona-free hamster eggs by these abnormal sperm has been reported[46,47] suggesting that they may in fact be capable of causing fertilization if placed in close proximity to the egg.

D. KINETICS

The assessment of sperm movement is not just a determination of the percentage of motile sperm. This value tells nothing of the quality of movement. Recent data suggests that determination of the speed and direction of travel of motile sperm can provide essential information concerning the fertility potential of the male partner. The analysis of kinetics, or perhaps more correctly kinematics, can be made by subjective or, more recently, by objective measurements.

1. Subjective Determination

An indication of sperm kinetics can be made by a subjective grading system. This grade is assigned during the wet prep analysis in the same way as subjective motility assessment is made. The grade can consist of either a numerical value or descriptive words (Table 5). The numerical score is useful if the calculation of the motility index is employed (see below). As in all subjective grading systems, experience is needed to ensure reproducible reports.

2. Objective Determination

The advent of MEP and especially CASA techniques has allowed objective assessment of sperm movement in a way heretofore not possible. Not only can one now accurately measure the speed of sperm travel but can also quantitatively define sperm movement characteristics. Data from these instruments provide information on straight line velocity, curvilinear velocity, average path velocity, linearity, straightness, wobble, amplitude of lateral head displacement (ALH), and beat/cross frequency (BCF). These terms are defined and explained in detail in Chapter 6. The methods utilized to derive these values and the clinical relevance of these measurements are also described in that chapter and will therefore not be discussed in detail here.

3. Motility Index

This parameter, first described by MacLeod,[48] is an attempt to characterize the movement of sperm by a single parameter. This calculation takes into account both the quantity (motility) and quality (kinetics) of sperm movement.[49] When using subjective methods, the motility index is defined as the product of sperm motility and kinetics. As an example, an ejaculate with a good kinetics (numerical score of 3) and 75% motility would have a motility index of $3 \times 75 = 225$.

Objective motility indices have also been presented in the evaluation of sperm movement.[32-34,36] Using CASA and MEP methodologies, the motility index is defined as the product of the velocity and the percent motility. As an example, an ejaculate with a sperm velocity of 25.3 μm/s and a motility of 78% would have a motility index of 25.3 × 0.78 = 19.7. The actual predictive value of this parameter is still being debated. However, studies have shown that the motility index is higher in fertile men compared with infertile men,[36] is increased significantly after *in vitro* capacitation,[32] and provides the best positive predictive value for sperm penetration into bovine cervical mucus.[33] The importance of this parameter to the infertility evaluation awaits further documentation.

4. Normal Values

Normal values for sperm kinetics (or kinematics) depends upon whether subjective or objective methods were utilized in determining the value. For subjective methods, a kinetic value of 2 (fair) should be considered the lower limit of normal. Using this value, the lower limit of normal for the motility index is 120 (2 × 60%) considering 60% motility as the lower limit using subjective methods.

The normal values for objective determination of kinematics are somewhat dependent upon the methodology used (see Chapter 6 for more detail). The parameter used to evaluate kinematics (velocity, ADH, BCF, etc.) will also determine what values are used. In our laboratory, using MEP methodology (which measures straight-line velocity), and room temperature, we have set the lower limit of normal velocity at 20 μm/s[33,34] (Table 2). Values will be slightly higher if measured at 37°C. In agreement with our cut-off values, recent data from another laboratory has shown that a linear velocity value of 22 μm/s is the best in dividing fertile and infertile male groups.[50] Our lower limit values for motility index are set at 8 μm/s (20 μm/s × 40%/100). Using CASA methodology (measuring curvilinear velocity), Mathur has suggested that 30 μm/s may be considered to be a discriminating value between fertile and infertile men,[36] a value also suggested by Holt et al.[35] Others have set a minimum value of 25 μm/s.[5] These same investigators have observed that MEP methodology yields slightly lower velocities than the videomicrography methods used in most CASA systems.[5] Thus, the lower limit values depend upon the system utilized.

5. Abnormal Results

Many of the same causes for asthenozoospermia can also result in poor kinetics. Clearly, ejaculates demonstrating poor kinetics should be evaluated for collection/transport errors initially. If these causes fail to explain the poor result, then pathological causes may be explored. We are just beginning to understand the correlates between poor qualitative sperm movement and fertility. It is clear that fertile men are associated with faster, more unidirectional swimming sperm than their infertile counterparts. However, the exact causes for poor sperm kinematics, relationships to infertility, and methods for improving these parameters awaits further investigation.

E. COUNT

The vast majority of laboratories performing semen analyses utilize the improved Neubauer Counting Chamber (hemocytometer) for determining the concentration of sperm in the ejaculate (Figure 7). This chamber has several advantages including low cost, ready availability, and is familiar to most clinical laboratory technicians. However, it also has several distinct disadvantages, the most serious of which deals with its relative inaccuracy due to within and between technician variation. A large part of this error is introduced during dilution of the sample prior to loading the chamber.[51] This dilution error has been attributed to the use of a standard WBC pipette. This has led others to suggest that more accurate results can be obtained by using an automatic micropipette rather than the WBC pipette.

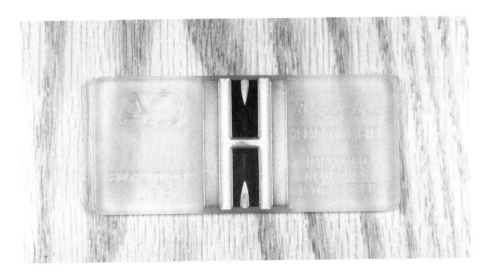

FIGURE 7.   An improved Neubauer Counting Chamber.

The use of the Makler chamber is more advantageous because dilution of the specimen is not required. Several other chambers and techniques have been introduced to measure sperm numbers, each with its inherent advantages and disadvantages (see Chapter 6).

1. Hemocytometer Method

1.   After complete liquefaction, mix the specimen thoroughly.
2.   Prepare a 1:20 or a 1:10 semen dilution:
    a. If greater than 50 sperm/hpf, make a 1:20 dilution by:
        (1) using a WBC pipette, draw semen up to the 0.5 mark and water up to the 11 mark, or
        (2) using a micropipette, add 0.1 ml semen to 1.9 ml water.
    b. If less than 10 sperm/hpf, make a 1:10 dilution by:
        (1) using a WBC pipette, draw semen up to the 1.0 mark and water up to the 11 mark, or
        (2) using a micropipette, add 0.1 semen to 0.9 ml water.
3.   Mix the dilution thoroughly. If using a WBC pipette, discard the first few drops from the pipette.
4.   Fill both sides of the counting chamber. Allow to settle for several minutes.
5.   Count all sperm within five of the red blood cell squares (Figure 8). Include in this count those sperm which lie across the outermost lines at the top and right sides, but not the bottom or left sides.
6.   Count both sides of the chamber and average the two.
7.   Calculate the total number of sperm/ml;
    a. If a 1:20 dilution was used, add six zeros to the number obtained from counting the five block area. In other words, the number of sperm counted in the five block area is equal to the sperm count in millions/ml ($\times 10^6$/ml).
    b. If a 1:10 dilution was used, divide the number obtained from counting the five block area by two and add six zeros ($\times 10^6$/ml).
8.   If rare sperm are observed on the wet prep analysis, prepare a 1:10 dilution and load the chamber as above. Count all the sperm in 25 red blood cell squares. For the sperm count/ml, add five zeros to the number obtained. If no sperm are noticed on wet prep analysis, the specimen must be centrifuged and the pellet checked for the presence of sperm (see below).

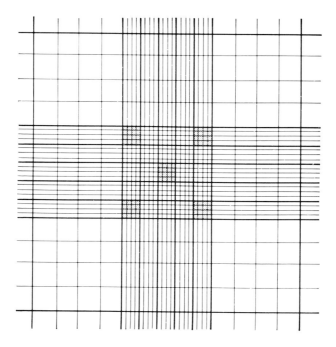

FIGURE 8.   Diagrammatic representation of one of the grids on an improved Neubauer Counting Chamber. The five shaded areas in the center of the grid are the red blood cell squares which are used for counting sperm.

9.   Diluents used to dilute semen are designed to immobilize sperm and will vary with the laboratory. Several different types of diluents have been suggested including buffered formaldehyde, chloramine T, and triphenyltetrazolium chloride. However, we[9] and others[2,4] have found that distilled water is adequate and very convenient.

2. Makler Chamber Method

1.   Clean and dry the chamber completely.
2.   Mix specimen well, place one drop (8 to 10 μl) onto the center of the lower disk.
3.   Place the cover glass on the four posts. Semen should spread over the entire area of the lower glass disk. Avoid adding excess semen which will flood over the four posts.
4.   Lift the chamber by the handles, place on the microscope stage and view using a ×20 objective and ×10 eyepiece.
5.   Count the number of sperm within a strip of 10 squares (Figure 3). Repeat this count from 2 to 3 other strips and average the counts. Reliability of counts can be improved by repeating the above using several different drops.
6.   Add six zeros to the average number of sperm counted in a 10 square area to give sperm count in millions/ml ($\times 10^6$/ml).
7.   If sperm are highly concentrated it may be difficult to count the motile sperm. Sperm can be immobilized by heating an aliquote at 50 to 60°C for 5 min. A drop of the immobilized sperm is placed onto the chamber and the total number of sperm are counted as above. Alternatively, the sperm can be immobilized by placing the loaded chamber at −20°C for 10 min and then proceeding with the count.

3. CASA Methodology

The determination of sperm numbers can be determined by CASA methodology in much the same way as motility (see above). The videomicroscopy systems used for determining sperm count are described in Chapter 6. Our laboratory uses a microcomputerized MEP system for semen analysis. This system, described above for motility determination, utilizes a multiple-exposed Polaroid instant photograph and a graphics tablet linked to a microcomputer. The sperm observed on the photograph are counted with the aid of the graphics tablet and computer. The magnification of the resulting photograph is such that the number of sperm counted from two pictures is equal to the concentration of sperm in millions/ml. The photograph can be saved as a permanent record of the analysis.

4. Motile Density

Perhaps the single most important value obtained from the semen analysis is the number of motile sperm. This value has been termed the motile density. It is calculated by the product of the sperm count and the motility. As an example, a specimen with a sperm count of 120×10^6/ml and a 45% motility will have a motile density of 54×10^6/ml (120×0.45). This value provides information on the number of sperm which have the potential for progressing from the site of semen deposition to the site of fertilization. This value is important not only for characterizing an ejaculate as normal or abnormal, but is also used in preparing the number of sperm needed for IVF and other related procedures.

5. Normal Values

Normal sperm counts are generally considered to be 20×10^6/ml or greater (Table 2). Patients are considered to be oligozoospermic if the count is less than 20×10^6/ml. Fertility appears to be significantly compromised if counts fall much below 10×10^6/ml. Normal motility densities are considered to be 8×10^6/ml (product of the normal motility of 40% and the normal sperm count of 20×10^6/ml).

6. Abnormal Results

a. Polyzoospermia

Excessively high sperm concentrations are occasionally observed. Reasons for this condition are obscure. It is usually not associated with a reduced semen volume and may or may not be accompanied with poor motility. Although the absolute relationship between polyzoospermia and fertility is not clear, in many cases markedly increased sperm concentrations are associated with diminished rather than increased fertility. Furthermore, it has been reported that the spontaneous abortion rate is increased in couples with this condition.[4] Polyzoospermia with associated poor sperm motility can also result in infertility. Dilution of the ejaculate with 5% dextrose in lactated Ringer's solution, followed by artificial insemination, has been reported to improve pregnancy rates in these patients.[52]

b. Oligozoospermia

As with many abnormal results, the possibility of a collection error must be ruled out when oligozoospermia is observed. This is particularly true if a reduced volume is also observed, suggesting that the first portion of the ejaculate may have been lost during the collection. Short-term abstinence can also result in reduced sperm counts. Once the patient has confirmed that this is not the case, and oligozoospermia is observed on repeat analysis, pathological causes must be explored. Endocrine profiles including serum testosterone, follicle-stimulating hormone (FSH) and luteinizing hormone (LH) may provide information concerning gonadal status. In cases of severe abnormalities of the endocrine system, exogenous hormone treatment is sometimes beneficial. However, if the hormonal levels are normal, exogenous hormone treatment is seldom helpful. For these patients, *in vitro* sperm preparation procedures (see Chapter 11) and artificial insemination can often result in increased pregnancy rates. The possibility of freezing and combining several ejaculates for insemination has been attempted. However, the results of such procedures have been disappointing, primarily due to the poor postthaw recovery of motile sperm in these samples.

c. Azoospermia

The etiology of azoospermia can be related to either testicular dysfunction, ejaculatory duct obstruction or retrograde ejaculation. If no sperm are noticed on the initial analysis of the semen, the specimen must be centrifuged and the pellet examined:

1. Transfer the ejaculate to a 15 ml conical centrifuge tube.
2. Centrifuge the specimen at $1000 \times g$ for 10 min.
3. Decant the supernatant (seminal plasma) and suspend the pellet in a small volume (approximately 200 μl) of seminal plasma (there is usually approximately this volume remaining after decanting the supernatant).
4. Place a drop of the resuspended pellet on a glass slide, cover with a cover slip, and examine for the presence of sperm.
5. If no sperm are observed, report on the analysis form that no sperm were observed on the original and centrifuged specimen. The specimen is then classified as azoospermia. If sperm are observed, the specimen is classified as severe oligozoospermia.

If sperm are present in the centrifuged specimen, total ductal obstruction is disproved. If no sperm are observed, a qualitative seminal fructose test should be performed as described below:

1. Add 50 mg of resorcinol to 33 ml of concentrated HCl. Dilute to 100 ml with distilled water.
2. The reagent may be stored in an amber bottle away from light at 4°C for 1 year.
3. Mix 0.5 ml well-mixed fresh semen with 5.0 ml reagent.
4. For controls, mix 0.5 ml distilled water (negative control) or 0.5 ml of 2 mg/ml fructose standard in distilled water (positive control) with the reagent.
5. Thoroughly mix and bring to a boil by placing tubes into a beaker of boiling water.
6. An orange-red color will appear within 60 s after boiling if fructose is present. If fructose is absent, the solution will remain colorless.

Fructose is secreted from the seminal vessicles. If congenital absence of the vas deferens is present, the seminal vesicles will also be absent and fructose will not be present. The semen volume will also be reduced. The presence of seminal fructose will rule out ejaculatory duct obstruction but not blockage of the vas deferens or epididymis. Localization of this blockage and confirmation of tubal patency requires open scrotal exploration and venography. If sperm are observed in the ejaculate, qualitative seminal fructose measurement provides little useful information with regard to decreased sperm count.

Azoospermia associated with severely reduced semen volume or complete aspermia is often associated with retrograde ejaculation. This condition is easily ruled out by examination of a postejaculation urine specimen. If large numbers of sperm are observed in the urine, especially after centrifugation of the specimen, the diagnosis of retrograde ejaculation is confirmed. Sperm can be harvested from this urine specimen and used for insemination of the wife.

If fructose is present in an azoospermic ejaculate, an endocrine evaluation of the male is indicated.[9] In a recent treatise dealing with the evaluation of the infertile male, Lipshulz and Howards[9] recommend measuring serum FSH as an initial screen for testicular dysfunction. If the FSH level is greater than two times normal, severe damage of the germinal epithelium is suggested and scrotal exploration is usually unnecessary. In these cases, measurement of testosterone and LH may aid in the diagnosis of primary testicular failure or hypothalamic-pituitary disease.[53] If, on the other hand, the azoospermic patient has normal FSH levels and no evidence of ductal obstruction, testicular biopsy is indicated.

F. MORPHOLOGY

Abnormalities in sperm morphology should be assessed by examining a stained preparation of semen. A number of staining procedures have been suggested, each with advantages and disadvantages. Several of these staining methods are presented in Appendix I. The optimal staining procedure is one that is easy, inexpensive, and differentiates between the various morphological abnormalities of sperm. An excellent atlas of sperm morphology has recently become available.[53a] This atlas provides photomicrographic examples of normal and abnormal forms of sperm stained by several techniques.

1. Normal and Abnormal Sperm Morphology

A number of morphological forms of human sperm have been identified. These forms fall into one of four main categories: normal forms, abnormal head, abnormal tail and immature germ cells (IGC).

a. Normal Forms

The normal spermatozoa have oval-shaped heads, intact midpiece, and an uncoiled, single tail (Figure 9A). The head is approximately 4 μm long and 2 μm wide. The tail is approximately 45 μm in length.

b. Abnormal Heads

A variety of head abnormalities are seen in semen. Large heads, termed macrocephalic, are >5 μm long and >3 μm wide. Small heads, termed microcephalic, are <3 μm long and <2 μm wide (Figure 9B). A complete absence of the sperm head can also be observed (sometimes referred to as "pinhead"; Figure 9C). Tapering sperm heads exhibit a diminishing head width in relation to head length[10] (Figure 9D). Pyriform head refers to an obvious teardrop shape coming to a point just above the midpiece. Duplicate or double headed sperm are sometimes seen. Gross irregularities of the sperm head are often referred to as amorphous.

c. Abnormal Tails

Coiling of the tail (Figure 9E) and 90° bending of the tail (sometimes referred to as "bent head" or "hammer head"; Figure 9F) is often observed. Duplications of the sperm tail, including two (Figure 9G), three, or even four tails on a single sperm can sometimes be seen. Broken tails, less than half the normal length, should also be classified as abnormal. The presence of a cytoplasmic droplet, seen as a roundish particle attached to the head, midpiece, or along the tail, should be reported. Since this cytoplasmic remnant is normally removed during epididymal transport, the presence of the droplet is often used to characterize sperm as immature. However, this classification should be differentiated from IGC, since these latter cells have not reached the stage of development of those sperm containing the cytoplasmic droplet.

d. Immature Germ Cells

It is often difficult to distinguish IGCs from polymorphonuclear WBCs on stained smears and virtually impossible on unstained wet mounts. Because of the potential diagnostic importance of WBCs in semen (pyospermia), it is important to differentiate between these two forms. It is also important to estimate the severity of pyospermia, if present. In our laboratory, if a significant number of "round cells" are observed on the wet mount analysis we will prepare an additional slide for possible PAP staining. If after morphological examination using our routine staining procedure (Rapid Wrights-Gram Stain, Appendix IA) we observe 10% or more "round cells", we will have the additional slide processed by PAP stain. This can be accomplished by sending the specimen to any pathology laboratory or by staining the slide in house using the procedure outlined in Appendix ID. Morphological

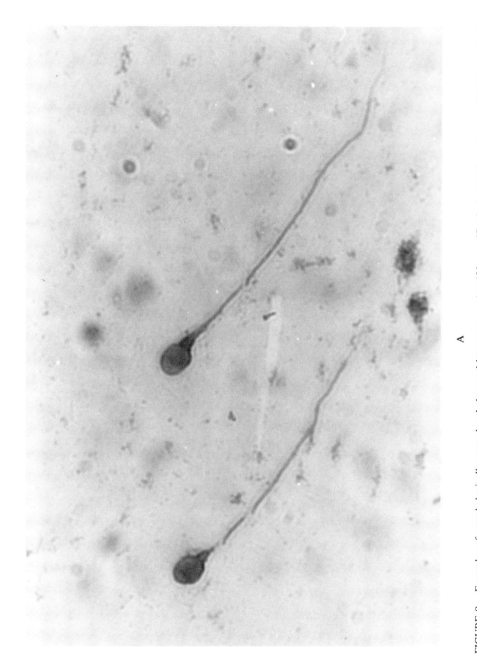

A

FIGURE 9. Examples of morphologically normal and abnormal human sperm ($\times$ 400 magnification). (A) Normal sperm. (B) Microcephalic sperm (center). (C) No head (center) superimposed over a normal sperm. (D) Tapering head sperm. (E) Coiled tail sperm. (F) Bent head, 90° bending of the sperm tail (note immature germ cell adjacent). (G) Double-tailed sperm (center). (H) Polymorphonuclear white blood cell seen in semen. (I) Immature germ cell. (J) Immature germ cell with eccentric nuclei.

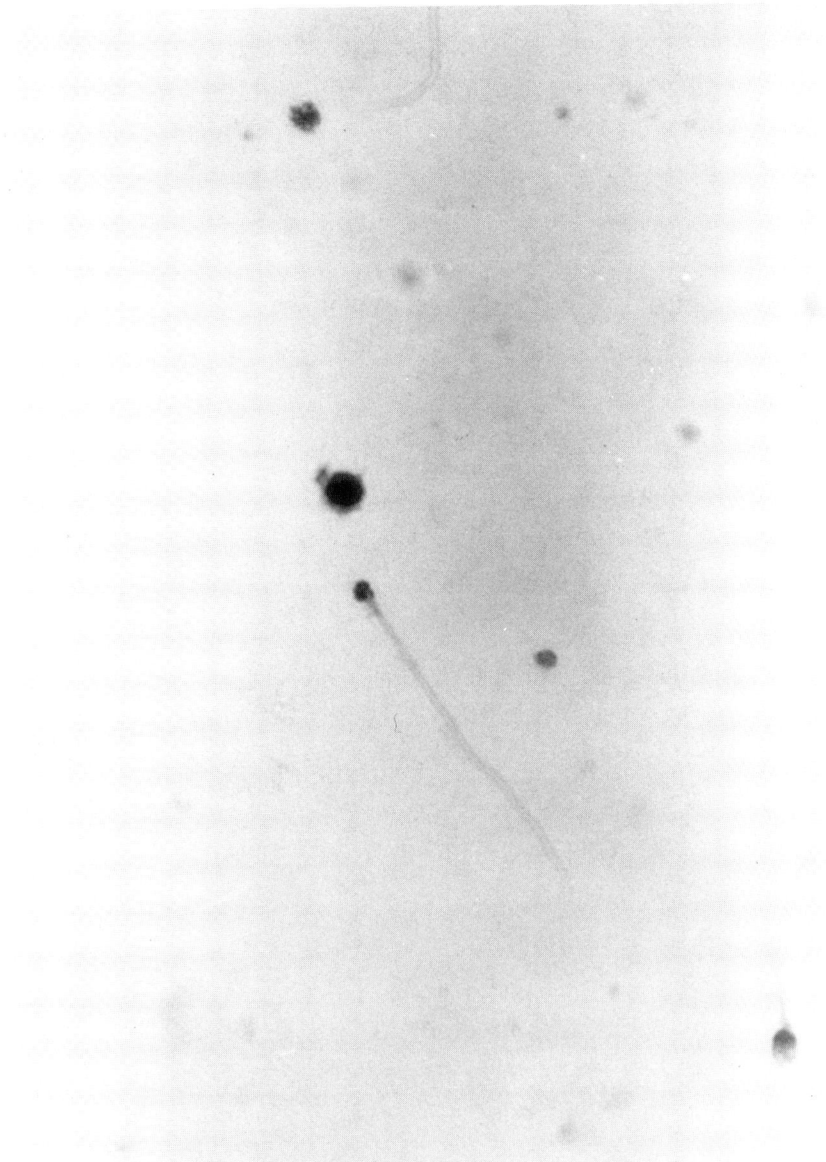

FIGURE 9B.

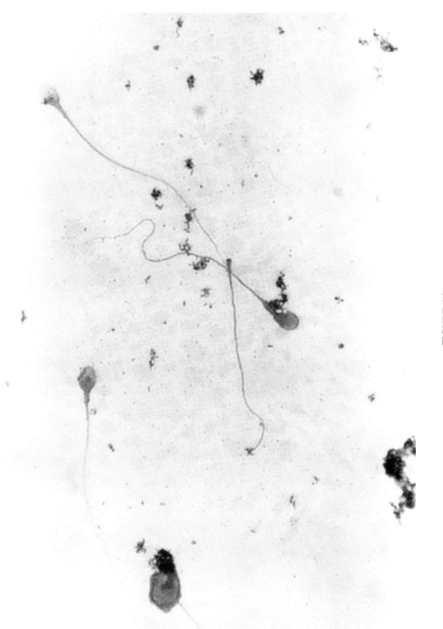

FIGURE 9C.

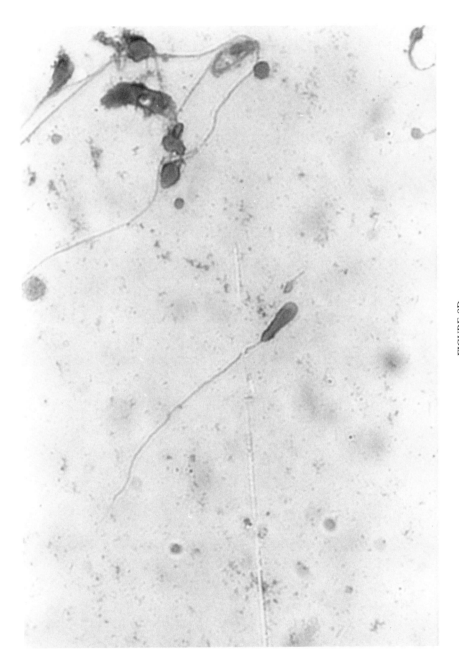

FIGURE 9D.

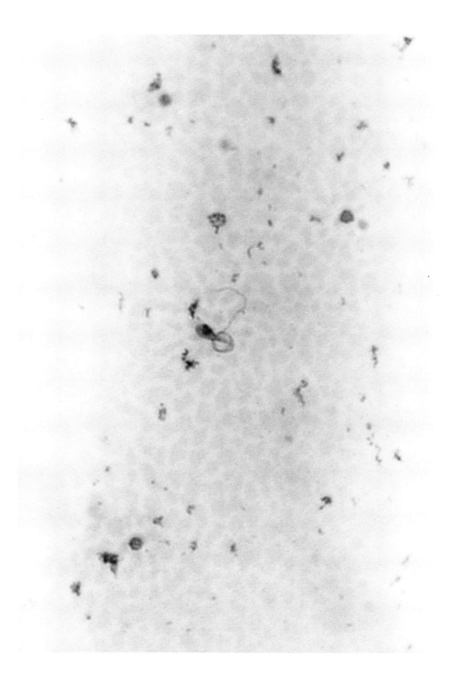

FIGURE 9E.

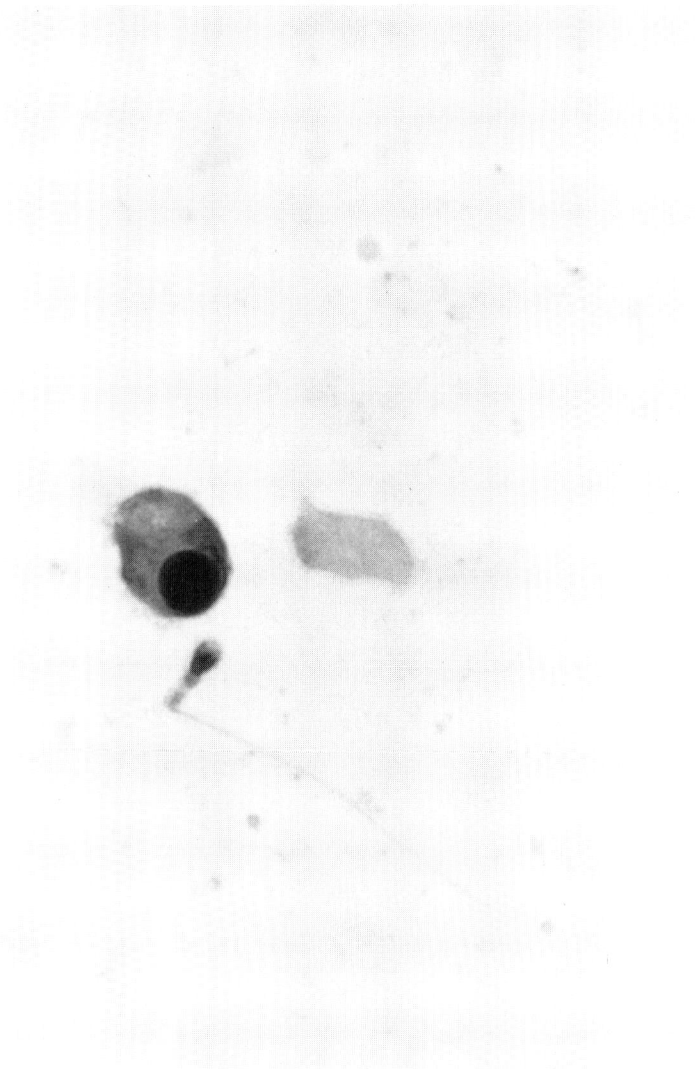

FIGURE 9F.

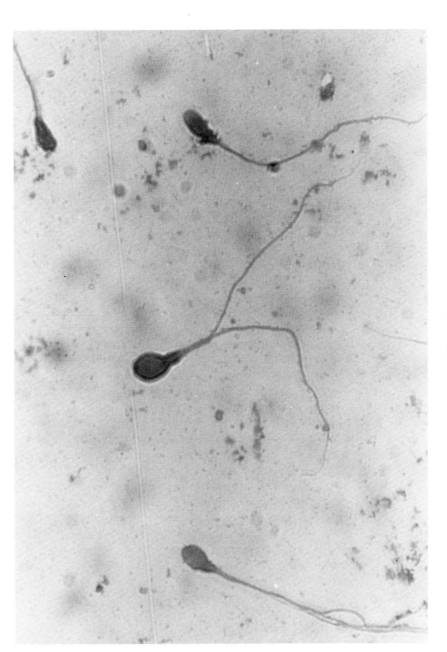

FIGURE 9G.

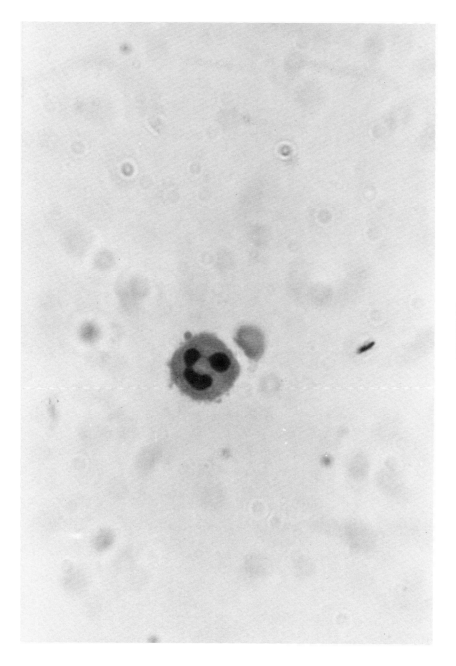

FIGURE 9H.

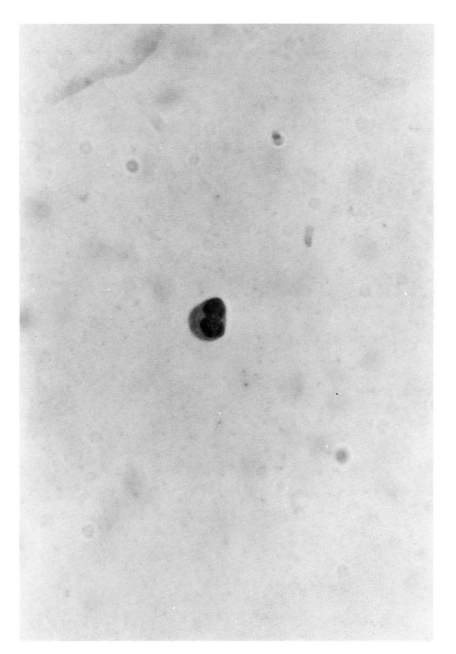

FIGURE 91.

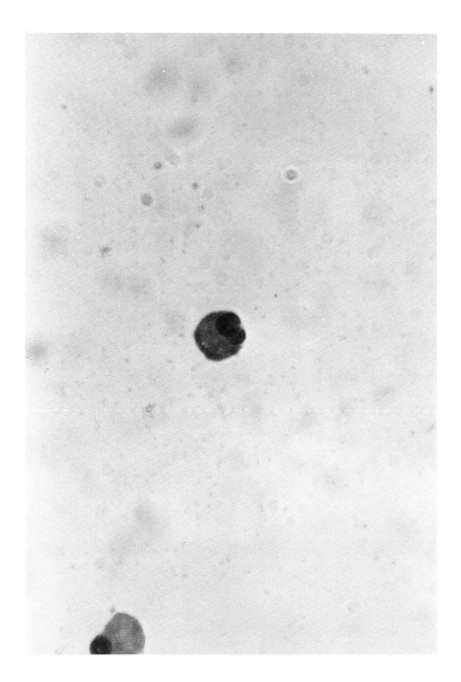

FIGURE 9J.

differentiation can then be made between the two cell types. A recent report has also described the use of antileukocyte monoclonal antibodies and immunohistologic methods to identify seminal leukocytes.[54]

Using the PAP stain method, polymorphonuclear leukocytes have a granular cytoplasm. The nuclei of these cells may or may not be connected by chromatic bridges (Figure 9H). The nuclei are often small, widely spaced, and irregular shaped. Small lymphocytes will have a nonhomogeneous, nonspherical shaped nucleus. In contract, IGCs have more spherical nuclei (Figure 9I). The nuclei to cytoplasm ratio is usually larger, and the nucleus is sometimes "polar" (eccentric), localized at one end of the cell (Figure 9J). Polynuclear IGC nuclei are usually spaced more closely together, and do not contain chromatic bridges.

If the ejaculate contains more than 10% "round cells", the number of WBCs should be calculated. This can be accomplished by performing the normal sperm cell morphological differential count while tallying the number of WBCs separately. The number of WBCs per 100 sperm observed is compared with the sperm concentration to achieve a number of WBCs per ml of ejaculate:

$$\text{WBC} \times 10^6/\text{ml semen} = (\text{sperm count} \times 10^6/\text{ml}) \times (\text{number WBCs}/100 \text{ sperm})$$

As an example, if 20 WBCs are counted per 100 morphologically recognizable sperm, and the original sperm concentration is 80×10^6/ml, the WBC count will be 16×10^6/ml.

2. Acrosome Staining

Before sperm are capable of fertilizing an egg they must become capacitated. The process of capacitation allows the sperm to undergo the acrosome reaction. The acrosome reaction is essential for mammalian fertilization because it allows for sperm penetration through the zona pellucida and for fusion with the oolemma.[55] Thus, the status of the acrosome region of the sperm is often important to examine. Several studies have evaluated methods for determining the acrosome status of human sperm. The more common assays include the triple stain method,[56] indirect immunofluorescence assay,[57,58] the chlortetracycline assay,[59] and the *Pisum sativum* agglutin-fluoroscein isothiocyanate assay.[55] Each of these assays has inherent advantages and disadvantages. Although each provides important information on the acrosome status, the use of these assays in routine clinical practice is at present limited. Clearly, as we learn more about the relationship of acrosome status and fertility, these assays will find there way into routine clinical laboratories in the near future.

3. Strict Criteria for Sperm Morphology

Recent evidence suggests that by applying strict criteria for classifying sperm as normal, sperm morphology is a good predictor of *in vitro* fertilization, and hence, fertility, out-come.[60-63] This new, strict criteria analysis utilizes an easy staining procedure and commercially available stain.[64] The results from these studies indicate that the fertility potential of male patients may be more accurately assessed using this new morphological criteria. Details of this procedure and its relationship to fertility potential are discussed in Chapter 4.

4. Normal Values

Most laboratories consider a normal ejaculate as one containing at least 60% normal forms (Table 2). If the ejaculate contains greater than 40 to 50% abnormal forms, including IGC, the specimen is termed teratozoospermic. There should be fewer than 4 to 5×10^6 WBC/ml of semen.

5. Teratozoospermia

Human seminal cytology provides a sensitive index of the germinal epithelium. Any significant alteration in sperm morphology is usually indicative of testicular insult which can result from one of several possibilities. A debilitating illness, viral infection, varicocele, radiation, and certain drugs may result in an increase in abnormal sperm morphology. Such an insult may result in what has been termed as a "stress pattern". This pattern is characterized by an increase in tapering sperm, amorphous heads, and immature forms. While this pattern was once thought to be associated with a varicocele, it has been shown more recently that the stress pattern is not pathognomonic for this condition.[5,60,61] Furthermore, with the possible exception of tail abnormalities and the presence of cytoplasmic remnants which seem to be related to epididymal dysfunction,[5,62] several investigators have not found the differential classification of abnormal forms to be useful clinically.[5,6] Clinical assessment of male fertility is then based on the overall percentage of normal forms. Isolated abnormalities of sperm morphology in the absence of other semen abnormalities is a rare and generally transient condition, usually indicating a limited and finite testicular insult.[2]

Abnormalities in semen parameters due to testicular insult may not become apparent until 30 to 70 d postinsult. This is due to the period of time required in the normal cycle of spermatogenesis from initiation of the process until the appearance of mature sperm in the vas deferens. Therefore, if testicular insult is suspected as the cause of teratozoospermia, repeat analysis should be postponed at least 2 to 4 weeks.

V. THE SEMEN ANALYSIS REPORT

A. THE REPORT FORMAT

Each laboratory should design its own report format to suit the laboratory's individual needs. We have found the form presented in Appendix V to be most useful. Regardless of the format used, several key pieces of information should be included.

First, the report should contain the patient's as well as his spouse's name. This is particularly important if the semen analysis report will be sent to the gynecologist's office who usually files charts under the female partner's name. The referring doctor's name, date of analysis, and period of abstinence should also be included. It is sometimes helpful to indicate the type of analysis performed (whether the analysis is a routine procedure, or part of another procedure, such as IVF, IUI, sperm penetration assay, retrograde ejaculation, etc.).

Certain laboratories may also require an accession code number for each sample analyzed. Our laboratory assigns a consecutive number for each sample received. This code number is then logged and is used to identify the specimen, any slides made from the specimen, the report form, the computer data base location and any subsequent information pertaining to the specimen.

Second, each analysis report form should contain normal values or the normal range of values for each semen parameter measured. These normal values should be printed adjacent to the observed values to aid in comparison of the patients results to the normal ranges. We have also found it convenient to have space for initial observations as well as posttreatment observations (such as pre- and postcryopreservation, pre- and postwash and rise, etc.). Our laboratory performs bovine mucus penetration studies on a routine basis, and the results of this analysis are placed on the semen analysis form (see Chapter 8 for more information on this test). Since different nomenclature is often used to describe sperm morphology (such as "no head", "pinhead", "microcephalic", etc.) we and others[3] have found it helpful to record sperm morphology on a chart which provides illustrations of the various types of forms recorded in our laboratory.

Last, space for comments should be provided. Comments should be made concerning collection errors, specimen condition, abnormal macro- and microscopic findings, or any other unusual result. In our laboratory, each semen analysis is signed by the technician performing the analysis and reviewed by the andrologist. This review system often detects errors in the report or accidental deletion of information prior to reporting to the clinician. This review also allows the andrologist to make comments to the clinician. This review also allows the andrologist to make comments on the analysis, including the classification of the specimen (normospermic, oligozoospermic, asthenoteratozoospermic, etc.) and, if abnormal, suggestions for subsequent action.

B. NORMAL VALUES

What constitutes a "normal" semen analysis has been the topic of discussion for several decades. Clearly, one must differentiate between "normal", "average", and "adequate" semen values. If one had access to a large, unbiased population of proven fertile males, the average semen values could be determined.[2] These values would then represent the range and lower limits of values for a fertile (normal) population. These data are, however, often difficult for the routine semen laboratory to obtain. Furthermore, what may represent a "normal" value for one individual or population may be significantly greater than the values required for fertilization in another group of individuals. In other words, semen values less than those of a normal, fertile population may in fact be adequate for fertilization. Pregnancies can occur routinely in patients treated for hypogonadotropic hypogonadism who have sperm counts less than 5×10^6/ml.[2,5] However, in this population of patients the germinal epithelium is comparatively intact suggesting that relatively low numbers of high quality, *functional* sperm can result in pregnancy. With this in mind, care must be taken when describing an ejaculate as normal vs. abnormal.

Nevertheless, normal values, or perhaps more appropriate, reference values, for the semen analysis should be used by the laboratory and the clinician in classifying the male patient. The actual values used will depend upon the methods used for the analysis and the practical experience of the clinician. The reference values used in our laboratory are shown in Table 2. These reference values have been determined using the multiple exposure photography system described by Burke and Kapinos[32] and Keel et al.[33,34]

VI. SPECIAL PROCEDURES

A. POSTVASECTOMY EVALUATION

Vasectomy is a common and effective method of male contraception. However, sterilization is not complete immediately after the surgical procedure. As many as six to ten ejaculations postsurgery may be required to render the ejaculate free of residual sperm. Therefore, patients should have one or more semen analyses after the vasectomy to assure sterility.

The semen should be evaluated 2 months postvasectomy and after ten ejaculations.[8] After 2 to 3 d of abstinence the patient should collect a specimen for analysis as described above for the routine semen analysis. The semen should be evaluated by wet mount analysis. If no sperm are observed, the specimen should be centrifuged and the pellet examined. The presence of any sperm in the semen or centrifuged specimen should be reported. A patient is considered sterile when two sperm counts, one month apart, are negative for the presence of sperm.[8]

B. RETROGRADE EJACULATION
1. Diagnosis

Initially, seminal fluid is deposited into the prostatic urethra during emission by way of the prostatic ducts. Closure of the bladder neck and the propulsion of the seminal fluid occur simultaneously.[64] Failure of the bladder neck to close during this process causes retrograde flow of the seminal fluid into the bladder, resulting in retrograde ejaculation. A variety of clinical conditions may result in retrograde ejaculation including prostatic or bladder neck surgery, diabetes, and certain drugs (psychotropics, antidepressants, and antihypertensives).[64] This condition is associated with hypospermia or aspermia (''dry ejaculation'') and infertility. Any patient with infertility and chronic low or absence semen volume should be suspect.

The diagnosis of retrograde ejaculation is straightforward. The patient is instructed to urinate, masturbate, and to collect an immediate postejaculation urine specimen into a clean, dry contaier. The urine is observed before and after centrifugation by wet mount analysis. If significant numbers of sperm are observed in the urine the diagnosis is made. The relative number of sperm per hpf should be reported. It should be pointed out that a few sperm left in the urethra after normal antegrade ejaculation may also be observed in a postejaculation urine specimen. However, in this case, there should only be several thousand total sperm noted (rare sperm per hpf).

2. Treatment

The initial treatment of retrograde ejaculation, depending upon the etiology, may be the administration of alphasympathomimetic agents. However, if these drugs are unsuccessful or contraindicated, the recovery of motile sperm for artificial insemination can often lead to a pregnancy. Several procedures have been implicated.[65-68] One such approach is discussed in Chapter 11. Our laboratory has successfully used a modification of the procedures described by Zavos and Wilson[66] as follows:

1. Starting the day before collection, the patient alkalinizes his urine by taking one teasponful baking soda in water, by mouth, three times a day. The patient should have 2 to 3 d of sexual abstinence before collection.
2. Instruct the patient to completely empty his bladder, and then collect an ejaculate by masturbation as above. If any semen is collected, this specimen should be examined by wet mount for the presence of sperm.
3. Immediately after ejaculation, have the patient void into a clean 250 ml container containing 50 ml of TEST-Yolk buffer (see Appendix IIG) which has been equilibrated at 37°C.
4. Record the total volume. Report the volume of urine (total volume — 50 ml). Examine the urine specimen immediately by wet mount for the presence of sperm. Make subjective estimates of sperm numbers and motility.
5. Divide the specimen evenly among several 50 ml conical centrifuge tubes. Centrifuge the specimens at $100 \times g$ for 10 min.
6. Carefully decant the urine. Resuspend each pellet in 1.0 ml of Tyrode's buffer (for vaginal insemination; Appendix IIB) or sterile Ham's F-10 (for intrauterine insemination, IUI), 37°C.
7. Combine all into one 15 ml conical tube, centrifge and decant as above.
8. Resuspend the pellet in 1.0 ml Tyrode's or 0.5 ml Ham's F-10 (37°C), depending upon the type of insemination.
9. Maintain specimen at 37°C until insemination.
10. Perform routine semen analysis, taking care to maintain sterility if the specimen is to be used for IUI.

C. LONG-TERM CRYOPRESERVATION OF SEMEN FROM CANCER PATIENTS

Many patients with testicular cancer, Hodgkin's disease, or other disease requiring radio- or chemotherapy may choose to have semen cryopreserved for potential future use. When the diagnosis of the disease is made, many of these patients will already be severely oligozoospermic or azoospermic. Patients with severely reduced sperm numbers will often have poor postthaw recoveries of motile sperm. For this reason, some investigators have suggested that cryopreservation may be an unrealistic solution for fertility assurance for these patients.[69] However, others have demonstrated a 45% cumulative pregnancy rate in testicular tumor and Hodgkin's patients who have banked frozen semen for later use.[70] With the advent of IVF and its related assisted reproductive technologies, fertility may be possible for these patients using cryopreserved semen. For this reason, we have recommended that patients who are faced with radio- or chemotherapy be given the option of semen banking.

The decision to seek semen banking for these patients is often made late in the treatment plan. There is often an urgency in starting therapy very soon after the diagnosis is made. Semen to be cryopreserved in this group of patients should be obtained and frozen as soon as possible after the diagnosis of disease and the decision to treat with radio- or chemotherapy. This fact, coupled with the anxiety of the patient and the frequent finding of reduced sperm numbers, requires special attention and consultation with both the patient and his physician. We have adopted a program for this population of patients which has proven to be successful. This program consists of five steps: consultation, collection, analysis, decision, and cryo- preservation.

Once the ejaculate is collected, a wet mount analysis should be performed. Often, no sperm are seen or the ejaculate may be severely oligoasthenozoospermic. If sperm are observed, a routine semen analysis should be performed. Depending upon the results of this analysis, the patient may opt for cryopreservation. Since time is of the essence, this specimen should not be discarded after analysis and should be maintained at 37°C. If the patient decides to freeze, this initial specimen can be processed thus saving the patient from having to produce unnecessary specimens. In our laboratory, if motile sperm are present, we will immediately freeze the specimen after analysis. If the patient and his physician decide not to proceed with long-term storage, the specimen may be discarded. However, if the decision is made to bank the patients semen, considerable time and effort has been saved.

Once the results of the initial semen analysis are available, the patient and his physician must decide whether to proceed with long-term storage of the semen. Our belief is that if any motile sperm are present, unless severe oligoasthenozoospermia is observed, the patient should be given the option to freeze. This belief is based on the fact that even if a nominal number of sperm survive the freezing process, future fertility is possible, albeit remote in some cases. With IVF and related assisted reproductive technologies, as few as 50,000 total motile sperm can result in a viable pregnancy. Indeed, recent reports have suggested that using micromanipulation techniques, a single sperm injected into the human egg can po- tentially result in a viable embryo.[70] Advances made during the next decade (which is a realistic time frame for a young patient considering cryopreservation) may make these and other as yet undescribed procedures commonplace. Another consideration should be the psychological benefit to the patient of having at least some hope for fertility in the future, however remote. For these reasons, if motile sperm are present, we will often recommend cryopreservation for these patients. At the same time, if the specimen is severely oligo- or asthenozoospermic, we may not recommend proceeding. We may, however, suggest a repeat analysis in 3 d to confirm the severity of the condition.

If the decision is made to long term freeze the patients semen, the semen specimen is cryopreserved by standard procedures. The process of semen cryopreservation are discussed in detail in Chapter 13. If the clinic or laboratory does not have the capability of freezing sperm, a semen cryopreservation kit can be obtained commercially (Xytex Corporation, Augusta, GA). This kit is delivered to the clinic or laboratory and contains everything needed to freeze several ejaculates. Once frozen, the ejaculates can be shipped back to the bank for long-term storage. This kit allows the service of sperm banking to be offered even to remote locations. We recommend storing at least three specimens. This will provide for at least five to six inseminations, depending upon the initial semen volume, sperm motile density postthaw, and the methods used for insemination.

VII. CONCLUSIONS

The semen analysis is perhaps the most important test used in the diagnosis of male infertility. From a practical sense, it is a very simple test to perform. However, meticulous attention to details and technique must be made if an accurate and reproducible analysis is to be obtained. Even simple potential problems, such as specimen collection errors, if overlooked can dramatically effect the semen analysis resulting in false-negative findings. Historically, analysis of semen has been based on subjective techniques for the determination of sperm numbers and estimation of sperm motility. Recent advances in computerization and video/photomicroscopy have dramatically improved the objectiveness of the analysis and have allowed for the first time reliable and easily accessible information on sperm kinematics. It is becoming apparent that it is not only important to know how many sperm are present and moving, but it is also equally important to be able to characterize the sperm's velocity and direction or path of travel. Sperm quality and function, rather than quantity, is the key factor in determining male fertility. With the advent of the assisted reproductive technologies, such as IVF, a virtual knowledge explosion has occurred with respect to our understanding of reproductive function and dysfunction. We are now able to visualize fertilization of the human egg and observe early embryonic development. The knowledge gained from these procedures has greatly improved our ability to determine, and in many cases improve, the functionality of the human sperm. The next decade promises to be exciting and will no doubt enhance our ability to diagnose and treat male infertility.

ACKNOWLEDGMENTS

The author gratefully acknowledges the excellent technical assistance provided by Kris Zumbach-Lasley, Toni Kurz, Nancy Jabara, and Michelle McShane and secretarial assistance of Kendra Hall. I wish to thank Drs. John Black and Armand Karow for introducing me to the fascinating field of andrology, and to Drs. Bobby Webster and Daniel Roberts for giving me the chance to develop that field in Wichita. Research in the authors laboratory is sponsored by the Women's Research Institute and the Wesley Foundation, Wichita, KS.

REFERENCES

1. *INFERTILITY, Medical and Social Choices, Summary,* Congress of the United States, Office of Technology Assessment, Washington, D.C., May 1988.
2. **Lipshultz, L. I. and Howards, S. S.,** Evaluation of the subfertile man, in *Infertility in the Male,* Lipshultz, L. I. and Howards, S. S., Eds., Churchill Livingstone, New York, 1983, chap. 9.
3. **Zaneveld, L. J. D. and Polakoski, K. L.,** Collection and physical examination of the ejaculate, in *Techniques of Human Andrology,* Hafez, E.S. E., Ed., Elsevier/North-Holland Biomedical Press, 1977, chap. 6.
4. **Jequier, A. M. and Crich, J. P.,** *Semen Analysis — A Practical Guide,* Year Book Medical Publishers, Chicago, IL.
5. **Overstreet, J. W. and Katz, D. F.,** Semen Analysis, *Urol. Clin. North Am.,* 14, 441, 1987.
6. **Spark, R. F.,** *The Infertile Male, The Clinician's Guide to Diagnosis and Treatment,* Plenum Medical Book Company, New York, 1988.
7. **Glasser, L.,** Seminal fluid and subfertility, *Diag. Med.,* 4, 2, 1981.
8. **Sampson, J. H. and Alexander, N. J.,** Semen analysis: a laboratory approach, *Lab. Med.,* 13, 218, 1982.
9. **Keel, B. A.,** The semen analysis: an important diagnostic evaluation, *Lab. Med.,* 10, 686, 1979.

10. **Belsey, M. A., Eliasson, R., Gallegos, A. J., Moghissi, K. S., Paulsen, C. A., and Prasad, M. R. N.,** in *Laboratory Manual for the Examination of Human Semen and Semen-Cervical Mucus Interaction.* Belsey, M. A., Eliasson, R., Gallegos, A. J., Moghissi, K. S., Paulsen, C. A., and Prasad, M. R. N., Eds., Press Concern, Singapore, 1980.

11. **Poland, M. L., Moghissi, K. S., Giblin, P. T., Ager, J. W., and Olson, J. M.,** Variation of semen measures within normal men, *Fertil. Steril.,* 44, 396, 1985.

12. **Schwartz, D., Laplanche, A., Jouannet, P., and David, G.,** Within-subject variability of human semen in regard to sperm count, volume, total number of spermatozoa and length of abstinence, *J. Reprod. Fertil.,* 57, 319, 1979.

13. **Reinberg, A., Smolensky, M. H., Hallek, M., Smith, K. D., and Steinberger, E.,** Annual variation in semen characteristics and plasma hormone levels in men undergoing vasectomy, *Fertil. Steril.,* 49, 309, 1988.

14. **Levin, R. M., Latimore, J., Wein, A. J., and Van Arsdalen, K. N.,** Correlation of sperm count with frequency of ejaculation, *Fertil. Steril.,* 45, 732, 1986.

15. **Tulandi, T. and McInnes, R. A.,** Vaginal lubricants: effect of glycerin and egg white on sperm motility and progression in vitro, *Fertil. Steril.,* 41, 151, 1984.

16. **Zavos, P. M.** Seminal parameters of ejaculates collected from oligospermic and normospermic patients via masturbation and at intercourse with the use of a silastic seminal fluid collection device, *Fertil. Steril.,* 44, 517, 1985.

17. **Strickland, D. M. and Ziaya, P. R.,** Reduced sperm motility in plastic containers, *Lab. Med.,* 18, 310, 1987.

18. **Check, J. H., Shanis, B. S., Wu, C. H., and Bollendorf, A.,** Evaluating glass, polystyrene, and polypropylene containers for semen collection and sperm washing, *Arch. Androl.,* 20, 251, 1988.

19. **Jondet, M., Mailloux, G., Tea, N. T., and Scholler, R.,** A practical device for collecting human ejaculate, *Fertil. Steril.,* 48, 340, 1987.

20. **Mehan, D. J. and Chehval, M. J.,** A clinical evaluation of a new silastic seminal fluid collection device, *Fertil. Steril.,* 28, 689, 1977.

21. **Schoenfeld, C., Amelar, R. D., Dubin, L., and Skwerer, R. G.,** Evaluation of a new silastic seminal fluid collection device, *Fertil. Steril.,* 30, 319, 1978.

22. **Makler, A., Tatcher, M., Vilensky, A., and Brandes, J. M.,** Factors affecting sperm motility. III. Influence of visible light and other electromagnetic radiations on human sperm velocity and survival, *Fertil. Steril.,* 33, 439, 1980.

23. **Milligan, M. P., Harris, S. J., and Dennis, K. J.,** The effect of temperature on the velocity of human spermatozoa as measured by time-lapse photography, *Fertil. Steril.,* 30, 592, 1978.

24. **Makler, A., Deutch, M., Vilensky, A., and Palti, Y.,** Factors affecting sperm motility. VIII. Velocity and survival of human spermatozoa as related to temperatures above zero, *Int. J. Androl., 4, 559, 1981.*

25. **Tauber, P. F., Zaneveld, L. J. D., Propping, D., and Schumacher, G. F. B.,** A new technique to measure the liquefaction rate of human semen: the bag method, *Fertil. Steril.,* 33, 567, 1980.

26. **Upadhyaya, M., Hibbard, B. M., and Walker, S. M.,** Use of sputolysin for liquefaction of viscid human semen, *Fertil. Steril.,* 35, 657, 1981.

27. **Benson, G. S. and McConnell, J.,** Erection, emission, and ejaculation: physiological mechanisms, in *Infertility in the Male,* Lipshultz, L. I. and Howards, S. S., Eds., Churchill Livingstone, New York, 1983.

28. **Makler, A.,** The improved ten-micrometer chamber for rapid sperm count and motility evaluation, *Fertil. Steril.,* 33, 337, 1980.

29. **Makler, A.,** A new multiple exposure photography method for objective human spermatozoal motility determination, *Fertil. Steril.,* 30, 192, 1978.

30. **Makler, A.,** Use of the elaborated multiple exposure photography (MEP) method in routine sperm motility analysis and for research purposes, *Fertil. Steril.,* 33, 160, 1980.

31. **Katz, D. F. and Overstreet, J. W.,** Sperm motility assessment by videomicrography, *Fertil. Steril.,* 35, 188, 1981.

32. **Burke, R. K. and Kapinos, L. J.,** The effect of in vitro sperm capacitation on sperm velocity and motility as measured by an in-office, integrated microcomputerized system for semen analysis, *Int. J. Fertil.,* 30, 10, 1985.

33. **Keel, B. A. and Webster, B. W.,** Correlation of human sperm motility characteristics with an in vitro cervical mucus penetration test, *Fertil. Steril.,* 49, 138, 1988.

34. **Keel, B. A., Webster, B. W., and Roberts, D. K.,** Effects of cryopreservation on the motility characteristics of human spermatozoa, *J. Reprod. Fertil.,* 81, 213, 1987.

35. **Holt, W. V., Moore, H. D. M., and Hillier, S. G.,** Computer-assisted measurement of sperm swimming speed in human semen: correlation of results with in vitro fertilization assays, *Fertil. Steril.,* 44, 112, 1985.

36. **Mathur, S., Carlton, M., Ziegler, J., Rust, P. F., and Williamson, H. O.,** A computerized sperm motion analysis, *Fertil. Steril.,* 46, 484, 1986.

37. **Ginsburg, K. A., Moghissi, K. S., and Abel, E. L.,** Computer-assisted human semen analysis sampling errors and reproducibility, *J. Androl.,* 9, 82, 1988.
38. **Mortimer, D. and Mortimer, S. T.,** Influence of system parameter settings on human sperm motility analysis using CellSoft, *Hum. Reprod.,* 3, 621, 1988.
39. **Knuth, U. A., Yeung, C., and Nieschlag, E.,** Computerized semen analysis: objective measurement of semen characteristics is biased by subjective parameter setting, *Fertil. Steril.,* 48, 118, 1987.
40. **Vantman, D., Koukoulis, G., Dennison, L., Zinaman, M., and Sherins, R. J.,** Computer-assisted semen analysis: evaluation of method and assessment of the influence of sperm concentration on linear velocity determination, *Fertil. Steril.,* 49, 510, 1988.
41. **Sokoloski, J. E., Blasco, L., Storey, B. T., and Wolf, D. P.,** Turbidimetric analysis of human sperm motility, *Fertil. Steril.,* 38, 1337, 1977.
42. **Levin, R. M., Greenberg, S. H., and Wein, A. J.,** Clinical use of the turbidimetric analysis of sperm motility: comparison with visual techniques, *Fertil. Steril.,* 35, 332, 1981.
43. **Keel, B. A. and Black, J. B.,** Reduced motility longevity in thawed human spermatozoa, *Arch. Androl.,* 4, 213, 1980.
44. **Dahlberg, B.,** Sperm motility in fertile men and males in infertile units: in vitro test, *Arch. Androl.,* 20, 31, 1988.
45. **Berthelsen, J. G.,** Vital staining of spermatozoa performed by the patient, *Fertil. Steril.,* 35, 86, 1981.
46. **Aitken, R. J., Ross, A., and Lees, M. M.,** Analysis of sperm function in Kartagener's syndrome, *Fertil. Steril.,* 40, 696, 1983.
47. **Moryan, A. I., Guay, A. T., and Tulchinsky, D.,** Normal penetration of hamster ova by human spermatozoa with dyskinetic motility, *Fertil. Steril.,* 45, 735, 1986.
48. **MacLeod, J.,** Semen quality in one thousand men of known fertility and in eight hundred cases of infertile marriage, *Fertil. Steril.,* 2, 115, 1954.
49. **Keel, B. A. and Karow, A. M.,** Motility characteristics of human sperm, nonfrozen and cryopreserved, *Arch. Androl.,* 4, 205, 1980.
50. **Hinting, A., Comhaire, F., and Schoonjans, F.,** Capacity of objectively assessed sperm motility characteristics in differentiating between semen of fertile and subfertile men, *Fertil. Steril.,* 50, 1988.
51. **Menkveld, R., Van Zyl, J. A., and Kotze, T. J. v. W.,** A statistical comparison of three methods for the counting of human spermatozoa, *Andrologia,* 16, 554, 1984.
52. **Quigley, M. M.,** Polyzoospermia With Poor Motility, in *Current Therapy of Infertility 1984—1985,* García, C. R., Mastroianni, L., Amelar, R. D., and Dubin, L., Eds., B. C. Decker, Philadelphia, and C. V. Mosby, St. Louis, London, 1984.
53. **Swerdloff, R. S. and de Kretser, D. M.,** in *Infertility in the Male,* Lipshultz, L. I. and Howards, S. S., Eds., Churchill Livingstone, New York, 1983, chap. 10.
53a. **Adelman, M. M. and Cahill, E. M.,** Eds., *Atlas of Sperm Morphology,* ASCP Press, Chicago, 1989.
54. **Wolff, H. and Anderson, D. J.,** Immunohistologic characterization and quantitation of leukocyte subpopulations in human semen, *Fertil. Steril.,* 49, 497, 1988.
55. **Liu, D. Y. and Baker, H. W. G.,** The proportion of human sperm with poor morphology but normal intact acrosomes detected with *Pisum sativum* agglutinin correlates with fertilization in vitro, *Fertil. Steril.,* 50, 288, 1988.
56. **Talbot, P. and Chacon, R. S.,** A triple stain technique for evaluating normal acrosome reactions of human sperm, *J. Exp. Zool.,* 215, 201, 1981.
57. **Wolf, D. P., Boldt, J., Byrd, W., and Bechtol, K. B.,** Acrosomal status evaluation in human ejaculated sperm with monoclonal antibodies, *Biol. Reprod.,* 31, 1157, 1985.
58. **Byrd, W. and Wolf, D. P.,** Acrosomal status in fresh and capacitated human ejaculated sperm, *Biol. Reprod.,* 34, 859, 1986.
59. **Lee, M. A., Trucco, G. S., Bechtol, K. B., Wummer, N., Kopf, G. S., Blasco, L., and Storey, B. T.,** Capacitation and acrosome reactions in human spermatozoa monitored by a chlortetracycline fluorescence assay, *Fertil. Steril.,* 48, 649, 1987.
60. **Rodriguez-Rigau, L. J., Smith, K. D., and Steinberger, E.,** Varicocele and the morphology of spermatozoa, *Fertil. Steril.,* 35, 54, 1981.
61. **Ayodeji, O. and Baker, H. W. G.,** Is there a specific abnormality of sperm morphology in men with varicoceles?, *Fertil. Steril.,* 45, 839, 1986.
62. **Pelfrey, R. J., Overstreet, J. W., and Lewis, E. L.,** Abnormalities of sperm morphology in cases of persistent infertility after vasectomy reversal, *Fertil. Steril.,* 38, 112, 1982.
63. **Freund, M. and Davis, J. E.,** Disappearance rate of spermatozoa from the ejaculate following vasectomy, *Fertil. Steril.,* 20, 163, 1969.
64. **Kaufman, D. G. and Nagler, H. M.,** Specific nonsurgical therapy in male infertility, *Urol. Clin. North Am.,* 14, 489, 1987.
65. **Mahadevan, M., Leeton, J. F., and Trounson, A. O.,** Noninvasive method of semen collection for successful artificial insemination in a case of retrograde ejaculation, *Fertil. Steril.,* 36, 243, 1981.

66. **Zavos, P. M. and Wilson, E. A.,** Retrograde ejaculation: etiology and treatment via the use of a new noninvasive method, *Fertil. Steril.,* 42, 627, 1984.

67. **Cameron, M. C. and Gillett, W. R.,** The recovery of sperm, insemination, and pregnancy in the treatment of infertility because of retrograde ejaculation, *Fertil. Steril.,* 44, 844, 1985.

68. **Urry, R. L., Middleton, R. G., and McGavin, S.,** A simple and effective technique for increasing pregnancy rates in couples with retrograde ejaculation, *Fertil. Steril.,* 46, 1124, 1986.

69. **Bracken, R. B. and Smith, K. D.,** Is semen cryopreservation helpful in testicular cancer?, *Urology,* 15, 581, 1980.

70. **Scammell, G. E., Stredronska, J., Edmonds, D. K., White, N., Hendry, W. F., and Jeffcoate, S. L.,** Cryopreservation of semen in men with testicular tumour or Hodgkin's disease: results of artificial insemination of their partners, *Lancet,* 31, 1985.

71. **Lanzendorf, S. E., Maloney, M. K., Veeck, L. L., Slusser, J., Hodgen, G. D., and Rosenwaks, Z.,** A preclinical evaluation of pronuclear formation by microinjection of human spermatozoa into human oocytes, *Fertil. Steril.,* 49, 835, 1988.

Chapter 4

CRITICAL EVALUATION OF SPERM MORPHOLOGY: COMPARISON WITH *IN VITRO* FERTILIZATION

Sergio Oehninger, Lucinda L. Veeck, Thinus Kruger, and Anibal A. Acosta

TABLE OF CONTENTS

I. INTRODUCTION

The critical evaluation of sperm morphology has taken on great importance in the Norfolk IVF program. Based on criteria used by Kruger and associates,[1,2] it has been found that this parameter has an excellent predictive value of fertilization success.

II. METHODS

A. STRICT CRITERIA USED FOR MORPHOLOGY EVALUATION

Spermatozoa are considered normal when the head has a smooth oval configuration with a well-defined acrosome involving 40 to 70% of the sperm head and an absence of neck, midpiece, or tail defects. (Figure 1) No cytoplasmic droplets of more than half the size of the sperm head should be present. The length of a normal sperm head should be 5 to 6 μm and the diameter 2.5 to 3.5 μm. A microscopic eyepiece micrometer is used to do routine measurements. In contrast to other methods, *borderline forms are counted as abnormal.* At least 200 cells are counted on each of two slides.

The amorphous head group is divided into two categories: slightly amorphous and severely amorphous. Slightly amorphous forms are those sperm with a head diameter of 2.0 to 2.5 μm with slight abnormalities in the shape of the head, but with a normal acrosome.

Severely amorphous heads are defined as those with no acrosome at all or with an acrosome smaller than 30% or larger than 70% of the sperm head. Completely abnormal shapes are also put into this category.

Neck defects are also classified into slightly amorphous and severely amorphous categories. The slight neck defect exhibits debris in the neck area or a thickness of the neck, but with a normally shaped head. Severe neck defects demonstrate a bend in the neck or midpiece.

All other abnormal forms — small, large, round, tapered, double head, double tail, coiled tail, cytoplasmic droplets — are classified according to standards set down by the World Health Organization classification.[3,4]

Spermatozoa with very long tails may represent an additional abnormal population incapable of normal fertilization. Although few references have been made to this aspect of sperm morphology in the literature, overly long tails have been observed, on occasion, in conjunction with failed fertilization (Veeck, unpublished data). Appleton and Fishel report a significant difference in the length of sperm tails in fertile vs. infertile males: 32.2 μm vs. 45.0 μm.[5]

B. TECHNIQUES

Two morphology slides are prepared for each sample and are stained by a quick-stain technique.[6] Special care is taken to clean the slides thoroughly with 70% ethyl alcohol before use, and no more than 5 μl of semen is placed on the slide in order to make the smears as thin as possible. Slides are then air-dried at room temperature, fixed for 15 s with Diff-Quik fixative (Diff-Quik AHS del Caribe, Inc. Aguada, PR 00602 also Baxter Healthcare Corp., Miami, FL) (1.8 mg/l triarylmethane in methyl alcohol), and then stained with Diff-Quik solution 1 (1 g/l xanthene in sodium azide-preserved buffer) for 10 s. Finally, slides are stained with Diff-Quik solution 2 (0.625 g/l azure A and 0.625 g/l methylene blue in buffer) for 5 s. In between the fixation step and each of the staining steps, excess solutions are drained from the slides by blotting the edges on bibulous paper. Slides are read and documented the same day. Morphology is evaluated by two independent observers. The inter-technician coefficient of variation and intratechnician variability are not significant.[2,4]

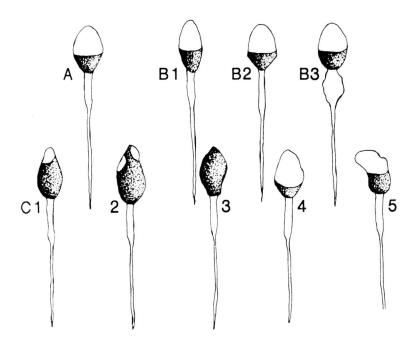

FIGURE 1. Diagrammatic representation of spermatozoa stained with the Diff-Quik technique. (A) Normal form. (B1,B2) Slightly amorphous heads. (B3) Slightly amorphous neck defect. (C1-5) Severely amorphous forms by strict criteria.

TABLE 1
Morphology vs. Fertilization and Pregnancy

	GROUP I (0—14%)	GROUP II (15—30%)	GROUP III (31—45%)	GROUP IV (46—60%)
No. cycles	22 (12%)	83 (44%)	67 (35%)	18 (9%)
% cycles with no fertilization	50%	7%	4%	6%
% oocytes fertilized	37%	81%	82%	91%
% pregnancy per transfer	0%	22%	31%	12%

From Kruger, T. F. et al., *Fertil. Steril.*, 46, 1118, 1986. With permission.

III. RESULTS

A. FERTILIZATION RATE VS. SPERM MORPHOLOGY

In 1986, Kruger and his clinical team from Capetown, South Africa, studied the relationship between percent normal morphology (based upon the strict criteria listed previously) and fertilization rates in 190 IVF cycles.[1] Based upon the percentage of morphologically normal spermatozoa, the patients were divided into four groups: I — normal forms between 0 and 14%; II — 15 to 30%; III — 31 to 45%; IV — 46 to 60%. In group I, 104 oocytes were retrieved of which 37% showed evidence of fertilization but no pregnancy resulted. In group II, 81% of 324 oocytes were fertilized with a pregnancy rate per transfer of 22%. In group III, 82% of 309 oocytes were fertilized with a 31% pregnancy rate, and in group IV, 91% of 69 oocytes were fertilized with a pregnancy rate of 12% (only 18 cycles). There was a clear threshold in normal forms at 14% (group I vs. groups II, III, IV), with lower fertilization and pregnancy rates below the 14% level (Table 1). In all cases, the inseminating concentration utilized was 50,000 motile sperm/ml/mature oocyte.

TABLE 2
Impaired Fertilization in Patients with Less than 14%
Normal Forms (Normal Values for Concentration and
Motility)

	<4% NF "P" PATTERN n = 13	4—14% NF "G" PATTERN n = 32
Average % normal forms	1.8%	7.7%
% slightly abnormal forms	18.0%	34.3%
Morphology index (normal plus slightly abnormal)	19.8%	42.0%
Concentration	63.3 × 10⁶/ml	83.3 × 10⁶/ml
Motility	45.6%	55.3%
% fertilization per oocyte	7.6%	63.9%
% pregnancy per transfer	7.6%	31.2%

From Kruger, T. et al., *Fertil. Steril.*, 49, 112, 1988. With permission.

B. THE NORFOLK EXPERIENCE

Kruger continued his andrology investigations in Norfolk, applying the same strict criteria for evaluation. He took special interest in the group of patients where <14% normal forms was discovered in the semen sample provided for IVF insemination, yet with acceptable sperm concentration (>20 × 10⁶/ml) and percent motility (>30%). Based upon his observations of the fertilizing potential of those patients with <14% normal forms, he further divided this group into two subgroups: poor prognosis pattern — <4% normal forms, and <30% normal and slightly abnormal forms; good prognosis pattern — 4 to 14% normal forms, and >30% combination normal and slightly abnormal forms. A morphology index of greater than 30% normal and slightly abnormal forms was significantly correlated with a positive fertilization result. Nevertheless, because "slightly abnormal" forms are difficult to assess and estimations are variable between readers, this index was largely disregarded. Excellent correlation continues to exist with the use of pure normal form gradings.

It was quite informative to discover that those patients exhibiting a "P" pattern (<4% NF) displayed a fertilization rate/oocyte of only 7.6% when inseminated with standard concentrations of 50,000 motile sperm/ml, while those with a "G" pattern (4—14% NF) had a significantly better rate of fertilization of 63.9% (p <0.0001) (Table 2). Patients during the same study period with normal forms >14% exhibited a >90% fertilizaton rate.[2]

C. PREGNANCY OUTCOME VS. SPERM MORPHOLOGY

There appears to be some degree of difference, even within various studies carried out in Norfolk, in evaluating the potential of live birth after fertilization with sperm samples of reduced quality. Kruger and Acosta reported that if fertilization occurs, the performance of the pre-embryos, as well as transfer and pregnancy rates, are no different from the general IVF population.[2,7] These initial studies were carried out either before critical morphologic criteria were applied to sperm evaluations or before the outcome of a large number of male factor pregnancies was known. Yovich reports much the same.[8] However, in a more recent study carried out by Oehninger and associates in Norfolk, it was pointed out that fertilization rates were significantly enhanced in the "P" pattern group of patients (<4% NF) by increasing sperm concentration around the oocytes up to 20 times the normal number. However, although fertilization rates improved by this practice, pregnancy outcome did not improve. The miscarriage rate was higher for women whose husbands displayed severe reduction in normal forms, and the ongoing pregnancy rate per cycle was extremely low.[9] It was concluded by this author that patients with sperm-head abnormalities have a lower ability to establish

TABLE 3
Ongoing Pregnancy vs. Sperm Morphology

	"P" PATTERN (<4% NF)		"G" PATTERN (4—14% NF)	NORMAL (>14% NF)
No. patients	43		144	41
No. cycles	47		144	41
% NF (avg)	1.4%		7.3%	18.4%
	50,000 sperm	>100,000 sperm		
% fertilization per oocyte	14.5%	62.6% (44.5%)	85.7%	94.3%
% pregnancy per cycle	6.6%	9.3% (8.5%)	33.3%	43.9%
% pregnancy per transfer	20.0%	12.5% (13.7%)	43.6%	43.9%
% ongoing pregnancy per cycle	6.6%	3.1% (4.2%)	19.4%	31.7%
% ongoing pregnancy per transfer	20.0%	4.1% (6.8%)	25.4%	31.7%

From Oehninger, S. et al., *Fertil. Steril.*, 50, 283, 1988. With permission.

successful pregnancies following IVF, and that even though fertilization may be achieved by corrective measures, overall reproductive potential appears to be poor (Table 3). More recent data from Norfolk involving 147 severe male factor patients (teratozoospermia alone or in combination with oligo- and/or asthenozoospermia) seems to substantiate this conclusion with an ongoing pregnancy rate of only 10.2%.

D. DOES A "SWIM-UP" PROCEDURE SELECT FOR MORPHOLOGY?

The standard "swim-up" technique employed by most IVF centers allows for the collection of a highly motile fraction of washed spermatozoa for oocyte insemination. While obviously selecting for sperm motility, this procedure also plays a role in the selection of normal forms. McDowell reported in 1986 that this technique provided a fraction of sperm with significant improvements in motility ($p < 0.001$) and improvements in morphology using old criteria ($p < 0.001$).[10]

More recent data generated in Norfolk utilized the methods of critical assessment to determine morphological improvements with the swim-up procedure. In a population of 73 consecutive IVF patients, the percent normal morphology improved 18.2% ($p < 0.05$) after the selection procedure.[7] Twenty-seven of these patients had a diagnosis of teratozoospermia (<14% normal forms), and 21 demonstrated significant improvement in the total percent of normal forms after processing, 6 demonstrated only slight improvement or no improvement at all, and no samples showed a decrease in normal forms.[11]

E. CORRELATION BETWEEN MORPHOLOGY AND RESULTS OF THE HAMSTER ZONA-FREE SPERM PENETRATION ASSAY (SPA)

Seventy patients with a sperm concentration $>20 \times 10^6$/ml, a motile sperm fraction >30%, and normal sperm morphology ranging from 1 to 39% were evaluated prospectively in the SPA.[12] BWW was utilized as the incubation medium and 3% bovine serum albumin (BSA) as the protein source during a short incubation (6 h) protocol.[13] Results showed a statistically significant relationship between the percent of sperm with normal morphology and penetration rate in the SPA ($p = 0.001$) (Table 4). Furthermore, the outcome of the SPA was correlated with *in vitro* fertilization, retrospectively, in 84 patients. Thirty-eight

TABLE 4
**Sperm Morphology as a Predictor of the SPA (Sperm
Concentration >20 × 10⁶/ml and Motility >30%)**

	GROUP 1 (41 pts.) (<14% normal forms)	GROUP 2 (29 pts.) (>14% normal forms)
SPA <10%	39/41 (95.1%)	4/29 (13.8%)[a]
SPA >20%	2/41 (4.8%)	25/29 (86.2%)[a]

[a] $p < 0.0001$ compared to group 1.

From Kruger, T. F. et al., *Int. J. Androl.*, 11, 107, 1988. With permission.

TABLE 5
Correlation Between SPA and IVF

	SPA <10%	SPA >10%
IVF: no fertilization	13/38 (34.2%)	8/46 (17.4%)
IVF: fertilizaiton	25/38 (65.8%)	38/46 (82.6%)

	SPA 11—19%	SPA 0%
IVF: no fertilizaition	1/8 (12.5%)	4/12 (33.3%)
IVF: fertilization	7/8 (87.5%)	8/12 (66.7%)

From Kruger, T. F. et al., *Int. J. Androl.*, 11, 107, 1988. With permission.

patients had an SPA <10%, with no fertilization *in vitro* in 13 patients (33.3%), and successful fertilization in 25 (66.7%). Forty-five had an SPA >10% with fertilization in 37 patients (82.2%), and no fertilization in eight (17.8%) (Table 5).

Based on these results, it was concluded that the SPA seems to have a good predictive value for IVF when it is normal, but is less reliable when results are <10%. Even patients with a sperm penetration assay of 0% had 66.7% fertilization in the human system. Overall, using the new criteria for sperm morphology and our SPA standards, morphology seems to be a better predictor of IVF outcome and a more useful adjunct for counseling patients.

F. FAILURE OF FERTILIZATION IN IVF: IMPACT OF ABNORMAL SPERM MORPHOLOGY

Hypothetically, failure of fertilization in IVF may be attributed to oocyte abnormalities (intrinsic and/or stimulation derived), sperm abnormalities (in quantity or in quality), or to technical factors. During Norfolk series 18 to 25, 1067 IVF attempts were performed in 583 patients; in 52 patients, failure of fertilization of mature oocytes occurred, representing 5.0% of attempts. We retrospectively examined these cases looking for possible causes that could explain the poor outcome. Additionally, we re-evaluated morphology slides applying the new, stricter criteria, and compared the results to the standard WHO classification. Interestingly, in more than 70% of the cases, sperm abnormalities could be detected, suggesting that these abnormalities could have played a significant role in the fertilization failure. Abnormal sperm morphology was involved in 69% of these cases.[4]

In addition, Franken et al., utilizing the hemizona assay (HZA), showed that semen samples classified as morphologically poor (<4% NF) exhibited a significant impairment of sperm binding to the human zona pellucida (Table 6).[14] Moreover, Oehninger et al. reported that IVF cases with poor fertilization rates (male factor patients) had lower sperm binding ability in the HZA as compared with patients with successful fertilization.[15]

TABLE 6
Number of Sperm Bound Tightly to Hemizonae During the HZA for Patients with Successful IVF vs. Patients with Failed IVF, and the Corresponding Group Semen Parameters

Parameter	Fertilization success (n = 27)	Fertilization failure (n = 9)
HZA: number of tightly bound sperm	36.1 ± 6.8	10.4 ± 3.6[a]
% normal morphology	12.7 ± 1.5	3.1 ± 0.9[a]
Sperm concentration ($\times 10^6$/ml)	74.2 ± 10.0	54.8 ± 7.8
% motility	45.2 ± 4.0	33.3 ± 6.2

[a] $p < 0.05$

From Franken, D. et al., *J. In Vitro Fertil. Embryo Transfer*, 6, 44, 1989. With permission.

Taken together, these data seem to indicate that abnormalities in spermatozoon morphology may be responsible for failed fertilization in some patients. Lower or abnormal binding to the zona pellucida, an early and critical step during the fertilization process, could be a significant cause for failure in some of these patients. However, other defects involving other steps of the fertilization process (oolemma binding, egg-sperm fusion, sperm nucleus decondensation, etc.) could also be responsible. Active research is being performed in this field which will hopefully elucidate this issue as well as provide information for the developing assisted reproduction technology.[16]

IV. DISCUSSION

When sperm morphology is evaluated by strict criteria, it proves to be a valuable tool in predicting a patient's chance to fertilize and reach the transfer stage. In an earlier study performed in Norfolk, 70 out of 71 patients with normal morphology greater than 14% reached the transfer stage, reflecting a high fertility in this group.[3] If normal morphology is less than 14%, fertilization potential is markedly impaired. Further results indicate that *severe* impairment occurs at levels less than 4%. By concentrating greater numbers of sperm with an oocyte (up to 1×10^6/ml/oocyte), rates of fertilization may improve, but ongoing pregnancy outcome may still be low as compared to patients with completely normal sperm parameters.[9]

REFERENCES

1. **Kruger, T. F., Menkveld, R., Stander, F. S. H., Lombard, C. J., Van der Merwe, J. P., Van Zyl, J. A., and Smith, K.,** Sperm morphologic features as a prognostic factor in in vitro fertilization, *Fertil. Steril.,* 46, 1118, 1986.
2. **Kruger, T., Acosta, A., Simmons, K., Swanson, R. J., Matta, J. F., and Oehninger, S.,** Predictive value of abnormal sperm morphology in in vitro fertilization, *Fertil. Steril.,* 49, 112, 1988.
3. **Kruger, T. F., Acosta, A. A., Simmons, K. F., Swanson, J. R., Matta, J. F., Veeck, L. L., Morshedi, M., and Brugo, S.,** A new method of evaluating sperm morphology with predictive value for IVF, *Urology,* 30, 248, 1987.

4. **Oehninger, S., Acosta, A. A., Kruger, T., Veeck, L. L., Flood, J., and Jones, H. W., Jr.,** Failure of fertilization in in vitro fertilization: the "Occult" male factor, *J. In Vitro Fertil. Embryo Transfer*, 5, 181, 1988.

5. **Appleton, T. C. and Fishel, S. B.,** Morphology and X-ray microprobe analysis of spermatozoa from fertile and infertile men in in vitro fertilization, *J. In Vitro Fertil. Embryo Transfer*, 1, 188, 1984.

6. **Kruger, T. F., Ackerman, S. B., Simmons, K. F., Swanson, R. J., Brugo, S., and Acosta, A. A.,** A quick reliable staining technique for sperm morphology, *Arch. Androl.*, 18, 275, 1987.

7. **Acosta, A. A., Chillik, C. F., Brugo, S., Ackerman, S., Swanson, R. J., Pleban, P., Yuan, J., and Haque, D.,** In vitro fertilization and the male factor, *Urology*, 28, 1, 1986.

8. **Yovich, J. L. and Stanger, J. D.,** The limitations of in vitro fertilization from males with severe oligospermia and abnormal sperm morphology, *J. In Vitro Fertil. Embryo Transfer*, 1, 172, 1984.

9. **Oehninger, S., Acosta, A. A., Morshedi, M., Veeck, L., Swanson, R. J., Simmons, K., and Rosenwaks, Z.,** Corrective measures and pregnancy outcome in in vitro fertilization in patients with severe sperm morphology abnormalities, *Fertil. Steril.*, 50, 283, 1988.

10. **McDowell, J. S.,** Preparation of spermatozoa for insemination in vitro, in *In Vitro Fertilization — Norfolk*, Jones, H. W., Jr., Jones, G. S., Hodgen, G. D., and Rosenwaks Z., Eds., Williams & Wilkins, Baltimore, 1986, 162.

11. **Scott, R. T., Oehninger, S. C., Menkveld, R., Veeck, L. L., and Acosta, A. A.,** Critical assessment of sperm morphology before and after double swim-up preparation for in vitro fertilization (IVF), *Arch. Androl.*, 23, 125, 1989.

12. **Kruger, T. F., Swanson, R. J., Hamilton, M., Simmons, K., Acosta, A. A., Matta, J. F., Oehninger, S., and Morshedi, M.,** Abnormal sperm morphology and other semen parameters related to the outcome of the hamster oocyte human sperm penetration assay, *Int. J. Androl.*, 11, 107, 1988.

13. **Swanson, R. J., Mayer, J. F., Jones, K. H., Lanzendorf, S., and McDowell, J.,** Hamster ova/human sperm penetration assay: correlation with count, motility, and morphology for in vitro fertilization, *Arch. Androl.*, 12, 69, 1984.

14. **Franken, D., Oehninger, S., Burkman, L., Coddington, C. C., Kruger, T. F., Rosenwaks, Z., Acosta, A. A., and Hodgen, G. D.,** The hemizona assay (HZA): a predictor of human sperm fertilizing potential in IVF treatment, *J. In Vitro Fertil. Embryo Transfer*, 6, 44, 1989.

15. **Oehninger, S., Coddington, C. C., Scott, R., Franken, D., Burkman, L., Acosta, A. A., and Hodgen, G. D.,** Hemizona assay: assessment of sperm dysfunction and predictor of in vitro fertilization outcome, *Fertil. Steril.*, 51, 665, 1989.

16. **Acosta, A. A., Oehninger, S., Morshedi, M., Swanson, R. J., Scott, R., and Irianni, F.,** Assisted reproduction in the diagnosis and treatment of the male factor, *Obstet. Gynecol. Surv.*, 44, 1, 1989.

Chapter 5

BIOCHEMICAL ANALYSIS OF SEMINAL PLASMA AND SPERMATOZOA

L. J. D. Zaneveld and R. S. Jeyendran

TABLE OF CONTENTS

I. INTRODUCTION

The ejaculate consists of a mixture of spermatozoa and the secretions from the epididymis and the accessory sex glands. Together, these secretions are called seminal plasma. The human spematozoon is approximately 50 μm long and consists of a head and tail. The sperm organelles are covered by the plasma membrane. Approximately 65% of the head is composed of chromosomal material, tightly packed with nucleoproteins. Located over the anterior two thirds of the head is the acrosome. The acrosome is a lysosomal, bag-like organelle and contains lytic enzymes that are required for the acrosome reaction, and sperm binding to and penetration through the oocyte investments. The sperm tail possesses an axonemal complex which is a series of microtubules capable of sliding along one another, producing tail motion. The energy (adenosine triphosphate, ATP) for the activity of the contractile fibers is generated in the midpiece, located at the anterior end of the sperm tail. The midpiece contains elongated, helical mitochondria wound around the axonemal complex. A small amount of cytoplasm is present between the mitochondria and the plasma membrane.

The human accessory sex glands are the seminal vesicles, the prostate gland, the ampulla of the vas deferens and the Cowper's (bulbourethral) glands. Of these glands, the seminal vesicles are the largest and contribute approximately 75% of the ejaculate volume. The prostate provides another 20% and all other secretions as well as the spermatozoa make up approximately 5% of the ejaculate. During ejaculation, the Cowper's gland secretions are emitted first, representing a small drop of fluid. Subsequently, the prostatic and ampullary secretions as well as the majority of the spermatozoa are ejaculated, followed by the seminal vesicle secretions. By performing a split (partitioned) ejaculate, these secretions can roughly be separated.

Immediately upon ejaculation, the semen coagulates. Liquefaction usually occurs within 15 to 30 min, releasing the spermatozoa that are trapped in the coagulum. Sperm entrapment can hinder their transport into the cervix so that prolonged liquefaction times, e.g., more than 1 to 2 h, may result in subfertility, particularly if only a small number of spermatozoa are ejaculated. The coagulating proteins originate from the seminal vesicles and the liquefying enzyme(s) from the prostate gland.

Seminal plasma functions as a vehicle for sperm transport. Although a large number of components are present in seminal plasma, it remains to be established that any one of these components has an essential function in the fertilization process.[1-3] This is exemplified by the ability of washed spermatozoa to fertilize when placed in the female genital tract. Under optimal conditions, it is generally thought that the seminal plasma components are supportive to spermatozoa rather than being essential for their function. Under less than optimal conditions, some components may be essential for sperm function but it is not known exactly when such conditions prevail or which these components are. Evidence for a supportive function is, for instance, that seminal plasma from ejaculates containing a high percentage of motile spermatozoa can occasionally increase the motility of poorly motile spermatozoa. Additionally, seminal plasma from ejaculates whose spermatozoa effectively penetrate zona-free hamster oocytes, can at times enhance the penetrating capacity of poorly penetrating spermatozoa.[4] Seminal plasma also contains antibacterial and immunosuppressive factors, possesses sperm nutrients such as fructose, and contains acrosomal stabilizing agents such as the decapacitation factor.[1-3] Finally, seminal plasma has a slightly basic pH that serves to neutralize the acidic environment of the human vagina.

The following is an overview of the biochemical assays that can be applied to seminal plasma and spermatozoa for diagnostic purposes. Details of each assay can be found under Specific Methodology in the references and/or in the WHO Laboratory Manual for the Examination of Human Semen and Semen-Cervical Mucus Interaction.[5]. References have been kept to a minimum so that the quoted reviews on a specific subject should be consulted if more detail is desired.

II. SEMINAL PLASMA

Although the physiological role of seminal plasma and its components needs to be established further, there is little question that the biochemical analysis of seminal plasma can be useful for diagnostic purposes. The seminal vesicles and prostate gland secrete components that are quite specific for each gland[1,2,6] and can be used to determine glandular function. The epididymal secretions also contain some fairly specific components that can be useful for the same purpose. It should be remembered that these components are more than likely not essential for sperm function so that they are not directly useful as fertility indicators but only to assess the status of the accessory sex glands. The contributions of the accessory sex glands to the ejaculate vary from ejaculate to ejaculate even in the same person. Therefore, quantitative analyses have so far not been useful to determine the relative functional activity of an accessory sex gland, i.e., a gland has to be severely altered before the amount or concentration of its components in seminal plasma becomes noticably low. For the same reason, the concentration or total amount of an accessory sex gland component in seminal plasma is a rather insensitive indicator of the adrogenic status of the man although the secretory activity of the accessory sex glands requires testosterone stimulation.

Human seminal vesicle fluid contains high levels of proteins and reducing sugars, and has a basic pH. This gland also secretes the glycoproteins that form the seminal coagulum. Fructose is normally used as the indicator of the seminal vesicle contribution to the ejaculate. The most frequently used assay for fructose is the resorcinol assay.[1,5] Although this technique is satisfactory for most diagnostic purposes, it is rather nonspecific because it measures all reducing sugars. A more sensitive and specific assay is the enzymatic technique.[7]

Human prostatic fluid possesses high levels of acid phosphatase, zinc, citric acid, lipids, and polyamines (spermine and spermidine), has an acidic pH, and contains the enzyme(s) responsible for liquefaction of the ejaculate. Only one liquefying enzyme has so far been identified and was called seminin. The characteristic odor of semen is due to the oxidation of spermine and spermidine. Zinc, citric acid, and acid phosphatase are the most commonly used indicators of the prostatic contribution to the ejaculate and relatively simple assays are available for these components.[5,8]

The fructose assay is primarily used when the ejaculate contains no spermatoza. Absence of spermatozoa may be due to a blocked ejaculatory duct at the vas deferens-urethral junction, to a congenital absence of the vas deferens (associated with the absence of the seminal vesicles), to low testosterone levels causing cessation of spermatogenesis, or to a blockage of the testicular excretory ducts. In case of the first two conditions, no fructose will be present in the seminal plasma and the blood testosterone levels tend to be normal. Such ejaculates will also fail to coagulate, have a pH below 7.2 and possess relatively high levels of zinc, citric acid or acid phosphatase. By contrast, some fructose is usually present in the second two conditions. If the blood testosterone levels are low, the azoospermia may be caused by the cessation of spermatogenesis. If the blood testosterone levels are normal, the testicular ducts may be blocked.

Occasionally, only the excretory ducts of the seminal vesicles but not the vas deferens may be blocked. The sperm content of the ejaculate and the blood testosterone levels would be normal under these conditions but the volume of the ejaculate would be greatly reduced and no fructose is present. Thus, fructose analyses are also useful when the volume of the ejaculate is abnormally low.

Reduced amounts or absence of citric acid, zinc, or acid phosphatase are indicative of a prostatic abnormality. Such ejaculates may also be poorly able to liquefy the coagulum. Therefore, assays for these components are indicated when a prostatic abnormality is suspect as, for instance, in case of an infection. However, it should be noted that patients with acute or chronic bacterial prostatovesiculitis may show substantial decreases in these prostatic indicators for even a year after the infection has been successfully treated due to irreversible damage to the secretory epithelium. Occasionally, only a partial ejaculate is collected while attempting to masturbate a sample in a container. If the first fraction is absent, the collected sample may be oligozoospermic. In order to differentiate this situation from true oligo-zoospermia, citric acid, zinc, or acid phosphatase assays can be performed. In case the first fraction is mostly absent, only low assay values will be obtained.

Epididymal secretions are characterized by L-carnitine and glycerylphosphorylcholine (GPC) although the latter can also be produced by postepididymal sites in the human. Free L-carnitine levels in seminal plasma may reflect the secretory function of the epididymis[9] but the use of this assay is still controversial and has as yet not found much application for diagnostic purposes.

Many andrology clinics measure the pH of the ejaculate. This is done either by placing a drop of semen on pH paper or, more accurately, with an electric pH meter. The pH of semen usually varies from 7.6 to 8.0. Above 8.2 or below 7.2 can be considered abnormal. No good evidence exists that the pH of the ejaculate alone has an effect on fertility. The pH tends to decrease to 7.5 or less in cases of chronic inflammatory diseases of the accessory sex glands and to increase to above 8.0 in case of acute disease. Since prostatic fluid has an acidic pH and seminal vesicle fluid a basic pH, an abnormally low or high pH is an indication that one or the other of these glands is not functioning normally. Therefore, the detection of an abnormal seminal pH should be followed by one or more of the biochemical analyses mentioned above. Since the pH is not a sensitive indicator of glandular function, it should never be relied upon by itself.

Seminal plasma contains a large number of other inorganic and organic constituents, including a number of enzymes. As yet, there is no good evidence that any of these constituents are of diagnostic value.

III. SPERMATOZOA

A. INTRODUCTION

Diagnostically, the analysis of sperm function has primarily relied on physical indicators such as sperm number or concentration, sperm motility characteristics, and the morphology of the spermatozoa. It is becoming increasingly clear that these physical characteristics are not sufficient by themselves to interpret the fertility status of an ejaculate unless these indicators are at extremely low levels, e.g., less than 0.5 to 1.0×10^6 sperm/ml, less than 10 to 15% motile spermatozoa or less than 10 to 15% normally shaped spermatozoa. The reason for this is that the fertilization process involves a large number of biochemical events that are not measured by these physical parameters. Therefore, additional tests need to be used to indicate the functional activity of the spermatozoa. One such test is the zona-free hamster oocyte penetration assay (see Chapter 7) that primarily measures the ability of spermatozoa to become capacitated, acrosome react, and decondense. However, this test is rather difficult, time consuming, and costly, and is not readily performed in private practice settings. Simpler assays would be of much value. It is logical to assume that evaluation of certain biochemical characteristics of the spermatozoon which are important for its function, would aid in the diagnosis of fertility/infertility. Often, such biochemical tests can be simplified so that they can be performed under private practice conditions. More detailed knowledge of the problem(s) that cause(s) spermatozoa to be infertile should also aid in developing better treatment protocols.

It is impossible to measure all the biochemical processes that are involved in the functional activity of spermatozoa. Therefore, some indicators need to be selected which can serve as probes for the activity of an entire sperm organelle. Such organelles are (1) the sperm plasma membrane, (2) the acrosome, (3) the nucleus, (4) the midpiece, and (5) the contractile elements of the tail. The last is readily studied by observing the movement characteristics of the tail so that a biochemical assay is probably not necessary. A number of assays have been proposed for the organelles but only one, the hypoosmotic swelling (HOS) test for the sperm membrane, is finding clinical application at present. Assays for the acrosome (acrosin assay) and the midpiece (creatine phosphokinase assay) are in various stages of development (see further). The results obtained so far indicate that these assays are of diagnostic use so that these tests may reach the clinic in the near future. Assays for the integrity of the nucleus have also been proposed based on sperm chromatin heterogeneity. Encouraging results have been obtained with acridine orange staining for double- or single-stranded DNA in relationship to fertility[10,11] although some caution has been advised.[12]

The following is a brief review of the HOS test, the acrosin assay, and the creatine phophokinase (CK) assay. Since these tests are relatively new, some detail is provided regarding the evidence that is available for their ability as fertility indicators. Controversy regarding their diagnostic use will probably be present for quite some time because it is extremely difficult to prove the usefulness of a sperm test as evidenced by the argument that still surrounds the interpretation of the standard sperm parameters (sperm number, motility, and morphology). In addition, a single test (probe) will never be sufficient to determine the functional status of spermatozoa, i.e., a number of tests need to be taken into consideration before a diagnosis is reached.

It is recommended that a standard sperm analysis is performed (see Chapter 3). If one of the standard parameters is extremely abnormal (see above), it is clear that the patient has a fertility problem and no further tests are necessary. However, if the standard parameters fall into the less abnormal, suspect, or normal ranges, it would be useful to perform the following tests. If any one of these tests is abnormal, the fertility status of the patient is probably impaired. However, if a test is normal, no definitive diagnosis can be reached because other factors may be abnormal. As long as the percentage of false negatives is low, a single sperm test is valid, independent of the percentage of false positives.

B. HYPOOSMOTIC SWELLING (HOS) TEST

The hypoosmotic swelling (HOS) test[13] measures the ability of the sperm membrane to transport fluid. In case fluid transport does not occur, it can be assumed that the membrane is chemically inactive and that it cannot function in the fertilization process. A functional membrane is important not only for sperm motility but also for capacitation and the acrosome reaction. This assay differs from the live/dead (viability) stain that measures whether the sperm membrane is physically disrupted (broken) as a result of sperm death. Since a sperm membrane can be physically intact, i.e., exclude dye, but be chemically inactive, the HOS test is more inclusive than the live/dead stain. The term ''viability stain'' is a misnomer because the sperm membrane may be physically intact but the spermatozoa may still not be viable, i.e., able to function normally.

The HOS test is performed by incubating spermatozoa under hypoosmotic conditions. Water transport into the cell will occur if the membrane is functional. The membrane around the sperm tail is quite flexible so that the entry of water will cause distention (ballooning) of this membrane. The contractile fibers of the tail are under tension so that they will curl within the membrane when the membrane expands. Thus, spermatozoa with functional membranes will show curled tail fibers which can readily be detected by phase contrast microscopy.

The clinical application of the HOS test was reviewed recently.[14] The outcome of the tests varies independently of the standard, physical sperm characteristics. The occurrence of 60% or more HOS-reactive (''swollen'') spermatozoa in an ejaculate is designated as normal and less than 50% as abnormal. In between, represents a suspect area where no diagnosis of normal or abnormal can be reached. Using these cu -off points, the HOS test is 75 to 85% predictive of the outcome (normal/abnormal) of the zona-free hamster oocyte penetration assay. By itself, the HOS test is a better indicator of the outcome of human IVF than the physical sperm characteristics. Sperm populations obtained by a swim-up procedure usually contain a significantly higher percentage of HOS-reactive spermatozoa than the original ejaculate.

In vivo studies tend to support the diagnostic usefulness of the assay. Although some disagreement is present,[15] the majority of the investigators found that almost all of the ejaculates from presumably fertile men produce a normal or, at the worst, a suspect HOS test, whereas a significant percentage of presumably infertile men or men with abnormal physical sperm characteristics produce an abnormal HOS test.[16-20] It was also reported that with a few exceptions, pregnancies only occur when ejaculates produce a normal HOS test.[19,20] After tamoxiphen treatment, a number of subfertile men improved the HOS test values from abnormal to normal.[21,22]

The HOS test may also be useful when studying the effect of cryopreservation on spermatozoa[23] which is not surprising since the sperm membrane is particularly susceptible to cryoinjury.

C. ACROSIN ASSAY

The sperm acrosome has an essential function in the fertilization process since it contains enzymes that are involved in the acrosome reaction, sperm binding to the zona pellucida, and the penetration of the spermatozoon through the oocyte investment. For diagnostic purposes, it is essential to assure that the acrosome is intact. Physical integrity is assessed by use of the Papanicolaou stain. However, physical integrity does not guarantee that the acrosomal contents are biochemically active so that an indicator of biochemical integrity should also be used. The most widely studied acrosomal enzyme is acrosin. Acrosin is a serine proteinase that has similarites to trypsin but differs from this enzyme kinetically and in its inhibitor spectrum. Much evidence has been presented for a role of acrosin in the fertilization process. Data are also available to show that the acrosin levels are altered in case of morphological abnormalities of the human acrosome.[24-26] For instance, ejaculates have been identified with reasonable sperm motility but the spermatozoa lack acrosomes, have a very low acrosin content and do not penetrate zona-free hamster oocytes.[24,26] Thus, it is likely that this enzyme is a good probe for both the biochemical and physical integrity of the sperm acrosome.

Many assays are available to measure sperm acrosin levels. Most are either too complicated and/or time consuming, are not sufficiently sensitive (such as the gelatin plate assay), or measure acrosin content rather than activity (such as immunological techniques). The last is disadvantageous because an enzyme can be present but inactive. In addition, acrosin exists primarily in an inactive form called proacrosin. In order to measure the total acrosin activity available for sperm function, the assay has to incorporate proacrosin conversion to acrosin before the activity is measured. A simple, sensitive assay that measures the total available acrosin activity based on the benzamidine-sensitive amidase activity of the enzyme, was recently developed and can readily be applied clinically.[27]

The acrosin activity was shown to vary independently of the physical sperm parameters.[28] The ejaculate can be retained for 24 h at 5°C without loss of acrosin activity.[27] The presence of leukocytes in the ejaculate does not alter the assay results.[27] Data are also available that support the diagnostic usefulness of the acrosin assay. Spermatozoa selected by the swim-up technique possess two-to threefold higher acrosin activity than nonselected spermatozoa.[27] Spermatozoa obtained from normospermic or presumably fertile men average significantly higher acrosin levels than spermatozoa obtained from patients attending infertility clinics or presumably infertile men.[29,30] Using unselected sperm samples, i.e., no swim-up was performed, it was shown that ejaculates which fertilize human oocytes *in vitro* possess significantly higher acrosin activity than ejaculates that did not fertilize oocytes.[27] Based on the preliminary data obtained in this study, values of 25 μIU acrosin/10^7 spermatozoa or more were tentatively accepted as normal and values of 14 μIU or below as abnormal. Finally, it has been shown that the acrosin assay can be used to identify subpopulations of infertile men which would not be detected by the physical sperm parameters.[31]

The acrosin activity of spermatozoa may also be useful as an additional indicator of cryoinjury to spermatozoa.[32] Of the acrosomal enzymes tested, acrosin was the only one that showed a large decrease in activity when the spermatozoa were cryopreserved.[25]

D. ATP AND CREATINE PHOSPHOKINASE (CK) ASSAYS

The movement of the contractile fibers of the tail results in sperm motility and is fuelled by ATP. Therefore, it is not surprising that investigators have attempted to correlate ATP levels with fertility. Using whole semen ATP values, it was reported that significant differences existed between fertile donors and husbands with "normal" wives attending infertility clinics, and that the ATP levels were correlated with the relative fertility of men *in vivo*.[33] Subsequent studies did not confirm these observations, particularly once adjustments were made for sperm concentration.[34] However, the use of ATP as a measure of midpiece integrity is still intriguing and more consistent results may be obtained if the ATP level of the spermatozoa had been determined rather than that of the whole ejaculate. Recently, it was shown that oligozoospermic ejaculates have higher sperm dynein ATPase activity than normozoospermic ejaculates.[35]

A presently more successful midpiece fertility marker is creatine-*n*-phosphotransferase (creatine phosphokinase, CK) which is a key enzyme in the synthesis and transport of energy. Creatine phosphate can enhance the motility and velocity of human spermatozoa.[36] Sperm CK levels show a highly significant inverse correlation with sperm concentration, i.e., oligozoospermic ejaculates have much higher CK levels than normozoospermic ($>20 \times 10^6$ sperm/ml) ejaculates.[37,38] Also, selection of spermatozoa by a swim-up procedure results in a highly motile sperm population with relatively low CK levels.[37] There is no association between sperm CK activity and sperm motility or morphology, or with the seminal plasma CK levels.[37] Tentatively, less than 0.250 CK units per 10^8 spermatozoa is taken as normal. Using this cut-off point, it was shown that the success of intrauterine insemination is highly correlated with a normal CK value.[39] The isoforms of CK (B-CK and M-CK) may further aid in differentiating normal from abnormal spermatozoa. The B-CK levels are higher in spermatozoa from oligozoospermic men than normozoospermic men, where as the reverse is true for M-CK.[40] The concentration of M-CK in spermatozoa may be a marker of cellular maturity.

IV. SPECIFIC METHODOLOGY

The numbers after each heading indicate the reference from which the technique was taken or modified.

A. FRUCTOSE (COLORIMETRIC TECHNIQUE)[1]
Reagents

1. $ZnSO_4 \cdot 7 H_2O$ (5% in H_2O)
2. $Ba(OH)_2$ (0.3 *N* in H_2O)
3. HCl (30%)
4. Resorcinol solution (0.1% resorcinol in ethanol)
5. Fructose standard (200 mg% in H_2O)

Procedure — In this procedure, seminal plasma is deproteinized by treatment with zinc sulfate and barium hydroxide. Subsequently, the fructose of the deproteinized seminal plasma is reacted with acidic resorcinol to form a colored complex.

1.   Place 0.25 ml water (blank), 0.25 ml seminal plasma and 0.25 ml fructose standard in separate tubes. Add 1 ml of H_2O to each tube.
2.   Add 0.25 ml $ZnSO_4$ solution to each tube and mix thoroughly.
3.   Add 0.25 ml $Ba(OH)_2$ solution to each tube and mix thorougly.
4.   Let the tubes stand for 10 to 15 min and centrifuge at 1000 *g* for 20 min. Collect the supernatant solution (should be clear).
5.   To 0.25 ml of each supernatant in a glass tube with glass stopper, add 0.5 ml H_2O, 1.0 ml resorcinol solution and 3.0 ml HCl (30%).
6.   Mix and heat to 100°C for 7 min.
7.   Cool rapidly in ice water and read the absorbance at 410 nm against the blank within 30 min.

Calculation

$$\text{Fructose (mg\%)} = \frac{\text{Absorbance of seminal plasma}}{\text{Absorbance of fructose standard}} \times 200$$

Alternately, compare to fructose standards (see fructose: enzymatic technique).

B. FRUCTOSE (ENZYMATIC TECHNIQUE)[7]
Reagents (Prepared by R. A. Anderson, Rush Medical Center)

1. **0.5 *M* sodium phosphate**—Weigh out 6.90 g sodium phosphate, monobasic. Dissolve in approximately 75 ml water. Adjust pH of resultant solution to 6.80 with sodium hydroxide (≥ 1.0 *N*). Bring final volume to 100 ml. This solution can be stored indefinitely in a stoppered container at room temperature.

2. **200 m*M* beta-D-fructose**—Weigh out 36.0 mg/ml in water. This should be freshly prepared each time; 5 ml is more than enough for most purposes.

From the 200 m*M* fructose stock solution, prepare fructose solutions which will be used to generate a standard curve. For human seminal plasma, standard fructose solutions should range from 2.0 to 20 m*M*. Prepare 1.0 ml of each standard as follows:

[Fructose] (m*M*)	ml of 200 m*M* stock solution to be added	ml H_2O to be added
0.0	0.00	1.00
2.0	0.01	0.99
3.0	0.015	0.985
5.0	0.025	0.975
10.0	0.050	0.950
15.0	0.075	0.925
20.0	0.100	0.900

3. **0.5 mg/ml sorbitol dehydrogenase (SDH; from sheep liver)**—Weigh out approximately 2 mg of the enzyme preparation. The actual activity will vary from lot to lot, depending upon the content of nonprotein solids in the preparation. For example, information on the bottle supplied by Sigma may indicate the following:

● 10 mg protein
● 60 mg solid
● 28 U/mg protein
● 4.66 U/mg solid

In this case, 0.33 mg protein (9.3 Units of activity) is weighed out for each 2 mg solid weighed out. Dissolve in *cold* (4°C) 0.1 *M* sodium phosphate, pH 6.8 to give a final concentration of 0.5 mg/ml. This solution should be freshly prepared each time and kept on ice.

4. **1.5 m*M* Beta-nicotinamide adenine dinucleotide, reduced form (Beta-NADH)**— The exact amount of this material to be weighed out may vary from lot to lot, depending upon the purity, water and ethanol content of the preparation. For example, information on the bottle supplied by Sigma may indicate the following:

Anhydrous mol wt: 709.4
Assay: 98%
H_2O: 1.0/mol
Ethanol: 4% (by weight)

From the above information, the formula weight would be:

$$(709.4 + 18.0)/(0.98)(0.96) = 773.2$$

The number *18* is that fraction of the formula weight accounted for by water of hydration; *0.98* corrects for the assay of purity (98%); *0.96* corrects for the ethanol content (4%, by weight). With this particular lot, one would weigh out 1.6 mg/ml, dissolved in 0.1 *M* sodium phosphate, pH 6.8. The most accurate way to prepare this solution, is to weigh out approximately 2 mg of NADH, record the exact amount weighed, and add a sufficient volume of 0.1 *M* sodium phosphate, pH 6.8, such that the final concentration of NADH is 1.16 mg/ml (1.5 m*M*). This solution should be freshly prepared each time.

For both NADH and SDH, greater consistency from lot to lot can be obtained if the NADH is weighed out, correcting for water of hydration, purity and ethanol content, and if SDH is weighed out according to enzyme activity, rather than protein or solid content. However, since standard curves are constructed with each set of assays, it is not necessary to know the exact amount of either of these reagents in the reaction mixture.

Procedure—The principal of the assay is based upon an increase in enzyme (SDH) activity as a function of substrate (fructose) concentration, at less than saturating substrate concentrations. Under these conditions, the rate at which SDH catalyzes the reduction of fructose to sorbitol is proportional to the concentration of fructose in the reaction mixture. The reaction can be expressed as follows:

$$\text{Fructose} \xrightarrow[\text{SDH}]{\text{NADH} \quad \text{NAD}^+} \text{Sorbitol}$$

The reaction can be followed spectrophotometrically by measuring the rate of decrease in absorbance at 340 nm due to the oxidation of NADH to NAD^+.

1. Add 0.05 ml of each standard or seminal plasma to 0.45 ml H_2O in test tubes. Place tubes in a boiling water bath for 7 min, so as to inactivate enzyme activity which may be present. Centrifuge samples in a clinical centrifuge for 15 to 20 min to sediment precipitated material. Decant supernatant into clean, appropriately labeled tubes.
2. To a semi-microcuvette (sample cuvette), add the following reagents, in order:

   (1) 0.2 ml 0.5 *M* sodium phosphate, pH 6.8
   (2) 0.4 ml H_2O

(3) 0.1 ml 1.5 mM NADH
(4) 0.1 ml SDH (0.5 mg/ml)

Place this cuvette in the sample compartment of a recording spectrophotometer.
3. To a second semi-microcuvette (blank cuvette), add the following reagents, in order:

(1) 0.2 ml 0.5 M sodium phosphate, pH 6.8
(2) 0.5 ml H$_2$O
(3) 0.1 ml 1.5 mM NADH

Place this cuvette in the reference compartment of a recording spectrophotometer.
4. Mix the contents of each cuvette by either covering with parafilm and inverting several times, or by carefully aspirating the contents in and out of a Pasteur pipette 3 to 4 times (being careful not to scratch the optical surface of the cuvettes with the pipette tip).
5. Set the expansion scale on the recorder such that full scale is 0.1 or 0.2 absorbance units. Adjust the recorder pen with the offset control such that it reads approximately 80% of full scale.
6. Add 0.2 ml of the processed sample (either fructose standard or seminal plasma) to each cuvette, mix the contents of each cuvette, and record the change in absorbance at 340 nm. If fructose is present, and all reaction components are present, the absorbance in the sample cuvette should decrease relative to that in the blank cuvette, as a function of time. Determine the linear rate of decrease over the first 3 to 4 min of reaction. The data can be expressed as rates of change in absorbance per minute.

Calculation—The standard fructose solutions should be assayed first, to determine whether, in fact, the initial fructose concentrations are proportional to the rate of change in the absorbance at 340 nm. A linear curve should be obtained when the rate change in absorbance at 340 nm (Y axis) is plotted as a function of fructose concentration (X axis). In this instance, the fructose concentrations are 0.0, 2.0, 3.0, 5.0, 10.0, 15.0, and 20 mM (it may not be necessary to determine the rates of all of these fructose concentrations). If the rates of change in absorbance at 340 nm seem to be too large or too small, the amount of SDH added to the reaction mixture can be adjusted accordingly.

The concentration of fructose in the seminal plasma is determined directly from the standard curve, based upon the observed rate of change (decrease) in absorbance at 340 nm.

C. ZINC[41]
Reagents

1. **Buffer solution (pH 10.0)**—Dissolve 6 g ammonium chloride in 20 ml H$_2$O and add 57 ml of ammonia solution (25% concentrated). Mix and dilute to 100 ml with H$_2$O
2. **Magnesium masking solution**—Dissolve 10 g of dodecyl hydrogen sulfate sodium salt in 500 ml of water. Add 10 g of ammonium fluoride and dilute to 900 ml with H$_2$O
3. **Pan solution**—100 mg of 1-(2-pyridylazo)-2 naphthol in 100 ml of methanol.
4. **Reagent solution**—Add 100 ml buffer solution to 900 ml magnesium masking solution. Mix. To 980 ml of this mixture, add 20 ml Pan solution.
5. **Zinc standard**—10 mg/100 ml H$_2$O

Procedure—In this procedure, the magnesium in seminal plasma is masked by treatment with dodecyl hydrogen sulfate. Subsequently, the zinc is reacted with a naphthol reagent to form a colored complex.

1. Place 0.025 ml H$_2$O (blank), 0.025 ml zinc standard and 0.025 ml of seminal plasma in separate tubes.
2. Add 3 ml of reagent solution to each tube.
3. Mix well, allow the mixtures to stand at room temperature for 5 min and measure the absorbance within an hour at 560 nm against the blank.

Calculation

$$\text{Zn (mg\%)} = \frac{\text{Absorbance of seminal plasma}}{\text{Absorbance of zinc standard}} \times 10$$

Alternately, compare to zinc standards (dilutions from 1—53 mM)

D. CITRIC ACID[8]
Reagents

1. 50% trichloracetic acid (TCA) in H$_2$O
2. Anhydrous grade acetic anhydride
3. Dry, reagent grade pyridine

   Procedure—In this procedure, deproteinized seminal plasma is incubated with warm acetic anhydride and upon addition of pyridine, citric acid gives a carmine-red color.

1. Deproteinize the seminal plasma by addition of 1.0 ml seminal plasma to 1.0 ml of the TCA solution. Mix, cool on ice, and centrifuge at 700 g for 15 min. Collect the supernatant solution.
2. Prepare a blank by adding 1 ml H$_2$O to 1 ml of the TCA solution.
3. Add 8 ml of anhydrous acetic anhydride to 1 ml of the supernatant solution or blank. Stopper the tubes and heat for exactly 10 min at 60°C.
4. Add 1 ml of dry, reagent grade pyridine to the tubes. Restopper the tubes and incubate at 60°C for 40 min.
5. Place the tubes in an ice bath for 5 min.
6. Measure the absorbance of the solution at 400 nm against the blank.

   Calculation—A standard curve is constructed by utilizing the above procedure with 25 to 400 μg citric acid in 1 ml 25% TCA (in H$_2$O). The amount of citric acid present in the seminal plasma sample is estimated from the standard curve.
   Note—The chromophore produced by the above reaction is temperature sensitive and it is essential that the incubation temperature is kept at 60 ± 1°C. Once the color is produced, it is relatively stable, but should be read within 1 h after the reaction has been completed. If less than 1 ml seminal plasma is available for the assay, 25% TCA is added to bring the sample volume up to 1 ml. This dilution should be taken into consideration when calculating the amount of citric acid per ml seminal plasma.

E. ACID PHOSPHATASE[42]
Reagents (Prepared by R. A. Anderson, Rush Medical Center)

1. **0.5 M sodium citrate, pH 4.85**—Weigh out 10.51 g of citric acid monohydrate. Dissolve in approximately 70 ml H$_2$O. Adjust pH to 4.85 with NaOH ($\geqslant$1.0 N). Bring volume to 100 ml with water. This buffer is stable for at least 1 month, stored stoppered at room temperature.

2.   **50 mM p-nitrophenylphosphate (disodium, hexahydrate)**—Weigh out and dissolve 18.6 mg/ml in H_2O. This should be freshly prepared each time.

3.   **6.0 N NaOH**—Weigh out 24.0 g NaOH pellets. Dissolve in approximately 80 ml H_2O. Due to the exothermic nature of this process, temperature should be controlled by placing the vessel in an ice bath. After all the NaOH has gone into solution, allow vessel to come to room temperature. Adjust volume to 100 ml with H_2O. This solution can be stored indefinitely in a capped plastic reagent bottle.

Procedure—Acid phosphatase activity is measured by quantifying the hydrolysis of p-nitrophenylphosphate at pH 4.8 to 5.0 as follows:

(1)   Label pairs of tubes "sample" and "blank", which correspond to each sample to be analyzed.

(2)   To each tube, add the following:

   0.50 ml 0.5 M sodium citrate, pH 4.85
   1.25 ml H_2O
   0.10 ml 50 mM p-nitrophenylphosphate

(3)   Place all tubes in a shaking water bath (37°C) for 5 min to allow for temperature equilibration.

(4)   Add 0.05 ml seminal plasma to appropriately labeled "sample" tubes, and incubate for 30 min.

(5)   Add 0.1 ml 6.0 N NaOH to all "sample" and "blank" tubes; mix well.

(6)   Add 0.05 ml seminal plasma to appropriately labeled "blank" tubes; mix well.

(7)   Prepare a reagent blank, consisting of the following:

   0.50 ml 0.5 M sodium citrate, pH 4.85
   1.30 ml H_2O
   0.10 ml 50 mM p-nitrophenylphosphate
   0.10 ml 6.0 N NaOH

(8)   Adjust the wavelength of a spectrophotometer to 410 nm. Zero the instrument with the reagent blank.

(9)   Read the absorbance at 410 nm of all "sample" and "blank" tubes. The absorbance due to the formation of p-nitrophenol is taken as the difference in absorbance at 410 nm of each "sample" tube and its corresponding "blank" tube.

Calculation—Acid phosphatase activity is calculated as micromoles p-nitrophenol released per minute per ml seminal plasma as follows:

$$[(Absorbance_{sample} - Absorbance_{blank})/(18.315)(30)(0.05)] \times 2.0$$

where *18.315* is the millimolar extinction coefficient for p-nitrophenol at 410 nm, *30* is the incubation time in minutes, *0.05* is the volume of seminal plasma used, and *2.0* is the total volume, in ml.

The most accurate estimate of enzyme activity is achieved when absorbance readings range from 0.2 to 1.0. If A_{410} due to the "sample" tubes fall outside of this range, adjust the volume of seminal plasma to either increase or decrease the amount of enzyme, as required.

F. HYPOOSMOTIC SWELLING TEST[13]
Reagents

1. Fructose (2.7 g in 100 ml of distilled water)
2. Sodium citrate. 2 H$_2$O (1.47 g in 100 ml of distilled water)
3. HOS solution: add 100 ml fructose solution to 100 ml sodium citrate solution (final volume: 200 ml) and mix. Pipette 1 ml aliquots of the HOS solution into separate test tubes; cap and freeze ($-20°C$) until use

Procedure

1. Thaw the test tube containing the HOS solution by incubation at 37°C for 10 min.
2. Add 0.1 ml of well mixed, fully liquefied semen to the HOS solution and mix.
3. Incubate the semen/HOS solution mixture for at least 30 min but no longer than 3 to 4 h at 37°C (preferably 2 h).
4. After incubation, place a drop of well mixed sample on a glass slide with a cover glass and observe under phase contrast ($\times 400$) for curling of the sperm tail (sperm swelling; HOS-reactive spermatozoa). A bright field microscope can be used but is less reliable.
5. If desired, the treated spermatozoa can be fixed with formaldehyde (18.5%, 0.1 ml) for evaluation at a later time (within 30 days).
6. Differentially count at least 100, preferably 200 spermatozoa per sample.

Calculation

$$\text{Percent HOS-reactive spermatozoa} = \frac{\text{number of reactive sperm} \times 100\%}{\text{total number of sperm counted}}$$

Note—Since some semen samples will have spermatozoa with curled tails before exposure to the HOS test, it is essential that an ejaculate is observed *before* exposure. The percent of spermatozoa with curled tails in the untreated sample should be subtracted from the percent obtained after treatment to obtain the actual percent of spermatozoa that reacted in the HOS test.

G. CLINICAL ACROSIN ASSAY[27]
Reagents

Solution A: Ficoll—11% Ficoll in 0.12 M NaCl, 0.025 M Hepes buffer at pH 7.4 to 7.6. The solution is prepared by dissolving 0.70 g NaCl, 0.60 g Hepes and 11.0 g Ficoll in approximately 90 ml of distilled, deionized water. The solution is adjusted to ph 7.4 to 7.6 (with HCl or NaOH as required) and then adjusted to a final volume of 100 ml with water. The Ficoll solution is stable for at least 3 days in the refrigerator and can be stored for extended periods in a refrigerator if sodium azide (0.1%, or 100 mg added to 100 ml of solution) is added as a preservative.

Solution B: Detergent buffer—0.01% Triton X-100 in 0.055 M Hepes, 0.055 M NaCl at pH 8.0. The solution is prepared by dissolving 1.31 g of Hepes, 0.32 g of NaCl and 1 ml of a 1% Triton X-100 stock solution (1 ml Triton in 100 ml water) in 95 ml of distilled, deionized water. The solution is adjusted to pH 8.0 (with 1 N NaOH as required) and then adjusted to a final volume of 100 ml with distilled, deionized water. The detergent buffer is stable for at least 3 days in the refrigerator and can be stored for extended periods in the refrigerator after addition of sodium azide (0.1%, or 100 mg added to 100 ml) as preservative.

Solution C: Benzamidine—500 mM in water. The solution is prepared by dissolving 87.3 g benzamidine-HCl in 1 liter distilled, deionized water. The solution can be stored in the refrigerator without any additives for at least 2 weeks.

Solution D: Substrate—23 mM BAPNA in DMSO. The solution is prepared by dissolving 25 mg *N*-benzoyl-*dl*-arginine para-nitroanilide-HCl (BAPNA) in 2.5 ml dimethylsulfoxide (DMSO). This should be prepared fresh on the day of the assay. Complete dissolution of the BAPNA in DMSO requires adequate vortexing.

Solution E: Substrate-Detergent Mixture—In a 50 ml Erlenmyer flask, thoroughly mix 22.5 ml of the detergent buffer (solution B) with 2.5 ml of the BAPNA/DMSO substrate solution (solution D). The assay solution is stable for only a short period of time. Optimally, it is prepared while the Ficoll centrifugation is taking place (see step 5 of the Procedure). Precipitates will appear if the BAPNA and DMSO (solution D) were not mixed well prior to the addition of the detergent buffer or if the solution is allowed to stand for several hours. Do not use the assay solution if such precipitates are present.

Note—If aberrant results are obtained, check the solutions or make fresh ones. Solutions D and E should always be made fresh.

Procedure—In this procedure, spermatozoa are extracted with Triton X-100 and the proacrosin and acrosin are released. The proacrosin is activated and the total acrosin activity is measured by hydrolysis of BAPNA.

1. Allow fresh semen sample(s) to liquefy completely. Measure the sperm concentration.
2. For each semen sample, calculate the volume (optimally no more than 250 μl) that will contain between 2 to 10 million spermatozoa total. For example, use 100 μl of a semen sample containing 80 million spermatozoa per ml (8 million total). For easier absorbance readings, it is preferable not to use less than 5 million spermatozoa. A volume above 250 μl should only be used in cases of severe oligozoospermia. When a volume above 250 μl is employed, it is useful to increase the volume of Ficoll (solution A; see step 3) to 750 μl.
3. Prepare 3 to 4 assay tubes per individual semen sample (1 control and 2 to 3 tubes for the test). Pipette 0.5 ml aliquots of the Ficoll (solution A) into 5 ml plastic, conical centrifuge tubes.
4. Thoroughly mix the ejaculate and layer the calculated volume of semen (see step 2 above) onto the Ficoll (solution A) in each assay tube (including the control tube), preferably with a pipettor. Note that the semen should "float" on top of the Ficoll, not mixed within that layer.
5. Centrifuge the assay tubes at $1000 \times g$ for 30 min at room temperature. During this time, prepare the substrate-detergent solution (solution E). Complete dissolution of the BAPNA in DMSO requires about 5 to 10 min.
6. After centrifugation, a sperm pellet will be visible at the bottom or streaked to the side of the tube. Carefully, so as not to disturb the sperm pellet, first remove the seminal plasma and then the Ficoll supernatant, preferably by suction through a thin stemmed (pasteur) pipette. As close to 0.1 ml as possible of the sperm pellet and Ficoll should be left behind in the tube.
7. Add 100 μl of the 500 mM benzamidine solution (solution C) immediately to the control assay tube. Mix well (vortex) immediately after addition of solution C.
8. To each tube, including the control, add 1 ml of the substrate-detergent (solution E) above and mix well, preferably using a vortexer.
9. Incubate the tubes at 22 to 24°C for exactly 3 h after the addition of the assay solution. It is optimal to mix the contents of the tubes periodically during the incubation period.
10. After exactly 3 h of incubation, add 100 μl of benzamidine solution (solution C) to all tubes except the control.

11. Centrifuge all the tubes at $100 \times g$ for 30 min to clarify the supernatants. Collect the supernatant solutions.

12. Adjust a spectrophotometer so that the substrate-detergent solution (solution E) has an absorbance reading of 0.0 at 410 nm. Read and record the absorbances of each supernatant solution at 410 nm. Use 1 ml cuvettes.

Calculation—The acrosin content of each sample series is calculated as follows:

μIU acrosin per million spermatozoa

$$= \frac{[(\text{mean OD}_{test}) - \text{OD}_{control}] \times 10^6}{1485 \times \text{number of sperm (in millions layered over the Ficoll)}}$$

Note—The control should show no or almost no absorption. If significant absorption occurs in the control, the centrifugation (step 11) was most likely inadequate or the benzamidine solution was inadequately prepared. Although it is recommended that the spectrophotometric analysis of the supernatant solutions is performed immediately, the supernatants can be stored for up to three days in the refrigerator. Changes in absorbance may occur over time but these are nullified by subtracting the control from the test absorbance readings (see Calculation). Trypsin can be used as enzyme control. As Substrate Control, 100 μl of 1 N NaOH can be added to 1 ml of Solution E, incubated for 3 h and the A_{410} determined (see Reference 27).

H. CREATINE-N-PHOSPHOTRANSFERASE (CREATINE PHOSPHOKINASE; CK)

(Prepared by G. Huszar, Yale School of Medicine)

Sperm Preparation Procedure—The sperm is washed with 10 to 15 volumes of PBS or similar isotonic buffer ($2000 \times g$, 20 min) to remove seminal fluid which also contains CK. The higher than usual speed is necessary to assure that all sperm of the ejaculate sedimented. If the test cannot be run within 3 h of collection, the sperm pellet should be overlaid with 0.2 ml homogenization solution: phosphate buffer-normal (0.15 M) saline, pH:7.0; 10% glycerol, 20 mM DTT, 0.1% Triton, and the sample may be stored refrigerated for 3 days or frozen ($-20°C$) up to 2 months. Repeated freezing and thawing will inactivate the CK-enzyme.

CK activity determinations—CK catalyzes the reversible phosphorylation of either ADP or creatine to ATP or creatine phosphate. The CK activity measurements in the direction of ATP-synthesis are based on a three-step reaction. In the first step, CK catalyzes the synthesis of ATP from creatine phosphate and ADP. In the second step, the ATP is utilized for glucose-6-phosphate synthesis in the presence of hexokinase. In the third step, the glucose-6-phosphate is oxydized to 6-phosphogluconate with reduction of NADP to NADPH with an optical density change at 340 nm and an increase in fluorescence.

Isoform Concentration Measurements—The sperm proteins, including the CK-isoforms, are subjected to electrophoretic separation on agarose-gels. The relative concentrations of the CK-isoforms are detected by their enzymatic activity. Commercially available CK kits (e.g., the Corning Creatine Kinase Isoenzyme kit) contain all the necessary reagents for these procedures. The NADH fluorescence is quantified on the electrophoretic film by a scanning fluorometer.

Electrophoresis procedure

1. Gently peel the agarose electrophoresis plate from its hard plastic cover.
2. Apply aliquots of the samples to the wells. Samples should be applied using a quan-

titative microliter dispenser and disposable sample tip. After sample application, allow the sample to diffuse into the agarose for one minute.

3. Insert the loaded agarose film into the electrophoresis cell, agarose side down.
4. Turn on power, adjust it to provide adequate current, typically 90 V (in case of the Corning system) and allow 20 min for the electrophoresis.

Visualization of the CK-isoform bands

5. Following electrophoresis grasp the agarose film by its edges and remove it. Place the film, agarose side up on a flat counter top.
6. Evenly dispense 1 ml of CK-substrate onto the agarose surface. To spread the substrate, slowly push the pipette across the agarose film.
7. Place the agarose film in the prewarmed incubator and incubate the plate at 37°C for 20 min.
8. Dry film for 15 to 20 min and scan agarose-film in an automated fluorometer/integrator which provides the relative concentrations of the B-CK and M-CK isoforms.

ACKNOWLEDGMENTS

The authors appreciate the manuscript preparation of Ms. N. Pabon. Unpublished results were supported by NIH HD 19555.

REFERENCES

1. **Mann, T.,** *The Biochemistry Semen and of the Male Reproductive Tract,* John Wiley & Sons, New York, 1964.
2. **Mann, T. and Lutwak-Mann, C.,** *Biochemistry of Seminal Plasma and Male Accessory Fluids: Application to Andrological Problems,* Springer-Verlag, New York, 1981.
3. **Polakoski, K. L. and Kopta, M.,** Seminal plasma, in *Biochemistry of Mammalian Reproduction,* Zaneveld, L. J. D. and Chatterton, R. T. Eds., John Wiley & Sons, New York, 1982, 89.
4. **Van der Ven, H. H., Binor, Z., and Zaneveld, L. J. D.,** Effect of heterologous seminal plasma on the fertilizing capacity of human spermatozoa as assessed by the zona-free hamster egg test, *Fertil. Steril.,* 40, 512, 1983.
5. *WHO Laboratory Manual for the Examination of Human Semen and Semen-Cervical Mucus Interaction,* Cambridge University Press, Cambridge, 1987.
6. **Beyler, S. A. and Zaneveld, L. J. D.,** The male accessory sex glands, in *Biochemistry of Mammalian Reproduction,* Zaneveld, L. J. D. and Chatterton, R. T., Eds., John Wiley & Sons, New York, 1982, 65.
7. **Anderson, R. A., Reddy, J. M., Oswald, C., and Zaneveld, L. J. D.,** Enzymatic determination of fructose in seminal plasma by initial rate analysis, *Clin. Chem.,* 25, 1780, 1979.
8. **Polakoski, K. L. and Zaneveld, L. J. D.,** Biochemical analysis of the human ejaculate, in *Techniques of Human Andrology,* Hafez, E. S. E., Ed., Elsevier/North Holland Biomedical Press, 1977, 265.
9. **Menchini-Fabris, A., Canale, D., Izzo, P. L., Olivieri, L., and Bartelloni, M.,** Free L-carnitine in human semen: its variability in different andrological pathologies, *Fertil. Steril.,* 42, 263, 1984.
10. **Evenson, D. P., Darzynkiewicz, Z., and Melamed, M. R.,** Relation of mammalian sperm chromatin heterogeneity to fertility, *Science,* 210, 1131, 1980.
11. **Tejada, R. I., Mitchell, J. C., Norman, A., Marik, J. J., and Friedman, S.,** A test for the practical evaluation of male fertility by acridine orange (AO) fluorescence, *Fertil. Steril.,* 42, 87, 1984.
12. **Hurst, R. E. and Roy, J. B.,** Acridine orange male fertility test, *Fertil. Steril.,* 43, 154, 1985.
13. **Jeyendran, R. S., Van der Ven, H. H., Perez-Pelaez, M., Crabo, B. G., and Zaneveld, L. J. D.,** Development of an assay to assess the functional integrity of the human sperm membrane and its relationship to other semen characteristics, *J. Reprod. Fertil.,* 70, 219, 1984.
14. **Zaneveld, L. J. D., Jeyendran, R. S., Krajeski, P., Coetze, K., Kruger, T. F., and Lombard, C. J.,** Hypoosmotic swelling test: results and discussion, in *Human Spermatozoa in Assisted Reproduction,* Acosta, A., Swanson, J., Ackerman, S., Kruger, T. F., van Zyl, J. A., and Menkveld, R., Eds., Williams & Wilkins, Baltimore, 1990, 223.

15. **Spittaler, P. J. and Tyler, J. P. P.,** Further evaluation of a simple test for determining the integrity of spermatozoal membranes, *Clin. Reprod. Fertil.,* 3, 187, 1985.

16. **Zaneveld, L. J. D., Jeyendran, R. S., De Castro, M. P. P., and Silvera, P. J. M.,** Analysis of prevasectomy ejaculates by the hypoosmotic swelling (HOS) test, *J. Androl.,* 8, 19P, 1987.

17. **Van Kooij, R. J., Balerna, M., Roatti, A., and Campana, A.,** Oocyte penetration and acrosome reactions of human sperms. II. Correlation with other seminal parameters, *Andrologia,* 18, 503, 1986.

18. **Kolodziej, F. B., Katzorke, T. T., and Propping, D.,** Der Schwelltest als Funktionstest der spermatozoen und seine Wertigkeit in der Andrologischen Diagnostik, in Physiologie and Pathologie der Fortplanzung, X. Veterinaer-Humanmedizinische Gemeinschaftung, Semm, K., Ahn, J., and Rohof, D., Eds., 1985, 36.

19. **Langenbucher, H., Ruck, S., Riedel, H. H., and Mettler, L.,** The importance of various in vitro sperm tests for the evaluation of ejaculate quality, 12th World Congress on Fertility and Sterility, Singapore, 1048, 1986.

20. **Check, J. H., Nowroozi, K., Wu, C. H., and Bollendorf, A.,** Correlation of semen analysis and hypoosmotic swelling test with subsequent pregnancies. *Arch. Androl.,* 20, 257, 1988.

21. **Nachtigall, M., Viehberger, G., Lunglmayer, G., Van der Ven, H. H., Szalay, S., and Aigner, H.,** The effect of tamoxifen on the sperm swell test, *Helv. Chir. Acta,* 53, 279, 1986.

22. **Perez-Pelaez, M., Jeyendran, R. S., Tarchala, S. M., and Damirayakhion, M.,** Possible role of tamoxiphen citrate in the therapy of oligospermic men, *J. Androl.,* 9, 36P, 1988.

23. **Jeyendran, R. S., Van der Ven, H. H., Perez-Pelaez, M., and Zaneveld, L. J. D.,** Nonbeneficial effect of glycerol on the oocyte penetrating capacity of cryopreserved lueman spermatozoa, *Cryobiology,* 22, 434, 1985.

24. **Jeyendran, R. S., Van der Ven, H. H., Kennedy, W., Heath, E., Perez-Pelaez, M., Sobrero, A. J., and Zaneveld, L. J. D.,** Acrosomeless sperm: a cause of primary male infertility, *Andrologia,* 17, 31, 1985.

25. **Mack, S. R. and Zaneveld, L. J. D.,** Acrosomal enzymes and ultrastructure of unfrozen and cryotreated human spermatozoa, *Gamete Res.,* 18, 375, 1987.

26. **Lalonde, L., Langlais, J., Antaki, P., Chapdelaine, A., Roberts, K. D., and Bleau, G.,** Male infertility associated with round-headed acrosomeless spermatozoa, *Fertil. Steril.,* 49, 316, 1988.

27. **Kennedy, W. P., Kaminski, J. M., Van der Ven, H. H., Jeyendran, R. S., Reid, D. S., Blackwell, J., Bielfeld, P., and Zaneveld, L. J. D.,** A simple clinical assay to evaluate the acrosin activity of human spermatozoa, *J. Androl.,* 10, 221, 1989.

28. **Goodpasture, J. C., Zavos, P. N., and Zaneveld, L. J. D.,** Relationship of human sperm acrosin and proacrosin. II. Correlations, *J. Androl.,* 8, 267, 1987.

29. **Mohsenian, M., Syner, F. N., and Moghissi, K. S.,** A study of sperm acrosin in patients with unexplained infertility, *Fertil. Steril.,* 37, 223, 1982.

30. **Goodpasture, J. C., Zavos, P. N., Cohen, M. R., and Zaneveld, L. J. D.,** Relationship of human sperm acrosin and proacrosin to semen parameters. I. Comparisons between symptomatic men of infertile couples and asymptomatic men, and between different split ejaculates, *J. Androl.,* 3, 151, 1982.

31. **Koukoulis, G., Vantman, D., Dennison, Z., and Sherins, R. J.,** Consistently low acrosin activity in sperm of a subpopulation of men with unexplained infertility, *J. Androl.,* 9, 46P, 1988.

32. **Jeyendran, R. S., Van der Ven, H. H., Kennedy, W., Perez-Pelaez, M., and Zaneveld, L. J. D.,** Comparison of glycerol and zwitter ion buffer system as cryoprotective media for human spermatozoa, *J. Androl.,* 5, 1, 1984.

33. **Comhaire, F., Vermeulen, L., Ghedira, K., Mas J., Irvine, S., and Callipolitis, G.,** Adenosine triphosphate in human semen: a quantitative estimate of fertilizing potential, *Fertil. Steril.,* 40, 500, 1983.

34. **Irvine, D. S. and Aitken, R. J.,** The value of adenosine triphosphate (ATP) measurements in assessing the fertilizing ability of human spermatozoa, *Fertil. Steril.,* 44, 806, 1985.

35. **Huszar, G. and Vigue, L.,** Oligo/asthenospermia and the activities of creatine kinase and dynein ATPase in human sperm, Am. Fertil. Soc. Annu. Meet., Toronto, 1986.

36. **Fakih, H., MacLusky, N., DeCherney, A., Walliman, T., and Huszar, G.,** Enhancement of human sperm motility and velocity in vitro: effects of calcium and creatine phosphate, *Fertil. Steril.,* 46, 938, 1986.

37. **Huszar, G., Corrales, M., and Vigue, L.,** Correlation between sperm creatine phosphokinase activity and sperm concentrations in normospermic and oligospermic men, *Gamete Res.,* 19, 67, 1988.

38. **Huszar, G., Vigue, L., and Corrales, M.,** Sperm creatine phosphokinase activity as a measure of sperm quality in normospermic, variablespermic and oligospermic men, *Biol. Reprod.,* 38, 1061, 1988.

39. **Huszar, G. and Vigue, L.,** Sperm CPK activity is a predictor of fertilizing capacity of oligospermic men, Am. Fertil. Soc. Annu. Meet., Nevada, 1987.

40. **Huszar, G., Quevedo, L., Vigue, L., and Vigue, C.,** Ratio of B-type and M-type sperm CPK isoforms correlates with CPU activity and sperm quality in oligospermic and normospermic specimens, Am. Fertil. Soc. Annu. Meet., Atlanta, GA, 1988.

41. **Fuentes, J., Miro, J., and Riera, J.,** Simple colorimetric method of seminal plasma zinc assay, *Andrologia,* 14, 322, 1981.
42. **Anderson, R. A., Oswald, C., Willis, B. R., and Zaneveld, L. J. D.,** Relationship between semen characteristics and fertility in electroejaculated mice, *J. Reprod. Fertil.,* 68, 1, 1983.

Chapter 6

OBJECTIVE ANALYSIS OF SPERM MOTILITY AND KINEMATICS

David Mortimer

TABLE OF CONTENTS

I. INTRODUCTION

Testicular spermatozoa of man, as for all other eutheria, are either motionless or very weakly motile. This immotility, which is true even if testicular spermatozoa are sampled by micropuncture and suspended in culture medium, is apparently due to the "immaturity" of the plasmalemma since demembranated spermatozoa can be induced, under appropriate conditions, to move almost as actively as mature spermatozoa from the cauda epididymidis.[1]

During passage through the epididymis spermatozoa undergo substantial maturational changes which result in the acquisition of fertilizing ability, including the development of motility.[2] However, while motile spermatozoa from the cauda epididymidis are capable of progressive motility when suspended in culture medium *in vitro*, they remain essentially immotile *in vivo*.[3] Only at ejaculation, when they are mixed with the secretions of the accessory glands, do spermatozoa undergo motility activation.

The motility of ejaculated spermatozoa has long been recognized as an extremely important functional characteristic that must be evaluated as an integral part of semen analysis.[4,5] More recently, major influences of sperm motility upon the cervical mucus penetrating ability and fertilizing potential of human spermatozoa have been demonstrated. However, it is not just the proportion of spermatozoa that are motile, nor even their concentration, that is of greatest importance. The objective and quantitative measurement of sperm movement characteristics derived from observations on individual cells has been found to be more predictive of functional ability, and hence a man's potential fertility.

Specific aspects of sperm movement such as the velocity of progression and the actual pattern of movement have been shown to be closely correlated with sperm penetration into cervical mucus,[6-9] the outcome of the heterologous zona pellucida-free hamster egg penetration test (HEPT)[10-12] and the results of *in vitro* fertilization (IVF) (see Section VII.B).[13] Consequently, in recent years increasing attention has been paid to the evaluation of sperm motility at more than the crude level of determining the proportion of motile spermatozoa.

Clearly, motility is a vitally important characteristic of spermatozoa which we need to measure objectively and accurately. Furthermore, it is apparent that we shall need to concentrate upon those approaches that provide reliable measurements of specific aspects of sperm movement, not just simple motility.

II. BASIC PRINCIPLES OF MEASUREMENT

A. PREPARATION DEPTHS

While 10 μm deep chambers may not influence the motility of human spermatozoa in semen[14] many spematozoa in culture media, prepared for example by swim-up migration, move with appreciably greater lateral movements of the head.[15] Therefore, the use of deeper preparations (e.g., 20 μm) is obviously required for washed or migrated sperm populations. Various workers have used 10 μl volumes under 22 × 22 mm coverslips to give preparations of approximately 20 μm depth,[15-17] and recent studies on human sperm movement and hyperactivation have used preparations of 32 to 33 μm.[18,19]

In general terms, studies on human spermatozoa in seminal plasma should use preparations at least 10 μm deep, while those on spermatozoa in culture media should use at least 20 μm. The deeper the preparation that can be used for any given study the less will be the chance of any artifactual biasing of the results due to the spermatozoa being constrained by the preparation. One should, however, remember that the numbers of spermatozoa seen per microscope field of observation will increase in direct proportion to the increasing preparation depth. Consequently, if the number of spermatozoa per field of view is in any way limiting then specimen dilution will be essential.

1. Makler Chamber

This chamber, originally designed for determination of sperm concentration and percent motility on undiluted semen,[20,21] is precision manufactured and correspondingly expensive. It has a stated depth of 10 μm although it would appear that under conditions of routine use this may be somewhat greater (D.H. Douglas-Hamilton, personal communication). Two chambers were tested as for specimen loading by removal and replacement of the cover glass. The depth of the empty chamber, measured by laser interferometry, was found to be 12.5 ± 1.5 (SD) μm for one chamber and 12.2 ± 3.3 μm for a second chamber. Individual measurements ranged between 10.0 and 17.1 μm. Although an average discrepancy of 2.5 μm is very small in real terms it does represent a 25% increase in chamber depth, and hence specimen volume, and will therefore contribute significantly to methodological error.

Another important point when using a Makler chamber is the volume of specimen applied. Although a sample aliquot of 5 to 7 μl has been recommended, we have found that a maximum volume of 4 to 5 μl gives the lowest incidence of ''flow'' within the specimen. Some laboratories use as much as 30 μl which will clearly cause flooding of the specimen over the cover glass support pillars with a resultant increase in specimen depth dependent upon the viscosity of the specimen.

2. Horwell ''Fertility'' Semen Counting Chamber

This chamber was developed on the same principles as the Makler but is a much less expensive unit and again only 4 to 5 μl are used to load the chamber. However, the chamber uses a standard hemocytometer cover glass and, as a consequence of variations in the closeness with which the cover glass may be apposed to the chamber surface, we have found it difficult to ensure a constant preparation depth. Furthermore, hemocytometer cover glasses are of lower planarity than the Makler chamber cover glass. While a variation in planarity of, say, 2 μm only represents an error of 2% when the cover glass is used with a hemocytometer, it represents an error of 20% when used with a Horwell chamber.

3. Petroff-Hausser Counting Chambers

This is a bacterial counting chamber with Neubauer-type ruling. It has a depth of 20 μm and may therefore be used with washed sperm populations. A disadvantage for experimental studies is that the chamber is relatively expensive and difficult to clean and dry quickly.

4. Chartpak Slides

These disposable slides are prepared by pressing dry transfer circles (13 mm diameter, Chartpak #RDC49, Chartpak, Leeds, MA, U.S.) onto thoroughly cleaned ordinary microscope slides. A standard chamber depth of 32 to 33 μm is obtained by using 5 μl sample aliquots and an ordinary glass coverslip. The coverslip is applied firmly, forcing the sample aliquot to fill the chamber and spill over the sides of the O-ring.[18] These preparations have the advantage that they are essentially sealed, thereby minimizing drying out, and the chambers are disposable. If the glass surfaces have to be coated to prevent "sticking-to-glass" (see Section II.B) then this should be done before application of the Chartpak circles.

B. THE "STICKING-TO-GLASS" PHENOMENON

While spermatozoa in seminal plasma do not demonstrate a tendency to attach to glass surfaces, washed sperm populations do. This "sticking-to-glass" phenomenon may be minimized by inclusion of an adequate concentration of either serum albumin,[22] or polyvinyl alcohol,[23] in the medium or by the use of various glass coating agents.[24]

Since this phenomenon is time-dependent, observations on washed spermatozoa should be made as quickly as possible (probably less than 2 min) unless a highly effective glass coating agent is used. Unfortunately, many, if not all, of the glass coating agents can cause problems when preparations are being analyzed by videomicrography and digital image analysis.

C. TEMPERATURE

Whereas the proportion of motile spermatozoa may not change substantially between 37°C and ambient temperature (20 to 25°C), and one may therefore use the lower temperature for counting the proportion of motile spermatozoa at semen analysis,[25] sperm movement characteristics are temperature sensitive. Consequently, all studies of sperm motility which include evaluation of velocity must be carried out at the appropriate physiological temperature (37°C for human spermatozoa) thereby requiring the use of a heated microscope stage. In addition, the specimen chambers and any other materials used for handling the spermatozoa should also be kept at 37°C prior to use.

While the use of 37°C increases the rate at which preparations dry out, this should not be a problem if observation is concluded rapidly. Sealed preparations should be used when longer periods of observation are needed. The use of warm air curtain devices should be avoided in low humidity areas when working with unsealed preparations.

D. DILUTION

If a sperm suspension is too concentrated for observation by a particular method then it must be diluted. This is a simple matter for sperm suspensions in culture medium but presents a number of problems for studies on seminal spermatozoa.

Seminal spermatozoa must be diluted with homologous seminal plasma because culture medium will cause substantial alterations in movement characteristics. This cell-free seminal plasma should be prepared from another aliquot of the same semen sample by centrifugation (either 1000 g for 15 min in a bench top centrifuge or by a microcentrifuge). A preliminary evaluation of pooled seminal plasma that had been stored frozen prior to use showed it to be unsuitable for use in studies on sperm motility (D. Mortimer and M. A. Shu, unpublished observations).

If one is at all concerned with the concentration of spermatozoa, then dilutions must be made using positive displacement-type pipettes and not those automatic pipettes with disposable plastic tips which have a large air dead space. Thorough mixing is essential, but high speed vortexing must be avoided.

III. MOVEMENT CHARACTERISTICS

A. HISTORICAL

Over the years a plethora of terminology has appeared in the literature describing the

Velocities

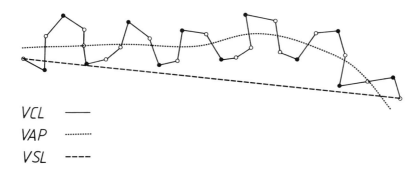

VCL   ——
VAP   ··········
VSL   ----

FIGURE 1.   Diagrammatic representation of a sperm track plotted at 30 frames/s. *Circles* denote head centroid positons (open circles = non-apex points, solid circles = apex points) and the *solid line* joining them is the actual path followed by the sperm head which is used to calculate *VCL*. The visually appraised average path used to calculate *VAP* is shown by the dotted line, and the broken line joining the first and last points of the track is the straight line path used to calculate *VSL*.

various movement characteristics of motile spermatozoa. Some terms are synonymous and describe the same characteristic, but sometimes essentially the same term has been used to describe different characteristics. This confusing and unacceptable state of affairs was addressed at a workshop on "Automated Sperm Motility Analysis" held at the American Society of Andrology's Annual Meeting in Houston (TX, U.S.) during March 1988. Terminology and abbreviations (and also appropriate numerical precision) were agreed upon for the three basic velocity measurements, the three ratios describing progression, and measures of the frequency and amplitude of lateral deviations of the sperm head. This terminology was subsequently accepted at an international symposium on "Human Sperm Movement and its Evaluation" organized by the Federation CECOS in Montpellier (France) in April 1988. The movement characteristics covered by these agreements are those derived from head centroid analysis (see below), and are of particular current significance since they are those provided by the automated motility analyzers now available.

B. CURVILINEAR VELOCITY (*VCL*)

VCL is calculated from the sum of the straight-lines joining the sequential positions of the sperm head along the spermatozoon's track (Figure 1). As such, *VCL* is essentially the two-dimensional projection of the true three-dimensional helical path of the spermatozoon as revealed by the time resolution of the imaging method used.

C. AVERAGE PATH VELOCITY (*VAP*)

This is the velocity along the "average" path of the spermatozoon (Figure 1). Because the average path can be derived in a number of ways (see Section IV.E.1) including visual interpolation, various mathematical smoothing techniques, or geometric construction, the precise method used for its derivation must always be stated.

D. LINEAR VELOCITY (*VSL*)

This is the straight line or "progression" velocity of the cell and is calculated as the straight line distance between the start and end of the observed track (Figure 1).

E. PROGRESSION RATIOS

Three progression ratios can be calculated from the three velocity measurements described above. They are

- "linearity" ($LIN = VSL/VCL \times 100$)
- "straightness" ($STR = VSL/VAP \times 100$)
- "wobble" ($WOB = VAP/VCL \times 100$)

F. AMPLITUDE OF LATERAL HEAD DISPLACEMENT (ALH)

This is calculated from the amplitudes of the lateral deviations of the sperm head about the axis of progression (average path). Different authors and commercial programs use either an average value calculated from the individual measurements made over the length of the track (or calculated from a minimum of three measurements at different places along the track) and/or the maximum value of all the measurements made along the track (see Section IV.E.2). Traditionally, ALH measurements are expressed as the width across the whole track, i.e., twice the average or maximum measurement.

Obviously in order to compare results between studies and/or analysis methods the derivation of ALH must be stated.

G. BEAT/CROSS FREQUENCY (BCF)

BCF is the number of times that the curvilinear track crosses the average path per unit time. In reality it is a derivation of the true flagellar beat frequency and the frequency of rotation (ROF) of the head.

Although it cannot be analyzed by the automated systems, the true head rotation frequency (ROF) is the number of times the sperm head rotates through $360°$ per unit time. A human spermatozoon swimming in seminal plasma will usually, but not always, rotate through $180°$ at the apex of each lateral deviation of the head about the axis of progression.[26]

H. NUMERICAL PRECISION

Values for VCL, VAP, VSL, ALH, and BCF (and ROF) should not be presented to more than one decimal place. The values for the three progression ratios are all expressed as integer percentages in the range of 0 to 100.

I. FLAGELLAR ANALYSIS

The most comprehensive description of sperm movement focuses on the detailed kinematics of flagellar beating since it is the generation and propagation of waves along the sperm tail that generate the actual propulsive force. While fundamental studies of the flagellar contraction mechanism require this level of analysis, there have been no decisions as yet regarding the most important or most appropriate flagellar parameters to measure.

Although the relationships are complex, analysis of sperm movement by following the head can provide a great deal of useful information on sperm movement. In view of the limited clinical interest in flagellar motion analysis this aspect of sperm kinematics will not be considered further at this time.

IV. METHODS OF MEASURING SPERM MOVEMENT

Early studies on the movement of mammalian spermatozoa used primarily time-lapse photomicrography,[27] or microcinematography,[28] although Harvey[29] measured the velocity of human spermatozoa by direct observation and a stop-watch. Over the last few years videomicrography has become the preferred method owing to its relative low cost and the elimination of delays caused by film processing.

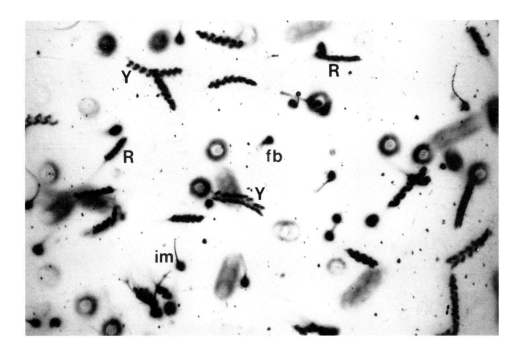

FIGURE 2.   A typical photomicrograph taken using the dark-ground timed-exposure photomicrographic (TEP) method. Immotile spermatozoa (im) are easily recognizable, while the blurred tails of the 'feeble beating' (fb) spermatozoa clearly distinguish them from the immotile cells. The dark "stripes" are the progressive spermatozoa of either the "rolling" (R) or "yawing" (Y) type.

A. TIMED-EXPOSURE PHOTOMICROGRAPHY (TEP)
1. Historical

The original work on time-lapse photomicrography, by which swimming spermatozoa left traces or "stripes" on a developed filmstrip negative (Figure 2), was used to relate velocity measurements of human spermatozoa to visually appraised subjective progressivity ratings.[30] These early studies derived velocity by measuring the lengths of the tracks left by the swimming spermatozoa during a 1 s exposure time. Further work produced a simple formula for the derivation of sperm velocity from the frequency with which the tracks of swimming spermatozoa crossed the diagonals drawn on an enlargement of the filmstrip frame.[31] A subsequent study using this "crossing diagonals" method of analysis demonstrated a 60 to 100% increase in the velocity of human spermatozoa between 25 and 37°C.[32]

With increased interest in the patterns of sperm movement in addition to their swimming speed, this approach, known as "timed-exposure photomicrography" (TEP), was developed as a system more amenable to routine clinical application.[16] Subsequently, measurement of *ALH* (originally described from microcinematographic studies of human sperm kinematics[26]) was incorporated.[10,11] Polaroid photographs have been used instead of film strips,[10,11] thereby eliminating the delays caused by film processing, although the images obtained in Polaroid photographs are appreciably smaller than those obtained by projecting filmstrips.

2. Movement Characteristics

TEP analysis of human sperm movement is able to provide reliable measures of *VSL* and *ALH*. Values for *BCF* cannot be determined reliably from TEP images since *BCF* measurements can only be made on tracks with large lateral head displacements (sometimes referred to as "yawing" spermatozoa, see Figure 2). In narrow tracks the head images are continually overlapped and the individual beats cannot be distinguished (sometimes termed "rolling" spermatozoa, see Figure 2). Because these latter spermatozoa may or may not have the same distribution of beat frequencies, deriving a *BCF* value only from those spermatozoa with sufficiently wide tracks cannot be justified statistically.

Since the actual three-dimensional trajectory of the sperm head is a helix of elliptical cross-section, it is probable that "rolling" and "yawing" tracks probably only represent tracks seen perpendicular to the minor or major axes of the elipse, respectively. Consequently, no distinction is now made between "rolling" and "yawing" tracks since they do not necessarily reflect different patterns of movement.

3. Technical Aspects

Although most workers who have used TEP employed a 1 s exposure time, periods of 0.5 and 2 s have been used in some cases. Because the fastest swimming spermatozoa will be more likely to leave the field during the period of observation and their tracks truncated, no velocity measurements can be made for these cells. There is therefore a significant risk of systematic bias in velocity measurements due to preferential exclusion of cells with higher velocities.

There is also the same likelihood of motile spermatozoa entering the field or leaving it during the period of observation. While this leaving/entering factor can be incorporated into determinations of percentage motility simply by counting only alternate tracks crossing the edge of the field as being part of the actual sample, no correction is possible for velocity distribution. It is therefore essential that the same exposure time be used in all studies whose data are to be compared, and 1 s has been accepted as the standard exposure time for TEP studies of human sperm kinematics.

For analysis, filmstrips are usually projected onto a sheet of white paper (or the active surface of a digitizer tablet for the semi-automated method,[33] see Section IV.A.4) and may be either measured directly or traced for subsequent measuring. Because measurements are made directly on Polaroid photographs, whose track images are substantially smaller than those obtained by filmstrip projection, this method has a lower precision, especially with regard to measurements of *ALH*.

VSL values are derived from TEP filmstrips or Polaroid photographs by measuring the straight-line distance between the two ends of the track using a rule (Figure 3). However, *ALH* has been measured in a number of ways. Usually the width of the track is measured at two or three places and these values averaged to give a mean value for the track (Figure 3). Measurements are made using a rule, sometimes with the aid of parallel rules,[15] or by superimposing a stencil of circles of various diameters.[13]

4. Semi-Automation

Semi-automated systems have been developed for analysis of TEP images[13,33] permitting the rapid, accurate measurement of track lengths and widths usually combined with computation of the mean values for the population of cells analyzed. One advantage of the Photomot semi-automated method[33] is that the track width is calculated as an average value integrated over the whole track since it is derived from the area of the projected track divided by a visually appraised average path length (Figure 4). Polaroid photographs can also be analyzed by the Photomot system with appreciably improved precision.

B. MULTIPLE-EXPOSURE PHOTOMICROGRAPHY (MEP)
1. Historical

In 1978 Makler[34] described an alternative photomicrographic method for the evaluation of human sperm motility using phase contrast microscopy in conjunction with stroboscopic illumination. This multiple-exposure photomicrographic (MEP) method provides a photographic record of the sequential positions of spermatozoa at $^1/_6$ sec intervals (Figure 5).

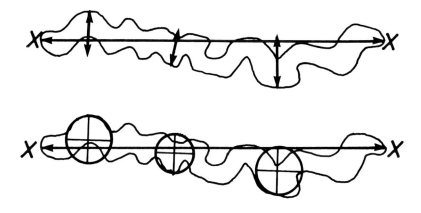

FIGURE 3. Manual analysis of a sperm track obtained using the TEP method. Having measured the length of the track (x—x) the width is measured at two or three places (arrows) either using a rule (upper figure) or a stencil of circles of different diameters (lower figure).

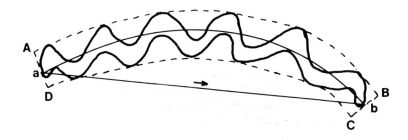

FIGURE 4. Diagrammatic representation of the derivation of trajectory parameters from a TEP track by the Photomot semi-automated method.[33] The trajectory of progression, used to calculate *VSL*, is the straight line joining a and b. The area of the rectangle ABCD is divided by the length of its midline, the curved line joining a and b to give its average width, which in turn is used to calculate *ALH*.

These "six-ringed chains" are used to differentiate between motile and immotile spermatozoa and to calculate the velocity of individual motile spermatozoa. Because this method uses the Makler chamber sperm concentration can also be determined.

It was from the validation of this system that a 1 s measurement period was found to be adequate for determination of the velocity of the human seminal spermatozoa.[35]

Numerous studies have used the MEP system[36-38] which has also been developed as a semi-automated method[39,40] including some commercial systems (e.g., "Sperm Works" by Zygotek, Springfield, MA, U.S.;[41] and "Spermamat" by Softool Microelectronics SA, Losone, Switzerland). It has also been implemented using Polaroid photomicrography.[42]

2. Movement Characteristics

From the semen analysis standpoint, MEP can provide values for sperm concentration (within the limitations of the Makler chamber, see above) and the percentage of motile spermatozoa. In terms of movement characteristics, only values for *VSL* can be obtained by measuring the straight-line distance between the first and last positions of the sperm head in the "six-ringed chains". An approximation of *VAP* can be derived by summation of the straight-line distances joining the head images in the "six-ringed chains", but unfortunately MEP provides neither a sufficiently integrated or sufficiently frequently sampled track for measurement of *VCL, ALH,* or *BCF*. In view of the apparent physiological and clinical significance of ALH measurements TEP is clearly a superior approach.

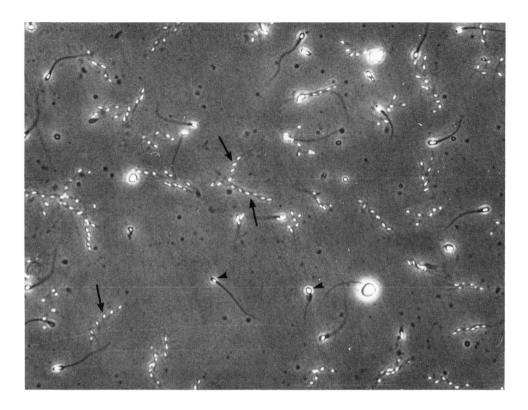

FIGURE 5. A typical image produced by the multiple-exposure photomicrographic (MEP) method. Immotile spermatozoa are visible as single images (arrowheads) while progressive spermatozoa leave a "six-ringed" chain of images of the sperm head (arrow). (Photomicrograph courtesy of Amnon Makler, M.D.)

C. MICROCINEMATOGRAPHY

1. Historical

This method has been used for studying sperm motility for almost 4 decades. Classic papers by van Duijn[43] using low-speed microcinematography (16 frame/s) and Phillips[44] using high-speed cine (500 frames/s) heralded the qualitative analysis of the human sperm kinematics. The derivation of specific movement characteristics from moderate speed (50 frames/s) microcinematographic studies on human spermatozoa was described by David et al.[26] and these have formed the basis of essentially all subsequent work on human sperm movement characteristics.

2. Movement Characteristics

Although there was for some time a debate as to whether the head-midpiece junction or the centroid of the sperm head should be used when reconstructing trajectories from cine film (or videotape) the majority of workers have used the head centroid. This would certainly seem to be the most appropriate approach, especially if digital image analysis techniques are employed for the reconstruction and analysis of sperm tracks from cine film[45,46] as well as videotapes (see Section IV.D.4).

Although both the image and temporal resolution that can be obtained by microcinematography is better than that currently available using videomicrography the high operating costs associated with microcinematography (even at moderate framing rates) has resulted in its more or less total replacement by videomicrography. Consequently, the analysis of movement characteristics from cine films will not be considered in detail.

D. VIDEOMICROGRAPHY

1. Historical

In 1981 Katz and Overstreet reported the first use of videomicrography for the assessment of human sperm motility.[47] This method, which relied upon manual playback and analysis of the videotapes, provided values for the percentage of motile spermatozoa and *VSL*. Simultaneous evaluation of the morphology of the individual spermatozoa was also found to be possible by this method, and demonstrated that (1) spermatozoa with abnormal morphology were more often immotile or weakly motile than were those with normal morphology in the same semen sample; and that (2) morphologically normal spermatozoa in ejaculates from infertile men were less likely to be motile, and tended to swim more slowly, than were those in ejaculates from fertile men.[48]

2. Semi-Automation and Automation

Computer-assisted semi-automated video tracking has been reported[49] for analyzing swimming human spermatozoa, but semi-automation has had its largest application in the calculation of movement characteristics from manually reconstructed sperm tracks.[50] Although automated methods have been developed for the assessment of human sperm morphology[51] it has not yet been possible to use it in conjunction with automated motility analysis to provide "morphility" assessments.[48]

More recently, a number of automated systems employing digital image analysis of video signals, either "live" from a camera or from a videocassette recorder (VCR), have appeared. The prediction that the routine use of video/computer systems would become a practical reality for routine evaluation of sperm motility[35] has certainly now come true. These systems have essentially rendered semiautomated methods more or less redundant except for their usefulness in validating the commercial automated systems and also in laboratories which do not have access to costly automated analyzers.

3. Technical Aspects

a. Television Standards

One confounding factor with video is that there are a number of different television broadcast and recording standards around the world. These fall into three major groups, each with their own subsets of minor variations. The National Television Standards Committee (NTSC) system has 525 lines and scans at 60 Hz which, with a 2:1 interlace, gives images at the rate of 30 frames/s. The phase alternating line (PAL) and *sequential couleur avec memoire* (SECAM) systems both have 625 lines and 50 Hz scan rates giving 25 frames/s. Although there are differences between PAL and SECAM in the method of color or chrominance encoding in the signal, making them incompatible as color television standards, when only monochrome images are used (as for digital image analysis) they can be considered essentially the same. The NTSC standard is used in Canada, Chile, South Korea, Taiwan, and the U.S., among other countries. Those using the PAL standard include Argentina, Australia, Austria, Belgium, Brazil, Denmark, Finland, West Germany, Hong Kong, Iceland, India, Israel, Italy, North Korea, the German part of Luxembourg, The Netherlands, New Zealand, Norway, Pakistan, Singapore, South Africa, Spain, Sweden, Switzerland, Turkey, The United Arab Emirates, The United Kingdom, and Yugoslavia while SECAM countries include Egypt, France, East Germany, Greece, Iran, Iraq, the French part of Luxembourg, Poland, and the USSR.

These differences in television standards have a very obvious consequence in that frame-by-frame analysis performed in the various countries will be performed at either 25 or 30 frames/s. Although this will not make enormous differences to movement characteristics, differences will exist especially in *VCL* measurements (see Section IV.E.3).

b. Video Standards

A number of different VCR standards also exist. The Sony Corporation has been responsible for the U-Matic and Beta systems and while the former is largely restricted to broadcast and serious research applications, the latter is widely used domestically, most recently as the SuperBeta variant. Three speeds (I, II, and III) are available for Beta standard VCRs and while almost all machines can play all three speeds, usually only "professional" machines record in Beta-I and domestic machines often only record in Beta-II and -III. The new Beta-IS is now available on some machines and these tapes can only be played on other machines compatible with this new standard. Video 8 and compact VHS or VHS-C are of little interest since these standards are essentially restricted to domestic camcorders. The VHS system also has multiple speeds: standard play (SP) and long play (LP) in PAL and SECAM countries plus a third speed, extended play (EP) or super long play (SLP), under the NTSC standard. A new high resolution Super-VHS (VHS-S) standard has recently become available although at high cost. All VCRs will function according to the television standard of the country for which they were manufactured and must be used in conjunction with an appropriate camera.

For image analysis purposes one should always use the fastest speed available to give the highest quality image for digitization, i.e., Beta-I or -II, or VHS in SP mode. To minimize the risk of tape deterioration or stretching during repeated play-back, videotape with the thickest base should be used, e.g., Beta L-250 or VHS 60 min tapes (T-60 in NTSC areas and E-60 in PAL/SECAM areas).

c. High Speed Systems

Two systems are available for working at high frame rates, the MHS-200 system (NAC Incorporated, Tokyo, Japan) which operates at 200 frames/s using a high sensitivity and high resolution camera, and the CTS-200 system, also capable of frame rates up to 200 Hz (Motion Analysis Corporation, Santa Rosa, CA, U.S.).

d. Calibration and Sample Identification

For calibration and/or identification purposes, time/date generators and character or text generators are used. These units encode additional text/numeric characters into the camera output before it is recorded. For research purposes we use the For-A VTG-33 time/date generator (For-A Company, Tokyo, Japan) whereas for routine purposes we have found the cheaper Panasonic Model WJ-810 (Panasonic Industrial Company, Matsushita Electric Corporation, Tokyo, Japan) to be perfectly adequate. We have also used a text imager (Model VTI-800, Vistek, Santa Barbara, CA, U.S.), which allows the use of free text, not just time/date information.

e. Microscope Optics

For manual track reconstruction both positive-low (PL) and negative-high (NH) phase contrast optics and Nomarski (differential interference contrast) optics have been used. PL-phase contrast optics are the most commonly used but, while the image is perfectly adequate for visual analysis, we have found NH-phase contrast provides much better images for digital image analysis and should probably be used for all recordings to be analyzed using "machine vision". Nomarski optics give a quasi-three-dimensional image which can be particularly useful when analyzing flagellar movement. There is, however, the disadvantage that a more powerful light source and/or a more sensitive video camera are required.

When making video recordings, as with photo- or cinemicrography, it is always advisable to work with the lowest power objective possible since this gives brighter images with a greater depth of focus. Providing resolution is not a problem it is often better to use a lower power objective in combination with immediate magnification (camera ocular). While this

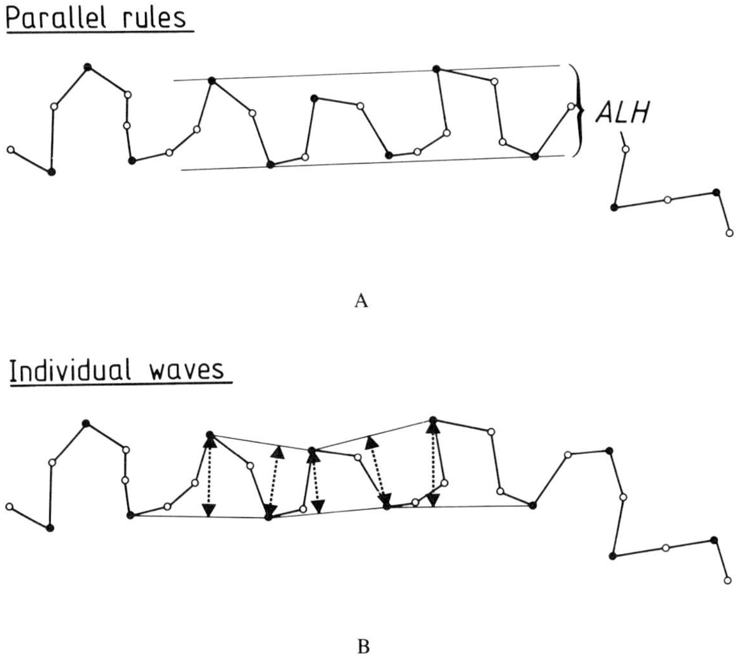

Parallel rules

A

Individual waves

B

FIGURE 6.   Diagrammatic representation of a sperm track plotted at 30 frames/s; circles denote head centroid positions (open circles = non-apex points, solid circles = apex points); (A) shows the traditional manual measurement of ALH using parallel rules while (B) shows the measurement of each wave to provide a mean *ALH* value for the whole track. Clearly the average of the measurements denoted by the double-headed arrows (B) will be smaller than the track width obtained using parallel rules.

does not eliminate the problem of adequate illumination it does provide a larger image without loss of depth of focus.

4. Movement Characteristics

Analysis of sperm motility and movement characteristics from video recordings has progressed a long way from the original "bullseye" method of Katz and Overstreet.[47] Motile spermatozoa are now tracked frame-by-frame to reconstruct movement over a period of time. Manually reconstructed tracks are analyzed by essentially the same methods as developed for microcinematography with the measurements being performed by either manual or semi-automated methods. Computerized sperm motility analysis systems (see Section V) automatically reconstruct the tracks and derive movement characteristics.

Manual measurement (see Figure 1) of the curvilinear track length is made using a curvimeter or map-measurer (Burnat Model No. 54, Berty, Paris, France) with the track being measured starting from both ends and the two values averaged. A curvimeter can also be used to measure the length of a visually integrated track midline or average path. The straight-line track length is calculated from the distance between the first and last points on the track measured using a rule.

ALH measurements can be made using either parallel rules at, usually three places along the reconstructed track (Figure 6B), or by measuring the distance from the apex of a lateral deviation of the sperm head on one side of the average path to the line joining the apices of the lateral deviations immediately before and after it on the opposite side of the average path (Figure 6A). This is repeated for every wave along the reconstructed track and the measurements then either averaged to provide a mean value for *ALH* or the largest value is

5-point smoothing

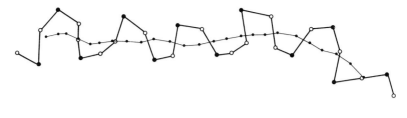

A

Geometric method

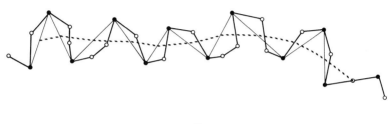

B

FIGURE 7.   Diagrammatic representation of a sperm track plotted at 30 frames/s; circles denote head centroid positons (open circles = non-apex points, solid circles = apex points). The average path used to calculate *VAP* is shown as derived by either a 5-point running average smoothing (A) or by the geometric method (B) whereby the midpoints of the thin solid lines joining adjacent pairs of apex points are connected by the dashed line.

taken and used as the maximum *ALH*. If *ALH* values are derived from measurements of the distances between apices of lateral head displacement and the average path then the mean or maximum value is doubled to represent the whole track width.

BCF is calculated from the number of times that the curvilinear path crosses the average path per unit time.

Various methods have been used for deriving the average path including geometric construction[50] and 5-point running average smoothing[52] (see Section IV.E.1)

E. METHOD DEPENDENCY OF MOVEMENT CHARACTERISTICS
1. Average Path Velocity

Because the path of a swimming spermatozoon is not absolutely straight and symmetrical, its average path can be derived in several ways. In TEP images (Figures 2 and 3) the track midline is visually appraised[33] as for centroid-reconstructed tracks being analyzed manually[26,50] (Figure 1). However, (semi-)automated systems require a mathematical derivation. Calculation of a 5-point running average has been the most widely used although this method will not always be appropriate for every track (Figure 7A).

Curvilinear velocity is not the same for all cells, not even for all cells with the same *VSL* or *VAP* due to variations in *BCF* and *ALH*.[26,53] However, it is *VCL*, in conjunction with the frame rate, that determines the spacing and location of the track points. While 5-point smoothing has been found to be the best alternative for human seminal spermatozoa analyzed at a 30 Hz frame rate,[52] it will not be for tracks sampled at higher frame rates[53] nor for washed or hyperactivated cells whose *VCL* values are much higher than those of seminal spermatozoa.[19] Consequently, we have been interested in using a method for deriving the average path of progressively motile human spermatozoa based on geometric principles which is neither *VCL*- nor frame rate-dependent[50,53] (Figure 7B).

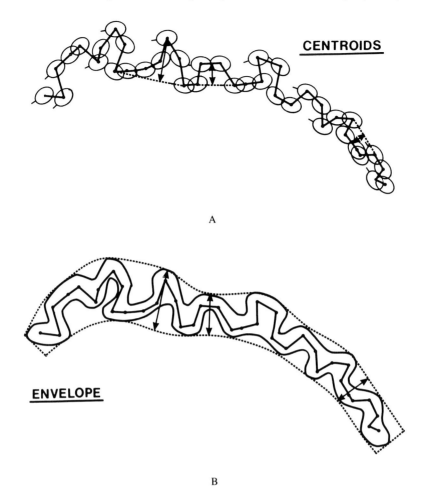

FIGURE 8.   Diagrammatic representation of a sperm track plotted at 30 frames/s showing how the use of head centroids (A) produces smaller values for *ALH* than does the "envelope" type (B) of image produced by timed-exposure photomicrography. The double-headed arrows denote three examples where *ALH* measurements are appreciably different between the two analysis methods. The dotted lines denote the edges of the track as defined by each method in their derivation of *ALH* measurements.

2. Amplitude of Lateral Head Displacement

In TEP images the track width, and hence mean *ALH,* is measured over the outside edges or the "envelope" of the track "stripe" on the projected filmstrip or Polaroid photograph[33] (Figure 8B). Obviously centroid analysis, because it uses the center of the sperm head and not its outside edge, will produce smaller values for *ALH* (Figure 8A). This difference, which is of the order of 3 to 4 μm,[54] is of no real importance other than for the confusion it causes for those not experienced in the various methods used for sperm movement analysis.

When a manually reconstructed track is measured for *ALH* determination it is usually done with parallel rules applied at several (usually three) places along the track. This method does not therefore take into account all the individual lateral deviations of the head, many of the smaller ones are ignored (c.f. Figure 6). However, (semi-)automated analysis of centroid-reconstructed tracks will measure each and every lateral wave and use all these values to calculate the average *ALH* for the track. Consequently, manual analysis will usually give slightly larger values for a track's mean *ALH.* A further problem is that at relatively

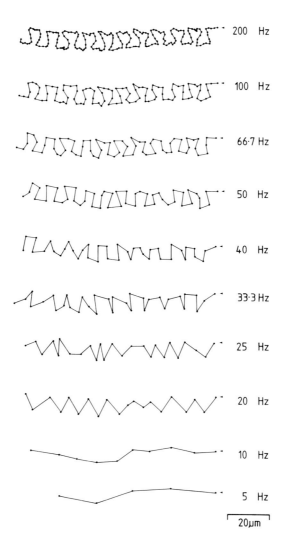

FIGURE 9. Influence of decreasing image sampling frequency upon the perceived track of a typical progressively motile human sperm track originally plotted at 200 frames/s. (From Mortimer, D., Serres, C., Mortimer, S. T., and Jouannet, P., *Gamete Res.*, 20, 313, 1988. With permission.)

low sampling frequencies such as 30 Hz the true apex of a lateral deviation may be missed; this would cause underestimation of the mean *ALH* by inclusion of artificially small individual wave measurements. The existence of these sources of error has resulted in the "definition" of a maximum *ALH* value of "*ALHMAX*" for a track which is simply twice the largest deviation measured to either side of the average/smoothed path (or the maximum width measured by the geometric method). As yet there is no evidence to suggest that this is either more representative of any particular spermatozoon's movement or that it is a more useful as a predictor or discriminant variable with regard to sperm functional ability.

3. Frame Rate Dependency of Movement Analysis

The image sampling frequency has profound effects upon the perceived movement characteristics of swimming spermatozoa.[53] While *VSL* remains constant, since it only requires a sampling frequency of 2 Hz, *VCL* is extremely frame rate-dependent (Figures 9 and 10). *VAP* remains more or less constant if derived by the geometric method, but would

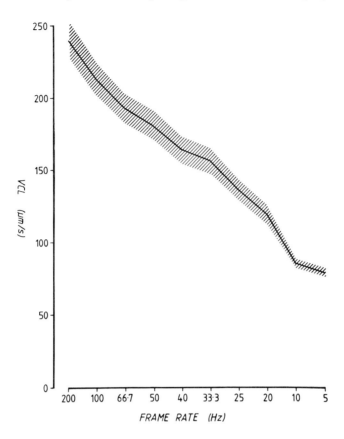

FIGURE 10. Mean ± SEM values for *VCL* of the same group of 30 sperm tracks of progressively motile human spermatozoa analyzed at image sampling frequencies of 200 to 5 frames/s. (From Mortimer, D., Serres, C., Mortimer, S. T., and Jouannet, P., *Gamete Res*, 20, 313, 1988. With permission.)

be expected to show great variability if standard, nonoptimized smoothing techniques were used at high frame rates.

There is also a significant problem in determining *BCF* values. When the image sampling frequency is about the same as, or less than, the real beat/cross frequency of a cell the observed value is constrained to be less than or equal to the frame rate. This problem of aliasing will always exist[55] and while its influence upon the movement analysis of seminal human spermatozoa will be rather small, it could easily cause appreciable error when analyzing washed spermatozoa.

Finally, because *VCL* is so frame rate-dependent its use to define subpopulations of cells (e.g., motile vs. immotile) will probably result in the identification of slightly different subpopulations. For example, if one analysis is performed at 30 Hz while another, perhaps using a PAL standard video system, is performed at 25 Hz then differences in the proportion of motile cells, as well as in the values for *VCL* and *LIN* (and also *WOB*), will exist. Standardization of the image sampling frequency, or the use of different *VCL* threshold values at different frame rates, must be used to avoid such discrepancies between analyses.

V. COMPUTER-ASSISTED SPERM MOTILITY ANALYSIS

A. GENERAL CONSIDERATIONS

In the past few years several commercial systems have appeared for the automated analysis of sperm concentration sperm motility, and sperm movement characteristics, opening

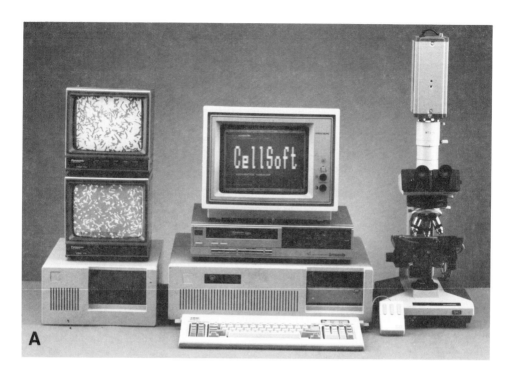

FIGURE 11.   Illustrations of typical hardware configurations of three CASA/CASMA systems. (A) is the CellSoft System 3000, (B) is the Hamilton-Thorn HT-M2030 system, and (C) is the Motion Analysis System CTS-30. (Photographs are courtesy of the manufacturers.)

up a new area of andrology which has come to be known as CASA (computer-assisted semen analysis). In order to distinguish between their use for semen analysis and the specific analysis of sperm movement characteristics, it is has been proposed that the latter procedure, which does not necessarily relate to semen analysis, be known as CASMA (computer-assisted, or computer-automated, sperm motility analysis), a distinction that will be made in this chapter. However, this terminology is by no means definitive, particularly in that it ignores other situations such as (1) CASA when human spermatozoa are studied under conditions other than semen analysis (e.g., concentration and percentage motility of washed spermatozoa); (2) "computer-assisted sperm analysis" applied to other species under any observation conditions; and (3) other facets of sperm analysis such as morphology or even "morphility" (see Section IV.D and Addendum).

Three major commercial systems are currently available (Figure 11): CellSoft (Systems 2000 and 3000: Cryo Resources Inc., New York, NY, U.S.), the HT-M2030 (Hamilton-Thorn Research, Danvers, MA, U.S.) and the CTS-30 system (Motion Analysis Corporation, Santa Rosa, CA, U.S.). Other systems include VICOS-SPERM (Mitec GmbH, Hofolding, West Germany) and LABSCAN VI (TS Scientific, Perkasie, PA, U.S.) while yet another system is under development at the University of Rennes (France). A system developed at the Oregon Regional Primate Research Center[56] is also to be commercialized.

Although similar basic principles underly the operation of all CASA/CASMA systems (e.g., those of digital image analysis[57]), appreciable differences exist in the optical systems used, image capture techniques, sperm identification techniques, track reconstruction algorithms, movement analysis algorithms, and in data analysis. Obviously anyone intending either using one of these systems or even using the data produced by one of them must be familiar with both the basic principles of sperm movement analysis and also with the specific system. It is clearly both inappropriate and impossible to provide a detailed description of

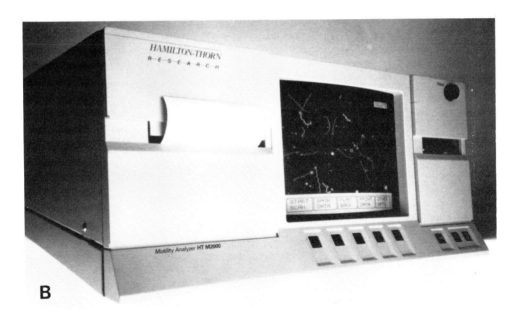

FIGURE 11B.

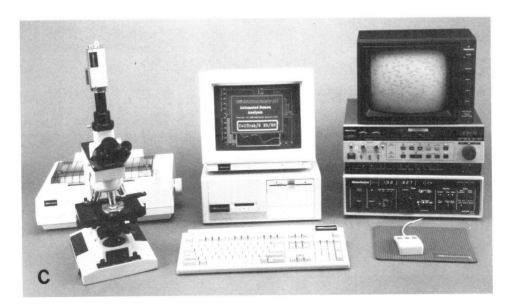

FIGURE 11C.

all facets of operation of any of these systems in this chapter. However, several of the more important characteristics and differences will be discussed. In no way is this intended to replace a User Instruction Manual and the reader must remember that often significant changes and improvements will be made to software, and even hardware.

B. EFFECT OF COLLISIONS

Of obvious significance is that if two swimming spermatozoa collide they will interfere with each other's movement. A similar problem would also exist if a swimming spermatozoon collided with an immotile one or with a large piece of debris or another cell (e.g., leukocyte). In fact, because the beat envelope of a sperm tail is at least as wide as the apparent track width as measured by *ALH*, spermatozoa do not need to actually collide for their movement to be altered. Dealing with this has been a difficult problem for all those working on movement analysis.[57] CellSoft stops tracking an object when its circle of maximum likelihood, or area of next possible position, includes a second object that has been classified as a spermatozoon. The radius of this circle, which is dependent upon the maximum velocity value set in the system parameters, is basically the anticipated maximum distance that a cell could have moved between video frames. If the tracks of two motile objects overlap then both are dropped from the analysis. While this is the safe approach to avoid possible corruption of a track due to collision, if the track is too short for movement analysis (according to the minimum requirement set in the system parameters, which should be 15 frames, or 0.5 s) then it is lost from the analysis of the sample's movement characteristics. While the HT-M2030 and CTS-30 systems do not exclude collisions, and as a result are not so concentration-dependent (see below), it still has to be proven whether their mean movement characteristics for sperm populations are free of significant bias. In general terms, we do not know the actual effect of collision on an individual spermatozoon's movement characteristics.

C. CONCENTRATION DEPENDENCY

A consequence of the sophistication of CellSoft's tracking algorithms is that the system is very concentration-dependent. Optimum movement analysis can only be performed on samples with less than 40×10^6 spermatozoa/ml using a maximum velocity setting of 200 μm/s.[58] Higher concentrations result in increased loss of tracks from movement analysis in a manner that is dependent not only upon the sperm concentration but also the proportion of motile cells and their velocity distribution. With higher maximum velocities, such as for washed spermatozoa (usually 300 or 400 μm/s), or deeper preparations the maximum analyzable concentration will be reduced.

D. COMMERCIAL CASA/CASMA SYSTEMS

1. CellSoft System 2000

This is essentially a simplified version of the CellSoft System 3000 intended as a "practitioner" system. Its analysis of basic semen characteristics such as sperm concentration and motility is the same as that for System 3000 except that a qualitative progressivity rating is provided. No movement characteristics are provided and consequently the system can be considered as having CASA but not CASMA capabilities. Its accuracy and precision as an automated semen analyzer is the same as that for the System 3000.

2. CellSoft System 3000

a. Basic Capabilities

The basic CellSoft hardware configuration (Figure 11A) comprises a monochrome video camera attached to an Olympus BH2-S microscope, two video monitors (one to display the real video image, the other the digitized image), an optional VCR, an 80286 or 80386-based MS-DOS microcomputer (optional, but recommended, math coprocessor), and a dot matrix printer. Specific hardware specifications are available from the suppliers. A heated microscope stage is also essential for movement analysis studies.

We have used the system successfully with both Makler and Petroff-Hausser chambers as well as with ordinary microscope slides and Chartpak slides; the Horwell chamber gave very disappointing images because of the thickness of its base.

This system has both CASA and CASMA capabilities and can be used either "live" from the camera or from video recordings. Currently recommended system parameter settings are given in Table 1 although each user is recommended to determine their own optimum settings by comparison with standard semen analysis methods (see Section VI).

TABLE 1
Suggested CellSoft System Parameter Settings for Version 3.x

System parameter	Units	Semen[d]	Swim-up
Image sampling frequency[a]	Frames/s	30	30
Number of frames analyzed[a]	—	30	30
Minimum sampling for motility	Frames	4	4
Minimum sampling for velocity	Frames	4	4
Minimum sampling for *ALH*	Frames	15	15
Threshold velocity	μm/s	20	20
Maximum velocity	μm/s	200	300[c]
Minimum linearity for *ALH*	—	2.5	0
Cell size range	Pixels	5—25	5—50
Magnification calibration[b]	μm/pixel	0.688	0.688

[a] For NTSC television standard systems, use values of 25 for PAL/SECAM.
[b] Assumes the standard Olympus BH2-S microscope with 10× objective and 6.7× camera ocular.
[c] A value of 400 is better but if it is used the histogram component of the Summary Report must be disabled.
[d] For the new "Forward Progression" version, the minimum samplings for motility, velocity, and *ALH* should be 1, 2, and 7 frames, respectively. The threshold and maximum velocities should remain at 20 and 200 μm/s with a minimum *LIN* for *ALH* measurement of 0. A *VSL* threshold of 10 μm/s should be used to define progressive cells.

b. CASA Capabilities

While CellSoft's precision, i.e., its consistency between two determinations on the same sample or between repeat analyses of the same sequence of videotape, are good,[59-61] there is disagreement in the literature as to its accuracy compared to traditional semen analysis methods.[58,62-64] The possible explanations for this disagreement cover a number of potential aspects of discrepancy and error.

First, CellSoft uses a Makler chamber which, as explained above (see Section II.A.1), may constitute a significant source of error in terms of sperm concentration. Comparison of CellSoft's sperm concentration values with those obtained by hemocytometry have revealed appreciable discrepancies.[58,63,64] A matter of major concern is the use of inappropriate and/or imprecise statistical procedures for data analysis in the majority of evaluations on CellSoft's (and other CASA systems') reliability in the automated determination of sperm concentration and percentage motile spermatozoa[64] (see Section VI).

Second, there are two potential sources of error originating in the digital image analysis technology: (1) the correct identification of all the spermatozoa in the field; and (2) the identification of motile as opposed to immotile cells. With regard to the first category, clumped spermatozoa (commonly seen in clinical material) will be digitized as a single image which, being too large for a sperm head according to the usual pixel size range set in the system parameters, would be rejected from the analysis. Even clumps of as few as two or three cells will be digitized as single objects and rejected if their area exceeds the maximum cell size (usually 25 pixels). This would simultaneously decrease the sperm concentration and, because mostly immotile spermatozoa are involved in clumping, increase the motile fraction. Furthermore, any debris or other cells of similar size and refractile appearance to a sperm head would appear to the system as valid cells and therefore be counted as immotile spermatozoa.

With regard to the motile vs. immotile question, CellSoft defines a motile object as one showing a curvilinear velocity which exceeds the pre-set threshold over the first (usually) four frames. To date, most workers have used a *VCL* threshold for motility of 10 μm/s. At

30 Hz this corresponds to a real movement between frames of 0.33 μm, therefore requiring the object centroid to move only 0.5 pixels between frames. Spurious motile objects could therefore be created easily by a small amount of specimen ''flow'' or by collisions or disturbances between motile spermatozoa at the start of the digitization grab period. Obviously this would further increase the motile fraction of the sample although a higher threshold velocity of 20 μm/s has been shown to improve CellSoft's determination of the proportion of motile spermatozoa as well as sperm concentration when used in conjunction with a requirement of motility being maintained over a larger number of frames.[65]

At low sperm concentrations, which may represent a majority of patients in some andrology laboratories, the incidence of refractile debris which machine vision can mistake for spermatozoa may be significant relative to the numbers of spermatozoa and thereby cause substantial increases in the apparent sperm concentration.[58,63]

c. CASMA Capabilities

With regards to sperm movement analysis, the values derived by CellSoft from a reconstructed track are accurate.[18] However, when mean values are presented for the whole population of motile cells in a sample they have caused concern.[65] When we investigated this problem it was found that there was often a substantial peak at the lower end of the velocity distribution (10 to 20 μm/s) sometimes as large as 30 to 40% of the motile spermatozoa. Examination of the Individual Cell Data printouts generated by CellSoft showed many of these spermatozoa to have extremely small *VSL* and *LIN* values. Although they had *VCL* values above the system threshold of 10 μm/s and were therefore considered to be motile cells, they clearly did not show any directional motility. Exclusion of these ''nonprogressive'' cells from the population, best achieved by defining a threshold *VSL* value for ''progressive motility'' did result in more representative mean movement characteristics for the population.[65] Insofar as seminal spermatozoa are concerned, such a definition of progressive motility is required to define those spermatozoa which are potentially functional.[6,9,12] As a consequence of this work a new ''forward progression'' version of CellSoft, which does employ a user-definable *VSL* threshold, is under development.

d. Files and Utilities

The standard CellSoft System 3000 output consists of a Summary Report and an Individual Cell Data Report. The data used to construct both these reports can be stored to disk immediately upon completion of an analysis although a utility for printing reports from the disk files is only currently available for Summary Reports. A number of experienced CellSoft users have developed, or are currently developing, utilities to allow printing of Individual Cell Data Reports from disk and these may be available in the future either from Cryo Resources or direct from their developers.

One facility that many users have found to be lacking from CellSoft is the ability to create several user-defined sets of system parameters selectable from a menu rather than by having to change individual parameter values through CellSoft's ''Set-Up Parameters'' option. The author has developed such a utility using a simple MS-DOS batch file and this may become generally available in the future.

Another option available in CellSoft is to store track data files. These files contain the individual x,y coordinates of the head centroid in each video frame for each of the sperm tracks identified. These files may then be examined and manipulated subsequently using the Research Module.

e. Research Module

The Research Module is a range of procedures which can be applied to track file data for the detailed study of sperm movement with respect to time and direction. The movement of either individual cells or groups of cells can be analyzed as a function of time providing information on acceleration, change of direction, rate of change in direction, and detailed analysis of *VCL* and *ALH* characteristics among others. This extra component of the CellSoft system is a powerful research tool for those working on sperm movement but presently lacks a track sorting option similar to that available for the HT-M2030 without using an expensive external statistics package.

f. Hyperactivation Module

The development of a highly active but nonprogressive ("dance") pattern of motility which has been termed "hyperactivation" now seems to be a ubiquitous concomitant of capacitation in the spermatozoa of eutherian mammals.[66] The precise pattern of hyperactivated motility varies between species at the flagellar level, and in some species it has a biphasic nature. For example, in the rabbit the nonprogressive "dance" pattern of movement is interspersed with periods of progressive "dashing" movement. Initially, human spermatozoa were not thought to demonstrate a real hyperactivated pattern of motility although appropriate changes in the pattern of motility displayed in capacitating media were recognized.[15,67] It is now possible to objectively classify the hyperactivation of human spermatozoa based upon their movement characteristics[19] using CellSoft. This work, which may become subject to a commercial patent, has led directly to the development of the "Hyperactivation Module" available as an add-on for the CellSoft System 3000.

3. Hamilton-Thorn HT-M2030
a. Basic Capabilities

The basic HT-M2030 system is a compact, self-contained unit with both CASA and CASMA capabilities (Figure 11B). It comprises a variable temperature-controlled specimen stage, integral optics and imaging system, and a dedicated 80286-based microcomputer. The single multifunction monitor serves as a user interface for system setup and operation, an imaging system and track viewing/editing display, as well as a results display. Control of the system is by eight buttons, three which control the specimen stage and five whose functions are under software control. An external keyboard may be attached giving access to a "Notepad" facility for entering patient/sample information. Hard-copy output is provided by an integral thermal printer allthough an external dot matrix printer (or plotter for track plots) may be attached.

Under normal conditions of use the HT-M2030 performs analyses and gives results printouts in "real time" although an external VCR (and even microscope) can be used. Reports and data can be sent to an external computer for subsequent retrieval (see below). Internal optical systems include infra-red, bright field and quasi-NH-phase contrast. Recent recommended system parameter settings are given in Table 2.

For human spermatozoa the phase optics give the best results although the infra-red system must be used when working with preparations in a rectangular cross-section glass capillary or "cannula" which is 200 μm deep (optimum concentration 0.05 to 2.0 × 10^6/ml). For more concentrated sperm suspensions and whole semen the HT-M2030 can use ordinary microscope/coverslip preparations as well as Makler, Horwell or Petroff-Hausser chambers (see Section II.A). Maximum analyzable sperm concentrations with each of these chambers depends on the magnification of the internal optical system.

An advantage of the HT-M2030's internal imaging system is that a frame rate of 30 Hz ("FAST/SPLIT" setting) can be used anywhere in the world. "European" models do exist using 220 to 240 V and 50 Hz AC power with either NTSC standard video (Model A: not compatible with locally bought VCRs or cameras) or a PAL/SECAM compatible video system (Model B). At the FAST/SPLIT setting a maximum of 20 track points (i.e., two thirds of a second) can be digitized; this may be a disadvantage for some applications.

TABLE 2
Suggested Hamilton-Thorn HT-M2030 System Parameter
Settings

System parameter	Negative phase[a]	Infra-red[b]
Minimum contrast	9	6
Minimum cell size (pixels)	7	3
Low size gate	0.6	0.4
High size gate	1.8	1.6
Low intensity gate	0.6	0.4
High intensity gate	1.8	1.6
Critical path velocity (μm/s)[c]	25	25
Critical linear index/straightness (%)[c]	90	90
Slow cells motile	NO	NO

[a] Settings for use with undiluted semen in a Makler chamber ($2.0\times$ magnification factor).

[b] Settings for use with a 200 μm cannula ($1.0\times$ magnification factor).

[c] Suggested values to define 'rapid/linear' progressive motility. Note, however, that *ALH* values will not be calculated for cells with lower values than that set. A value of 70% might be more useful for general purposes to obtain maximum information on movement characteristics.

Newer versions of the HT-M2030 software will include a menu-selectable series of user-definable system parameter sets for different types of material or analyses.

b. CASA Capabilities

Being a later arrival on the commercial market few critical studies have been published as yet evaluating the HT-M2030's performance as an automated semen analyzer in comparison to standardized traditional methods. However, preliminary reports indicate that the HT-M2030 performs comparably to CellSoft in measuring sperm concentration and percentage motility.[62] Our experience with an early model HT-M2030, fitted with infra-red optics only, supports this conclusion (D. Mortimer, M.A. Shu, and R. Swart, unpublished observations). Another comparison of the HT-M2030 and CellSoft concluded that the HT-M2030 was "clearly superior" although only very small numbers of semen donors and infertile patients were studied.[68]

Because it does not truncate tracks for collisions or near-misses the HT-M2030 is able to analyze samples with up to 150×10^6 spermatozoa/ml in a Makler chamber (see Section II.A.1) before a "too dense" warning is displayed and specimen dilution should be considered.

c. CASMA Capabilities

The HT-M2030 provides measurements of *VCL*, *VAP*, *VSL*, *LIN*, *STR*, and *ALH*. In addition, three other values are given which describe the proportions of cells in a sample which meet certain user-variable definitions of quality of progression ('progressive motility', 'critical', and 'anticrit').

Only preliminary evaluation studies of the movement characteristics provided by the HT-M2030 have been published so far. These studies have shown higher mean velocity and linearlity values for the HT-M2030 than obtained using CellSoft. Considering the possible effects of not having diluted the samples prior to CellSoft analysis in these studies (see Section V.D.2.b) the HT-M2030's values were probably closer to the truth. No information is yet available regarding the other movement characteristics measured by the HT-M2030, except that it should be noted that the *BCF* values reported in early versions should be multiplied by 2 to obtain values in accordance with the standard definition.

d. Files and Utilities

Results of an analysis can be sent to an external computer for subsequent retrieval and printing using the system's HREAD communications program, representing a significant advantage of the HTM-2030 over CellSoft. Users wishing to store data in special formats, store track centroid data, or to perform further manipulation of track data can use the optional HDATA utility.

e. Research Option

With this optional addition to the system the user is able to edit and sort track data and obtain multiple printouts of the results before and after re-analysis. The sort option can be used only on new data (i.e., immediately after an analysis has been completed) but not with data files previously stored to an external computer using the HDATA utility. This low-cost option has extensive research applications not possible using CellSoft without an expensive additional statistics package.

Single cell tracking (up to 1000 track points) can also be performed with subsequent track analysis in 20-point segments. Results are displayed by segment and averaged over the entire track. Such a feature is not currently available with CellSoft.

4. Motion Analysis CTS-30
a. Basic Capabilities

The CTS-30 system is a second generation development of Motion Analysis Corporation's successful cell biology CellTrak/S software specifically developed for CASA/CASMA applications.[69] The system includes its own camera, specially designed by Motion Analysis using the RS-170 standard (the monochrome component of the NTSC standard), the host MS-DOS microcomputer incorporating the video processor, and a dot matrix printer (Figure 11C). A VCR is not normally supplied but can be used. The system thoughtfully includes on-line 'Help' at any time within the system's menus and the computer's 'Print-Screen' key acts as a screen dump to provide hard copy of any information, including graphics displays, seen on the screen.

Specimen chamber depth is set in the system calibration although normally a Makler chamber is used for CASA applications. The CTS-30 allows 20 user-defined menu-selectable configurations in addition to the factory demonstration calibration set ('Set O'; see Table 3).

b. CASA Capabilities

No critical studies have yet been published on the CTS-30's performance as an automated semen analyzer but it must be expected to suffer from the same problems as all systems using a Makler chamber and machine vision. The system is considered useful up to 180×10^6 spermatozoa/ml without needing dilution because tracks are followed through collisions. Slight underestimations of sperm concentration and percentage motility will be expected since the program requires that all cells be tracked for the full duration of the analysis for them to be counted; hence those motile cells which leave the field during the analysis period will be lost.

c. CASMA Capabilities

The CTS-30, which has already been modified to use the recently agreed terminology, provides values for *VCL, VSL, LIN,* and *ALH*. Measurements of *BCF* and *VAP* or progression ratios derived from it are not currently provided except within the CellTrak Research option (see Section V.D.4.e). Clinical applications and evaluations of the CTS-30 system's performance compared to other CASMA systems or to the "gold standard" of manual track analysis have not been published. However, the system's track analysis capabilities are

TABLE 3
Suggested Motion Analysis CTS-30 System Parameter
Settings[a]

System parameter	Units	Human semen
Frame rate	Frames/s	30
Duration of data capture	Frames	30
Minimum motile speed	μm/s	20
Maximum burst speed	μm/s	250
Distance scale factor	μm/pixel	16.406
Camera aspect ratio[b]	—	1.023
ALH smoothing factor	Track points	5
Centroid X search neighborhood	Pixels	4
Centroid Y search neighborhood	Pixels	2
Centroid cell size minimum	Pixels	1
Centroid cell size maximum	Pixels	8
Path maximum interpolation	Frames	1 or 2
Path prediction percentage	%	0
Depth of sample	μm	10

[a] For undiluted semen in a Makler chamber.
[b] Depends upon the specific video camera used.

derived from the Motion Analysis 'ExpertVision' system, which has been used in fundamental studies on sperm movement analysis,[52,69] and should consequently provide reliable values for the parameters measured.

The software includes a variable path interpolation algorithm which is used to bridge gaps in broken tracks using linearly interpolated data. Therefore, in situations where a sperm head may be lost at digitization over one or two frames, the CTS-30 is able to reconstruct the track and keep the cell in the analysis. Some errors may arise if a different cell is picked up, e.g., if a cell leaves the field at a point very close in time and space to where another cell enters.

d. Files and Utilities

Results of an analysis can be stored and subsequently retrieved for printing new or updated semen analysis reports. Track data are also stored for use with the CellTrak Research option.

e. CellTrak Research Option

This option is a development of the well-established ExpertVision software which has been used extensively for studies at all levels of cell motility including fundamental studies on sperm movement.[52,70] It uses a sophisticated command language whose instructions can be linked as programs to perform multiple data manipulation tasks automatically. This Research Option is probably the most powerful available for CASMA research, especially when used in conjunction with the high frame rate CTS-200 system. Its disadvantage is that it requires greater user computer familiarity than do the CellSoft Research Module or the HT-M2030 Research Option.

VI. QUALITY CONTROL

A. GENERAL CONSIDERATIONS

Any laboratory method has two potential sources of error: random (e.g., sampling error) and systematic (e.g., observer bias). The magnitude of both these components must be known in order to evaluate laboratory test results.[70]

Random error is usually described in terms of a result's precision and can be calculated from repeated measurements on the same sample. Values are often presented as the mean ± standard deviation (SD) but, because the variance is usually proportional to the absolute size of the mean, a relative measure of dispersion may be more appropriate. This is the Coefficient of Variation or "CV" and is calculated as the SD ÷ mean multiplied by 100 to give a percentage value.

The term (in)accuracy is normally used to described systematic error and defined as the real deviation between the estimated and true value for an observation. The accuracy of a new method, such as CASA, is determined either by comparison with results obtained by another, well-established method of accepted precision and accuracy, or by verifying the addition or removal of known quantities of what is being measured.

The accuracy of a CASA system can be determined by mixing various proportions of semen and cell-free seminal plasma (see Section VI.B.1). This will result in proportionate decreases in the total concentration of spermatozoa but minimal decrease in the percentage motile. Fresh semen may also be mixed with various proportions of another aliquot of the same ejaculate which has been quench-frozen and thawed two or three times to kill all the spermatozoa. This will maintain a constant sperm concentration while decreasing the percentage motility. For both situations both standard hemocytometer counts of the sperm concentration and visual motility counts should be performed using methods of known accuracy and precision.[71]

B. SPECIFIC PROBLEMS
1. Accuracy of Dilutions

Volumetric dilutions of aqueous solutions or suspensions can be made with both high accuracy and precision using modern measuring devices such as volumetric glassware, dispensers, and pipettes. However, these devices are calibrated for distilled water (at 20°C, although temperature variations can be ignored). When serological pipettes, even of the "to contain" or "blowout" types, are used to measure semen aliquots there will be significant loss of semen adhering to the inside of the pipette due to the viscosity of semen. All the adherent semen must be recovered to obtain an accurate aliquot. This same problem also exists when automatic pipettes, even such high precision instruments as those manufactured by Gilson (Gilson Medical Electronics SA, Villiers-Le-Bel, France, also Rainin Inst. Co., U.S.), are used. Semen will adhere to the inner (and outer) surfaces of the disposable plastic tips, although less if they are "non-wetting". However, these devices have an air dead-space inside the body of the pipette which is extremely large compared to the sampling volume. Increased viscosity will allow a disequilibrium between the air pressures inside and outside the pipette body and this will be exacerbated with very small aperture tips.

A simple solution to these problems of coating and air dead-space is to use positive displacement pipettes when measuring fixed volume aliquots of semen. These pipettes use disposable glass capillaries calibrated to contain, and deliver, a fixed volume irrespective of viscosity. They have a tight-fitting, easily cleaned Teflon-tipped plunger which is in direct contact with the sample so there is no space between the sample meniscus and the plunger. Numerous models are available from companies such as Gilson, SMI (Scientific Manufacturing Industries, Emeryville, CA, U.S.) and Drummond (Drummond Scientific Co., Broomall, PA, U.S.).

2. Magnification Calibration

Accurate measurements of sperm movement characteristics require that the exact magnification of the optical and imaging systems be known. This is extremely simple for all methods using a microscope: a photograph, cine film, or video recording is made of a stage micrometer and its scale (usually 1 mm subdivided into 100 and 10 μm units) measured in the final image. CASA systems usually incorporate a pixel (or ''picture element'') calibration from an image of a Makler grid (100 μm square boxes). Whenever a component of the optical system, including the camera, is changed the real magnification of the system must be recalibrated. Changing from a $6.7 \times$ camera ocular to a $3.3 \times$ will approximately half the magnification of the final image (giving four times the image area or field of view) but the precise figure must be determined. Different makes of microscopes will often have different real magnifications even when apparently the same power objective is used. Finally, the addition of intermediate magnification or a microscope ''tube factor'' will change the final image magnification substantially.

3. Temperature Control

Sperm motility is dependent upon cellular metabolism and will therefore be temperature-dependent. While changes in temperature may not cause appreciable changes in the proportions of immotile and motile, or nonprogressively motile and progressively motile spermatozoa, movement characteristics will be affected. Velocity is extremely temperature sensitive and may increase by 60 to 100% when the specimen temperature is increased from 25 to 37°C (see Section II.C).[32] Obviously all evaluations of sperm movement must be performed at 37°C, and this was accepted unanimously at the Federation CECOS Workshop (see Section III.A).

All chambers, sample vials, and pipette tips must be kept at 37°C prior to use and the microscope must be equipped with a heated stage.

4. Sampling Error

Thorough mixing of a semen sampling or sperm suspension is essential before an aliquot is taken for any quantitative procedure. Suitable mixing methods include fairly vigorous swirling of the sample around the collection container, very gentle vortex mixing, automatic cradling, or stirring with a disposable glass or plastic rod.[4] High-speed vortex mixing must not be used as it may affect sperm motility or movement characteristics.

Because extremely small aliquots are taken for use in chambers such as the Makler (see Section II.A) several preparations should be used for each observation. Several fields of view should then be evaluated from each aliquot to achieve a representative sampling of the total sperm population. The minimum number of fields to achieve stable values for an aliquot is between three and nine,[58] and we have found that, on average, three Makler preparations are needed to achieve reliable values for concentration and motility by visual counting (D. Mortimer and E. F. Curtis, unpublished observations). Another study has shown that optimum results using CellSoft are achieved by analyzing at least 225 spermatozoa from at least four fields with the analysis being done in triplicate.[61] CASA is clearly neither simple nor fast at the present time.

Reduced sampling will obviously increase the potential sampling error and, while this may not change a clinical diagnosis, the increased variability of the data as a whole will limit its usefulness in epidemiologic or research studies.

The consensus of opinion reached at the Federation CECOS Workshop in Montpellier (France) in April 1988 (see Section III.A) included recommendations for the minimum numbers of cells that needed to be analyzed by CASA/CASMA systems to achieve acceptable accuracy and precision. At least 200 cells must be analyzed from at least four different fields for calculation of the percentage motility. A minimum of 30 (and preferably 50) tracks should be used for calculation of population mean movement characteristics. This would increase to a minimum of 200 tracks if subpopulations are to be identified (e.g., studies on hyperactivation).

C. STATISTICAL METHODS

Linear regression analysis is of little use in determining the agreement between two methods of measurement. Presentation of "correlations" between two sets of readings using the correlation coefficient ("r") and its associated level of significance is meaningless. A significant r value only demonstrates that the paired data points lie sufficiently close to a straight line, there is no information about the slope or intercept of the line and therefore no information as to the actual relationship between the two sets of readings. For example, if the slope is not 1.0 (which can be tested) then the two methods of measurement are not related on a 1:1 basis. In an extreme case the slope may be zero and then the statistics have actually proved that the two sets of values are totally unrelated. Similarly if the intercept is significantly greater or less than zero then the two measurement methods are offset.

What we really need to know is whether the difference between the two methods is, on average essentially zero, or whether there is a systematic difference in one direction, which would be reflected in a positive or negative mean difference. Such an analysis is most simply achieved using the paired t test which tells us if the mean difference between the paired data is significant compared to the original data.

However, the situation could easily arise where the mean difference is more or less zero but there is a wide spread of actual difference values both sides of zero (i.e., positive or negative differences). Ideally we need to know the range of these variations and this can be calculated from the SD of the mean difference. Multiplying the SD by the appropriate value of t (taken from the $p = 0.05$ t-table for n-1 data pairs) and then adding this to, and subtracting it from, the mean difference gives the 95% range of the differences. In other words, in 95% of cases the difference between the two methods of measurement will fall within the 95% range, and in only 5% of cases will it be greater than the positive or negative 95% confidence limit.

Obviously the ideal mean difference is zero, but deciding what is an acceptable 95% range is more difficult. In most biological situations a range of $\pm 5\%$ relative to the measured value is adequate so that two readings will fall within a range of 10% of each other 95% of the time. For sperm concentration, which has a very wide range, the differences must be expressed as percentages relative to the average of the two readings; clearly a difference of $+/- 10 \times 10^6$/ml is of greater significance for a sample of 20×10^6/ml than for one of 100×10^6/ml.

The relevance of this approach has been demonstrated theoretically by Bland and Altman[72] and has been applied to an evaluation of the CellSoft CASA system.[64] However, when appreciable discrepancies between the "old" and "new" methods are apparent the use of the average of the two methods for calculation of percentage variation will give biased results and therefore the "old", presumably acceptably reliable, method values only should be used.

D. CONCEPTS OF "TRUTH"

Many clinicians, as well as the authors of many clinical research papers, appear to take the results generated by laboratories as absolute, true values and ignore the components of sampling and methodological error associated with any biological measurement. For example, classifying one man with 19×10^6 spermatozoa/ml as "oligozoospermic" and another with 21×10^6/ml as "normozoospermic" is ridiculous; both could fall into either category simply by a 10% error in determining sperm concentration. While it has long been accepted that standard semen analysis methods are prone to substantial methodological error and potential observer bias,[70,73] it is widely assumed that CASA systems, because they are "computerized", must be accurate and precise. Unfortunately, the majority of evaluation studies are showing this assumption to be false and that much more validation, as well as improvement, is required.[60-65,74,75]

Because computers calculate numbers to high precision we have developed the tendency to report numbers to the nth decimal place, regardless of the resolution of the measuring

TABLE 4
Suggested Definitions for Classification of Human Sperm
Motility According to WHO Guidelines[25]

Motility category	VCL	VSL	STR
Immotile	< 20 μm/s	—	—
Nonprogressively motile	≥ 20 μm/s	<10μm/s	—
Progressively motile	—	≥10 μm/s	—
Fast/linear	—	≥25 μm/s	≥90%
Slow or nonlinear	—	≥10 and <25 μm/s	<90%

and analysis systems. If the results were taken from analog displays (e.g., dials) then we would be happy to accept that the readings were subject to error and be content with a reasonable number of decimal places (DP). It is to combat this idea of false precision that measured movement characteristics should be presented to one DP and the derived progression ratios should be presented as integer percentages (see Section III.H).

VII. INTERPRETATION OF MOVEMENT CHARACTERISTICS

A. GENERAL CONSIDERATIONS

The need for standard terminology (see Section III) to describe sperm movement characteristics is obvious. But there is also a need for comparability in the values reported. For example, the CellSoft Summary Report presents a mean value for "Linear Velocity" along with a histogram. Only by reading the manual does one realize that this is *VCL* and not *VSL* or *VAP* as are presented by the HT-M2030 and CTS-30 systems. In fact neither of these other velocities is presented in the CellSoft Summary Report, although a mean value for *VSL* can be calculated from the mean 'Lin Vel' and 'Linearity' values. As a consequence of this there may well have been some confusion between the different velocities as reported by the different systems.

Another divergence between CASMA systems is the subpopulation of cells used for calculation of mean movement characteristics. Sections V.B and V.C have dealt with the effect of collision algorithms and the associated problem of concentration dependency. Section V.D.2.c has considered the need for some definition of progressive motility when presenting mean movement characteristics for seminal spermatozoa (this consideration is relevant to all systems, not just CellSoft).

B. CLINICAL RELEVANCE
1. Semen Analysis

The purpose of CASA systems is to provide values for sperm concentration and sperm motility more rapidly, and/or more accurately than those obtained using traditional semen analysis methods. For many small or nonspecialized laboratories where specially trained andrology technicians are not available this is not a difficult task. However, in a center providing tertiary level infertility services and following WHO recommended methods with appropriate standardization and quality control[4,25,70,71,73] CASA systems may not yet be sufficiently accurate for them to replace traditional methods.[58,60,63,65]

CASMA parameters should allow more precise classification of spermatozoa into the nonprogressive and progressively motile categories. It should also make the WHO recommended subclassification of spermatozoa into the 'rapid, linear', and 'slow or nonlinear' categories both practical and accurate using objective definitions (Table 4).

When comparisons are being made between clinical studies the movement analysis method used must be taken into consideration because of the method-dependent differences in absolute values obtained for some movement characteristics such as *ALH* (see Section IV.E). While the same qualitative relationships will be maintained, the specific quantitative relationships must be expected to vary.

The total sperm concentration is well known to have little diagnostic value;[5] it is the progressively motile spermatozoa in a semen sample (and their movement characteristics) that are of biological, and hence clinical, significance (see Sections VI.B.2—5). Therefore, these are the semen characteristics that ought to be measured (along with sperm morphology, vitality, etc.). It seems pointless expending great effort trying to use modern technology to make unreliable and inaccurate measurements of characteristics. The opportunity should be taken to apply modern technology to the assessment of sperm functional potential thereby making a significant advance in clinical andrology.

2. Sperm-Cervical Mucus Interaction

Several groups have demonstrated an influence of sperm movement characteristics upon the outcome of sperm-cervical mucus interaction.[6-9] Good progression (e.g., mean *VSL* $\geqslant$25 μm/s with large mean *ALH* (e.g., $\geqslant$7.5 μm using TEP) are important discriminators in predicting *in vitro* sperm-mucus interaction test (SMIT) outcome. Using these values in conjunction with a minimum concentration of progressively motile spermatozoa ($\geqslant$25 × 10^6 spermatozoa/ml with *VSL* $\geqslant$10 μm/s) we were able to show that 25/30 "good" semen samples produced normal SMIT results whereas all 13 samples that failed to meet these three criteria produced abnormal SMIT results.[9] In addition, a small number of men have been identified whose motile spermatozoa are permanently unable to penetrate into cervical mucus or migrate through it, a defect caused by extremely small *ALH*.[7]

Since penetration of cervical mucus is the first obstacle that spermatozoa must face if conception is to be achieved *in vivo*,[76,77] movement analysis of seminal spermatozoa will be of greatest significance in studies evaluating sperm functional potential when *in vivo* fertility prediction is the biological endpoint (see Section VII.B.5).

3. Hamster Egg Penetration Test

Aitken and colleagues have provided substantial evidence of a relationship between sperm movement characteristics and sperm fertilizing ability as evaluated by the zona pellucida-free hamster egg penetration test (HEPT).[6,10-12,78] The best discrimination between normal or abnormal HEPT results was obtained using movement characteristics of the washed, preincubated sperm suspension. Such sperm populations show higher *VSL* and larger *ALH* values than do seminal spermatozoa[15] and the apparent relationship between smaller mean *ALH* values and normal HEPT results cannot be explained physiologically — although its discriminant power is unquestioned.

No studies on sperm hyperactivation in relation to the HEPT have yet been performed. But since there is no biological requirement for hyperactivated motility in the case of sperm interaction with zona-free oocytes, because there are no egg vestments to penetrate, a clearly definable relationship may not be apparent. Because the HEPT is itself an indirect bioassay of human sperm functional potential one should expect relationships between it and other sperm function tests (e.g., laparoscopic sperm recovery[70]) or movement analysis. However, these correlations do not necessaily reflect the direct biological involvement since the parameters being assessed may themselves be secondary events. Increased intracellular calcium causes increased flagellar curvature[80] and it is flagellar curvature that determines *ALH*.[81] Calcium influx is associated with the later stage(s) of capacitation and induction of the acrosome reaction[66] and therefore one would expect to see (1) larger ALH values and (2) increased proportions of hyperactivated cells in capacitating and capacitated sperm populations.[15,19,67] Perhaps it is the cells with the largest *ALH* values that develop hyperactivated motility and thereby reduce the mean *ALH* of the progressive sperm population. Certainly the identification of hyperactivated cells is not easy using TEP.[15,33]

4. *In Vitro* Fertilization

Sperm motility is clearly essential for fertilization both *in vivo* and *in vitro*. In the *in vivo* situation motility is also necessary for successful sperm transport,[76] a step that is bypassed with *in vitro* fertilization (see Section VII.B.5). To date only one publication has documented a relationship between clinical *in vitro* fertilization (IVF) and sperm movement analysis. Jeulin et al.[13] reported that preincubated post-swim-up spermatozoa from men who fertilized ≤33% of human oocytes *in vitro* showed lower mean *ALH* values (analyzed using TEP) and more morphologically abnormal acrosomes.

Obviously this is an area in which we shall see a proliferation of papers over the next few years, hopefully leading to the establishment of clearly defined relationships between sperm movement characteristics, and their dynamic changes associated with capacitation, which can be used in clinical management.

5. *In Vivo* Fertility Prediction

The prediction of potential fertility *in vivo* is distinct from the diagnostic assessment of sperm fertilizing ability. Its biological endpoint requires the successful completion of sperm-mucus interaction, sperm transport, capacitation, penetration of the egg vestments, the acrosome reaction, and sygamy between the male and female gametes. However, both are opposite sides of the same coin assuming no medical intervention (e.g., IVF). Consequently, it should be possible to define an appropriate battery of sperm function tests, sometimes likened to a laboratory "assault course" for spermatozoa, which evaluate all the physiological processes involved in conception.

Most of these except for sperm transport could be achieved *in vitro*.[76,79,82] Because of its pivotal role in sperm-mucus interaction, sperm transport and fertilization, sperm motility — and, most importantly, sperm movement analysis — will clearly be a crucial component of such a testing protocol. Unfortunately the prospective clinical trials necessary for the validation of this approach will perforce take several years to complete, including an appropriate patient follow-up period. Before we embark upon projects of this magnitude we must be certain that all the laboratory procedures are perfected so as to minimize the confounding influence of methodological error. CASA/CASMA systems are not really ready for this: software upgrades and system modifications during the course of such a project could prejudice the ultimate statistical analyses.

VIII. CONCLUSIONS

CASA and CASMA are still in their infancy. The first commercial version of CellSoft appeared in mid-1985, and it, like other CASA systems is still undergoing frequent revisions and improvements. Computer and video technologies have advanced rapidly in recent years and will continue to do so for the forseeable future. This may help resolve the present limitations of machine vision and image analysis and so lead to further improvements in CASA/CASMA systems. The present dialogue between system developers, gamete biologists, and andrologists must continue, it is the only route whereby practically useful CASA/CASMA systems can be developed.

Ultimately, because of the vital role of sperm motility in the reproductive process, such systems will enable us to move into a new era of diagnostic andrology. The clinical management and treatment of infertile couples will become more precise and cost-effective. Identification of appropriate forms of therapy will be based on physiologically relevant characteristics thereby avoiding biologically inappropriate treatments.

ACKNOWLEDGMENTS

The author's own work on computer-aided sperm analysis has been supported by the

Nat Christie Foundation, the Alberta Heritage Foundation for Medical Research, and the Medical Research Council of Canada.

ADDENDUM

Unavoidable publishing delays, combined with the rapid developments in this field, make it impossible for a book such as this to be totally up-to-date. Consequently, it has been necessary to add at least some updates to this manuscript, written in September 1988, as an Addendum: including reference to an excellent technical review of automated semen analysis by Boyers et al.[83]

MICROCELLS

A new disposable, precision sperm counting chamber, the "μ-CELL", has recently been announced (Cyto Fluidics, College Park, MD, U.S.). It is expected to be available in several depths, including 20 μm, with a quoted tolerance of $\pm \leqslant 1$ μm, as a double chamber unit requiring approximately 10 μl per chamber.

VOLUMETRIC DILUTION OF SEMEN

A more detailed study has been published on the relative accuracies of positive-displacement and air-displacement pipettes.[84] It confirms the absolute need to use positive-displacement pipettes when taking volumetric samples of semen.

CASA

As an extra point of interest, discussion of this acronym should consider its proposition by Russ Davis and David Katz as "Computer-Aided Sperm Analysis" at a Biomedical Engineering Symposium held at the University of California (Davis) in 1986.[57] This term may be considered a better general description because the systems and methods used in CASA are also applicable to morphology, physiology, motility, or flagellar analysis — or for combinations of these four.[83]

CellSoft "Forward Progression" Version

This new version of CellSoft determines movement characteristics using only progressive cells (see Section V.D.2.c) and, in addition, gives values for *VAP* and *STR*. A WHO-style four-category motility classification[25] is also provided.

Hamilton-Thorn HT-M2030 Version 7.X

This new version of the HT-M2030 software includes multiple parameter sets (2 factory-set, 3 user-definable) and a 'SORT' function. The SORT function can be enabled as an 'AUTOSORT' so that a 'Sort Fraction' is provided for every analysis. Used in conjunction with suitable variables this feature allows hyperactivation analysis to be performed automatically on appropriate preparations.[85,86]

Motion Analysis CellTrak/S 3060

This new version of the CTS-30 system allows routine use of a 60 Hz frame rate which, it is suggested, should be considered more acceptable as a general standard for movement analysis studies on human spermatozoa, especially for washed or "swim-up" preparations. An integrated, rack-mounted version of the Motion Analysis system is also now available.

REFERENCES

1. **Mohri, H. and Yanagimachi, R.,** Characteristics of motor apparatus in testicular, epididydmal and ejaculated spermatozoa. A study using demembranated sperm models, *Exp. Cell Res.,* 127, 191, 1980.
2. **Bedford, J. M.,** Sperm transport, capacitation and fertilization, in *Reproductive Biology,* Balin, H. and Glasser, S., Eds., Excerpta Medica, Amsterdam, 1972, 338.
3. **Turner, T. T. and Reich, G. W.,** Cauda epididymal sperm motility: a comparison among five species, *Biol. Reprod.,* 32, 120, 1985.
4. **Mortimer, D.,** *The Male Factor in Infertility Part I. Semen Analysis. Current Problems in Obstetrics, Gynecology and Fertility Vol. VIII No. 7,* Year Book Medical Publishers, Chicago, 1985, 1.
5. **Collins, J. A.,** Diagnostic assessment of the infertile male partner, *Curr. Prob. Obstet. Gynecol. Fertil.,* 10, 173, 1987.
6. **Aitken, R. J., Sutton, M., Warner, P., and Richardson, D. W.,** Relationship between the movement characteristics of human spermatozoa and their ability to penetrate cervical mucus and zona-free hamster oocytes, *J. Reprod. Fertil.,* 73, 441, 1985.
7. **Feneux, D., Serres, C., and Jouannet, P.,** Sliding spermatozoa: a dyskinesia responsible for human infertility?, *Fertil. Steril.,* 44, 508, 1985.
8. **Aitken, R. J., Warner, P. E., and Reid, C.,** Factors influencing the success of sperm-cervical mucus interaction in patients exhibiting unexplained infertility, *J. Androl.,* 7, 3, 1986.
9. **Mortimer, D., Pandya, I. J., and Sawers, R. S.,** Relationship between human sperm motility characteristics and sperm penetration into human cervical mucus *in vitro, J. Reprod. Fertil.,* 78, 93, 1986.
10. **Aitken, R. J., Best, F. S. M., Richardson, D. W., Djahanbakhch, O., and Lees, M. M.,** The correlates of fertilizing capacity in normal fertile men, *Fertil. Steril.,* 38, 68, 1982.
11. **Aitken, R. J., Best, F. S. M., Richardson, D. W., Djahanbakhch, O., Mortimer, D., Templeton, A. A., and Lees, M. M.,** An analysis of sperm function in cases of unexplained infertility: conventional criteria, movement characteristics and fertilizing capacity, *Fertil. Steril.,* 38, 212, 1982.
12. **Aitken, R. J., Warner, P., Best, F. S. M., Templeton, A. A., Djahanbakhch, O., Mortimer, D., and Lees, M. M.,** The predictability of subnormal penetrating capacity of sperm in cases of unexplained infertility, *Int. J. Androl.,* 6, 212, 1983.
13. **Jeulin, C., Feneux, D., Serres, C., Jouannet, P., Guillet-Rosso, F., Belaisch-Allart, J., Frydman, R., and Testart, J.,** Sperm factors related to failure of human in-vitro fertilization, *J. Reprod. Fertil.,* 76, 735, 1986.
14. **Makler, A.,** The thickness of microscopically examined seminal sample and its relationship to sperm motility estimation, *Int. J. Androl.,* 1, 213, 1978.
15. **Mortimer, D., Courtot, A. M., Giovangrandi, Y., Jeulin, C., and David, G.,** Human sperm motility after migration into, and incubation in, synthetic media, *Gamete Res.,* 9, 131, 1984.
16. **Overstreet, J. W., Katz, D. F., Hanson, F. W., and Fonseca, J. R.,** A simple inexpensive method for objective assessment of human sperm movement characteristics, *Fertil. Steril.,* 31, 162, 1979.
17. **Talbot, P. and Chacon, R. S.,** Observations on the acrosome reaction of human sperm in vitro, *Am. J. Primatol.,* 1, 211, 1981.
18. **Mack, S. O., Wolf, D. P., and Tash, J. S.,** Quantitation of specific parameters of motility in large numbers of human sperm by digital image processing, *Biol. Reprod.,* 38, 270, 1988.
19. **Robertson, L., Wolf, D. P., and Tash, J. S.,** Temporal changes in motility parameters related to acrosomal status: identification and characterization of populations of hyperactivated human sperm, *Biol. Reprod.,* 39, 797, 1988.
20. **Makler, A.,** A new chamber for rapid sperm count and motility estimation, *Fertil. Steril.,* 30, 313, 1978.
21. **Makler, A.,** The improved ten-micrometer chamber for rapid sperm count and motility evaluation, *Fertil. Steril.,* 33, 337, 1980.
22. **Harrison, R. A. P., Dott, H. M., and Foster, G. C.,** Effect of ionic strength, serum albumin and other macromolecules on the maintenance of motility and the surface of mammalian spermatozoa in a simple defined medium, *J. Reprod. Fertil.,* 52, 65, 1978.
23. **Neill, J. M. and Olds-Clarke, P.,** A computer-assisted assay for mouse sperm hyperactivation demonstrates that bicarbonate but not bovine serum albumin is required, *Gamete Res.,* 18, 121, 1987.
24. **Chapeau, C. and Gagnon, C.,** Nitrocellulose and polyvinyl coatings prevent sperm adhesion to glass without affecting the motility of intact and demembranated human spermatozoa, *J. Androl.,* 8, 34, 1987.
25. World Health Organization, *WHO Laboratory Manual for the Examination of Human Semen and Semen-Cervical Mucus Interaction,* 2nd ed., Cambridge University Press, Cambridge, 1987, 1.
26. **David, G., Serres, C., and Jouannet, P.,** Kinematics of human spermatozoa, *Gamete Res.,* 4, 83, 1981.
27. **Rothschild, Lord,** A new method for measuring the activity of spermatozoa, *J. Exp. Biol.,* 30, 178, 1953.
28. **Gray, J.,** The movement of the spermatozoa of the bull, *J. Exp. Biol.,* 35, 96, 1958.
29. **Harvey, C.,** The speed of human spermatozoa and the effect on it of various diluents, with some preliminary observations on clinical material, *J. Reprod. Fertil.,* 1, 84, 1960.

30. **Janick, J. and MacLeod, J.,** The measurement of human spermatozoan motility, *Fertil. Steril.,* 21, 140, 1970.

31. **Katz, D. F. and Dott, H. M.,** Methods of measuring swimming speed of spermatozoa, *J. Reprod. Fertil.,* 45, 263, 1975.

32. **Milligan, M. P., Harris, S. J., and Dennis, K. J.,** The effect of temperature on the velocity of human spermatozoa as measured by time-lapse photography, *Fertil. Steril.,* 30, 592, 1978.

33. **Mortimer, D.,** A microcomputer-based semi-automated system for human sperm movement analysis, *Clin. Reprod. Fertil.,* 4, 283, 1986.

34. **Makler, A.,** A new multiple exposure photography method for objective human spermatozoal motility determination, *Fertil. Steril.,* 30, 192, 1978.

35. **Makler, A. and Blumenfeld, Z.,** Optimum measurement time for human sperm velocity determination, *Arch. Androl.,* 5, 189, 1980.

36. **Makler, A., Itskovitz, J., Brandes, J. M., and Paldi, E.,** Sperm velocity and percentage of motility in 100 normospermic specimens analyzed by the multiple exposure photography (MEP) method, *Fertil. Steril.,* 31, 155, 1979.

37. **Makler, A.,** Use of the elaborated multiple exposure photography (MEP) method in routine sperm motility analysis and for research purposes, *Fertil. Steril.,* 33, 160, 1980.

38. **Makler, A.,** Use of the multiple exposure photography (MEP) method to describe shaking movement of human spermatozoa, *Int. J. Androl.,* 4, 606, 1981.

39. **Makler, A., Tatcher, M., and Mohilever, J.,** Sperm semi-autoanalysis by a combination of multiple exposure photography (MEP) and computer techniques, *Int. J. Fertil.,* 25, 62, 1980.

40. **Makler, A., MacLusky, N. J., Chodos, A., Haseltine, F., and DeCherney, A.,** Rapid microcomputer-based analysis of semen characteristics from photographs taken by the MEP method, *Arch. Androl.,* 12, 91, 1984.

41. **Burke, R. K. and Kapinos, L. J.,** The effect of in vitro sperm capacitation on sperm velocity and motility as measured by an in-office, integrated, microcomputerized system for semen analysis, *Int. J. Fertil.,* 30, 10, 1985.

42. **Kamidono, S., Hamaguchi, T., Okada, H., Hazama, M., Matsumoto, O., and Ishigami, J.,** A new method for rapid spermatozoal concentration and motility: a multiple-exposure photography system using the Polaroid camera, *Fertil. Steril.,* 41, 620, 1984.

43. **van Duijn, C., Jr., van Voorst, C., and Freund, M.,** Movement characteristics of human spermatozoa analysed from kinemicrographs, *Eur. J. Obstet. Gynecol.,* 4, 121, 1971.

44. **Phillips, D. M.,** Comparative analysis of mammalian sperm motility, *J. Cell Biol.,* 53, 561, 1972.

45. **Amann, R. P. and Hammerstedt, R. H.,** Validation of a system for computerized measurements of spermatozoal velocity and percentage of motile sperm, *Biol. Reprod.,* 23, 647, 1980.

46. **Schoëvaërt-Brossault, D.,** Automated analysis of human sperm motility, *Comput. Biomed. Res.,* 17, 362, 1984.

47. **Katz, D. F. and Overstreet, J. W.,** Sperm motility assessment by videomicrography, *Fertil. Steril.,* 35, 188, 1981.

48. **Overstreet, J. W., Price, M. J., Blazak, W. F., Lewis, E. L., and Katz, D. F.,** Simultaneous assessment of human sperm motility and morphology by videomicrography, *J. Urol.,* 126, 357, 1981.

49. **Holt, W. V., Moore, H. D. M., and Hillier, S. G.,** Computer-assisted measurement of sperm swimming speed in human semen: correlation of results with in vitro fertilization assays, *Fertil. Steril.,* 44, 112, 1985.

50. **Mortimer, D., Curtis, E. F., and Ralston, A.,** Semi-automated analysis of manually-reconstructed tracks of progressively motile human spermatozoa, *Hum. Reprod.,* 3, 303, 1988.

51. **Schoëvaërt, D.,** Automated recognition and morphological analysis of human spermatozoa, in *Computers in Endocrinology,* Robard, D. and Forti, G., Eds., Raven Press, New York, 1984, 187.

52. **Katz, D. F. and Davis, R. O.,** Automatic analysis of human sperm motion, *J. Androl.,* 8, 170, 1987.

53. **Mortimer, D., Serres, C., Mortimer, S. T., and Jouannet, P.,** Influence of image sampling frequency on the perceived movement characteristics of progressively motile human spermatozoa, *Gamete Res.,* 20, 313, 1988.

54. **Mortimer, D., Curtis, E. F., Shu, M. A., Mortimer, S. T., and Brooks, J. H.,** Analysis technique-dependent differences in measurements of the lateral head displacement of progressively motile human spermatozoa, in preparation.

55. **David, R. O. and Katz, D. F.,** Harmonic analysis of sperm motion kinematics using real-time video edge images, *Proc. 31st SPIE International Technical Symposium on Optical and Optoelectronic Applied Scientific Engineering,* in press.

56. **Stephens, D. T., Hickman, R., and Hoskins, D.D.,** Description, validation, and performance characteristics of a new computer-automated sperm motility analysis system, *Biol. Reprod.,* 38, 577, 1988.

57. **Davis, R. O. and Katz, D. F.,** Computer-aided sperm analysis (CASA): Image digitization and processing, *Biomaterials, Medical Devices and Artificial Organs,* University of California, Davis, in press.

58. **Vantman, D., Koukoulis, G., Dennison, L., Zinaman, M., and Sherins, R. J.,** Computer-assisted semen analysis: evaluation of method and assessment of the influence of sperm concentration on linear velocity determination, *Fertil. Steril.,* 49, 510, 1988.

59. **Mathur, S., Carlton, M., Ziegler, J., Rust, P. F., and Williamson, H. O.,** A computerized sperm motion analysis, *Fertil. Steril.,* 46, 484, 1986.

60. **Knuth, U. A., Yeung, C.-H., and Nieschlag, E.,** Computerized semen analysis: objective measurement of semen characteristics is biased by subjective parameter setting, *Fertil. Steril.,* 48, 118, 1987.

61. **Ginsburg, K. A., Moghissi, K. S., and Abel, E. L.,** Computer-assisted human semen analysis. Sampling errors and reproducibility, *J. Androl.,* 9, 82, 1988.

62. **Mahony, M. C., Alexander, N. J., and Swanson, R. J.,** Evaluation of semen parameters by means of automated sperm motion analyzers, *Fertil. Steril.,* 49, 876, 1988.

63. **Knuth, U. A. and Nieschlag, E.,** Comparison of computerized semen analysis with the conventional procedure in 322 patients, *Fertil. Steril.,* 49, 881, 1988.

64. **Mortimer, D., Goel, N., and Shu, M. A.,** Evaluation of the CellSoft automated semen analysis system in a routine laboratory setting, *Fertil. Steril.,* 50, 960, 1988.

65. **Mortimer, D. and Mortimer, S. T.,** Influence of system parameter settings on human sperm motility analysis using CellSoft, *Hum. Reprod.,* 3, 621, 1988.

66. **Yanagimachi, R.,** Mammalian fertilization, in *The Physiology of Reproduction,* Vol 1, Knobil, E.,Neill, J. D., Ewing, L. L., Markert, C. L., Greenwald, G. S., and Pfaff, D. W., Eds., Raven Press, New York, 1988, 135.

67. **Burkman, L. J.,** Characterization of hyperactivated motility by human spermatozoa during capacitation: comparison of fertile and oligozoospermic sperm populations, *Arch. Androl.,* 13, 153, 1984.

68. **Gill, H. S., Van Arsdalen, K., Hypolite, J., Levin, R. M., and Ruzich, J. V.,** Comparative study of two computerized semen motility analyzers, *Andrologia,* 20, 433.

69. **Katz, D. F., Davis, R. O., Delandmeter, B. A., and Overstreet, J. W.,** Real-time analysis of sperm motion using automatic video image digitization, *Comput. Meth. Prog. Biomed.,* 21, 173, 1985.

70. **Eliasson, R.,** Analysis of semen, in *Progress in Infertility,* 2nd ed., Behrman, S. J. and Kistner, R. W., Eds., Little, Brown, Boston, 1975, 691.

71. **Mortimer, D., Shu, M. A., and Tan, R.,** Standardization and quality control of sperm concentration and sperm motility counts in semen analysis, *Hum. Reprod.,* 1, 299, 1986.

72. **Bland, J. M. and Altman, D. G.,** Statistical methods for assessing agreement between two methods of clinical measurement, *Lancet,* I, 307, 1986.

73. **Eliasson, R.,** Standards for investigation of human semen, *Andrologie,* 3, 49, 1971.

74. **Lorton, S. P.,** Sperm motion analysis, letter to the editor, *Fertil. Steril.,* 47, 885, 1987.

75. **Mortimer, D.,** Computerized semen analysis, letter to the editor, *Fertil. Steril.,* 49, 182, 1988.

76. **Mortimer, D.,** Sperm transport in the human female reproductive tract, in *Oxford Reviews of Reproductive Biology,* Vol. 5, Finn, C. A., Ed., Oxford University Press, Oxford, 1983, 30.

77. **Mortimer, D.,** *The Male Factor in Infertility Part II. Sperm Function Testing. Current Problems in Obstetrics, Gynecology and Fertility,* Vol. VIII, No. 8, Year Book Medical Publishers, Chicago, 1985, 1.

78. **Aitken, R. J., Best, F. S. M., Warner, P., and Templeton, A.,** A prospective study of the relationship between semen quality and fertility in cases of unexplained infertility, *J. Androl.,* 5, 297, 1984.

79. **Templeton, A. A., Aitken, R. J., Mortimer, D., and Best, F. S. M.,** Sperm function in patients with unexplained infertility, *Br. J. Obstet. Gynaecol.,* 89, 550, 1982.

80. **Lindemann, C. B., Goltz, J. S., and Kanous, K. S.,** Regulation of activation state and flagellar wave form in epididymal rat sperm: evidence for the involvement of both Ca^{2+} and cAMP, *Cell Motility Cytoskel.,* 8, 324, 1987.

81. **Serres, C., Feneux, D., Jouannet, P., and David, G.,** Influence of the flagellar wave development and propagation on the human sperm movement in seminal plasma, *Gamete Res.,* 9, 183, 1984.

82. **Templeton, A. A. and Mortimer, D.,** The development of a clinical test of sperm migration to the site of fertilization, *Fertil. Steril.,* 37, 410, 1982.

83. **Boyers, S. P., Davis, R. O., and Katz, D. F.,** *Automated Semen Analysis. Current Problems in Obstetrics, Gynecology and Fertility,* Vol. XII, No. 5, Year Book Medical Publishers, Chicago, 1989.

84. **Mortimer, D., Shu, M. A., Tan, R., and Mortimer, S. T.,** A technical note on diluting semen for the haemocytometric determination of sperm concentration, *Hum. Reprod.,* 4, 166, 1989.

85. **Mortimer, S. T. and Mortimer, D.,** Kinematics of human spermatozoa incubated under capacitating conditions, *J. Androl.,* 11, 1990, in press.

86. **Mortimer, S. T., Anderson, S., Robertson, L., and Mortimer, D.,** Human sperm hyperactivation analysis using the Hamilton-Thorn sperm motility analyzer, *J. Reprod. Fertil. Abstr. Ser.,* 3, 41, 1989.

Chapter 7

METHODOLOGY FOR THE OPTIMIZED SPERM PENETRATION ASSAY

Aron Johnson, Brenda Bassham, Larry I. Lipshultz, and Dolores J. Lamb

TABLE OF CONTENTS

I. INTRODUCTION

Nearly 20% of couples attempting a pregnancy for the first time are infertile. An abnormality in the male contributes to the infertility in about half of the cases. In the past, the only diagnostic tests for male factor infertility available to the physician were the routine semen analysis (sperm concentration, motility, forward progression, and morphology) and endocrine studies (circulating levels of sex steroids and pituitary hormones). While these tests provide valuable data, they yield no information concerning the functional competence of the sperm. In other words, they give no information about the ability of the sperm to penetrate and fertilize ova.

Although sperm-egg fusion normally occurs *in vivo*, the development of *in vitro* techniques has permitted precise analytical studies of the fertilization process. The sperm penetration assay (SPA) was developed to measure the functional properties of sperm. The SPA was initially developed following the observation that, upon the removal of the zona pellucida of hamster ova, the species specificity of fertilization[1-4] and the block to polyspermy are lost. In particular, heterologous penetrations between hamster ova and sperm from a variety of species, including humans has been observed.[4,5] Ideally, human ova should be used for this assay, but they are not widely available and there are ethical problems associated with their use. Therefore, hamster ova have provided a useful model for the measurement of humam sperm function.[6]

For fertilization to occur *in vivo*, the sperm must first be capacitated and have undergone the acrosome reaction. The physiology of sperm capacitation is not clearly defined. In particular, it is not known whether capacitated sperm which have gained the ability to penetrate human ova, have undergone the acrosome reaction or whether this occurs as a local event at the time of gamete fusion. Regardless, the SPA, which requires both capacitation and the acrosome reaction to occur, has proven to be a reliable technique for the evaluation of sperm fertilizing capacity.[7]

One of the inherent problems with a bioassay, such as the SPA, is interassay variability and the lack of quality control. Furthermore, results obtained in different laboratories have not been comparable due to distinct differences in protocol. Our laboratory has devised a standardized protocol which has been optimized for sensitivity and reproducibility.

A. THE SPERM PENETRATION ASSAY

We have optimized the SPA as described in the earlier studies of Yanagimachi and co-workers,[4-6] Rogers,[8] Overstreet,[9] Wolf,[10] and others. Each step in the procedure was investigated to increase assay sensitivity and reduce false-negative results. Although most laboratories report their results as percent of ova penetrated with a score of less than 10 to 15% of the ova penetrated as being abnormal, in our optimized SPA, normal fertile donors penetrate 100% of the ova with extensive polyspermy. The results are therefore expressed as the mean number of penetations per ovum which we have termed the "sperm capacitation index" (SCI).[7] Our normal range was determined based upon the results from 30 fertile donors. The value two standard deviations below the mean was calculated to have a lower limit of five penetrations per ovum.[7] Figure 1 (Panel A) shows the SPA results from 13 pregnancy proven donors with a mean SCI of 33.1 and a lower limit of 4.8 penetrations per ovum.[7] Note the wide range of normal SCI obtained for the fertile population. Panel B shows the results from an additional 17 normal fertile donors assayed 2 years later. The mean SCI was 37.4 with a lower limit of 5.3 penetrations per ovum. These values confirm our earlier results for the definition of our normal range and emphasize the consistancy of our results over time. Clearly, this normal range should be verified in each individual laboratory.

A patient with a SCI of <5 will have a lower probability of achieving penetration in

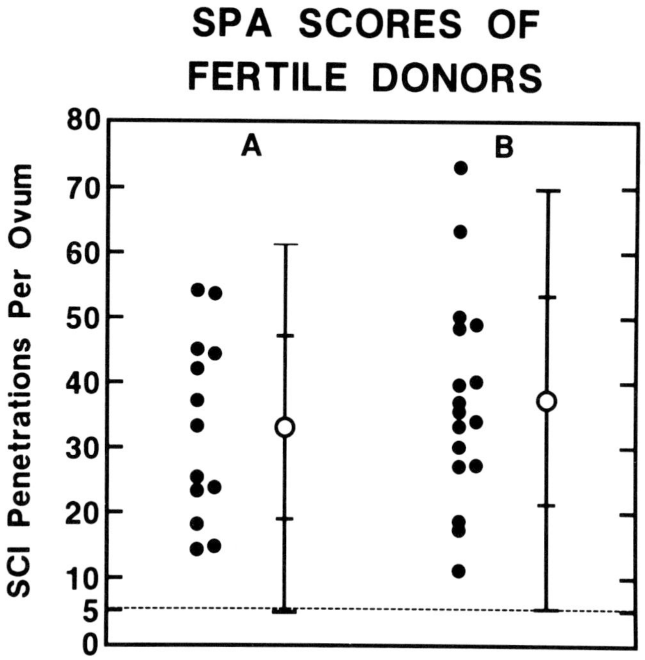

SPA SCORES OF
FERTILE DONORS

FIGURE 1.   Determination of normal fertile range for the optimized sperm penetration assay. The SPA was performed on 13 pregnancy proven donors (Panel A) and the range of sperm capacitation indexes (SCI) plotted. Panel B shows the range of SCI obtained for pregnancy-proven donors assayed two years after Panel A. The mean value ±2 standard deviations is also plotted. The lower limit of the normal fertile population (2 standard deviations below the mean) was 4.9 in Panel A and 5.3 in Panel B, emphasizing the remarkable consistency of our assay over time.

IVF and this probability is directly correlated to the number of penetrations per hamster ovum. A SCI of zero is clearly abnormal. Correlation of the SCI with *in vitro* fertilization has shown that a positive SCI is highly predictive of a positive IVF outcome.

We describe in detail below the protocol developed by our laboratory for the optimized SPA.

II. METHODOLOGY

A. MEDIA PREPARATION

A 500 ml bottle of Biggers, Whitten, and Whittingham's (BWW) media (Irvine, #9086) must be supplemented with 1.8 ml Na lactate syrup (Sigma, #L1375) and 5.0 ml Pen.-Strep. solution (Gibco, #600-5140), as well as 1.5 g human serum albumin (HSA) (Sigma, #A-1653), 1.05 g NaHCO$_3$, and 0.014 g pyruvic acid (Sigma, #P-2256) which may be pre-weighed and stored at $-20°C$. The modified BWW-0.3% HSA also contains 40 mM Hepes and can be used with confidence for 1 week when kept refrigerated. This concentration of Hepes successfully maintains the pH at 7.4 during the assay.

B. SPERM PREPARATION
1. Semen Analysis

The ejaculate is collected in a wide-mouth cup and allowed to liquefy for 30 min at 37°C. The specimen is transferred to a 15 ml graduated tube (Lux, #4106) to measure the volume. A standard semen analysis is then performed (see Chapter 3 for more details).

SPA Semen Processing

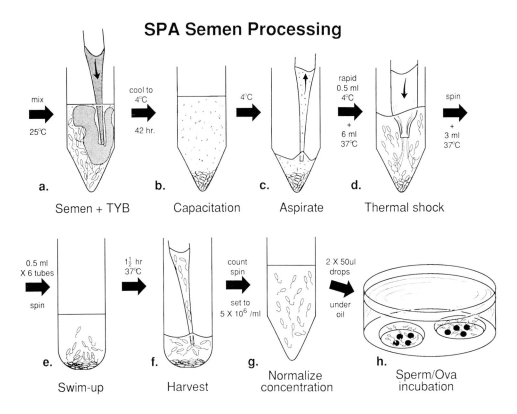

FIGURE 2.   SPA semen processing. Summary of the protocol for sperm treatment for the SPA.

Using a 50 μl pipette, 5 μl of semen is placed on a pre-warmed microscope slide and covered with a cover glass. Fifty microliters of semen is mixed with 0.95 ml H_2O (1:20 dilution) in a 12 × 75 mm glass test tube. The diluted semen is loaded into a hemocytometer counting chamber and set aside. Sperm quality is assessed by viewing the slide of undiluted semen on a 37°C warmed stage at 400× magnification under phase-contrast. The percent motility and quality of forward progression is determined. The use of computer assisted semen analysis systems (CASA) for quantitation of sperm concentration and percent motility is not recommended. The sperm should be counted in a hemocytometer after they have settled to the same focal plane of the counting grid. Multiply the final count by the percent motility and multiply this produce by the ejaculate volume to yield the total number of motile cells per specimen. [Sperm count ($×10^6$ cells/ml) × % motility × volume (ml) = total number of motile cells/ejaculate].

2. Addition of TYB and Cooling

The semen is then diluted with an equal volume of room temperature sterile TEST-YOLK buffer (TYB) (Irvine, Refrigeration medium #9972) and mixed with the aid of a pasteur pipette (Figure 2A). This semen/TYB mixture is gradually cooled by immersing the tubes in a container of room temperature water and placing this in the refrigerator. Not more than 1 h should elapse from the time the sample is collected until the start of the cooling process in the refrigerator. The samples should remain undisturbed for 42 h (Figure 2B).

3. Preparation of Sperm for Incubation with Ova

Upon removing the samples from the refrigerator at 8:00 A.M. of the 4th day a visible sperm pellet will have settled in the conical tube (Figure 2B). Aspirate the TYB seminal plasma supernatant (Figure 2C) to 0.5 ml leaving the visible pellet. *Immediately* add 6.0 ml of 37°C BWW-0.3% HSA and thoroughly resuspend this pellet by passing this solution in and out of a pasteur pipette three times (Figure 2D). These last three procedures should be performed in rapid sequence on individual samples to assure the same temperature shock to all samples (0.5 ml sperm @ 4°C + 6.0 ml buffer @ 37°C). We refer to this step as "thermal shock", and it is an important step for maximizing sperm ova penetration rates.

Centrifuge all tubes for 10 min at 600 × g. Aspirate the supernatant and resuspend the pellet with another 3.0 ml of BWW-0.3% HSA. Divide the resuspension equally into six 12 × 75 mm tubes (Falcon, #2027) and cap. Spin for 5 min at 600 × g and place the tubes in a 37°C heat block for 60 to 90 min to allow motile sperm to "swim-up" into the clear supernatant (Figure 2E). By aliquotting the sample into six tubes instead of one or two for the swim-up procedure, the surface area is effectively increased resulting in an improved yield of motile sperm.

Again, using a pasteur pipette, aspirate the supernatants from each set of tubes taking care not to disturb the sperm pellets and pool the supernatants in another 15 ml graduated tube (Figure 2F). Determine the sperm concentration using a hemocytometer. Since these sperm concentrations are lower than in the original semen, it is necessary to dilute a 50 μl aliquot into 200 μl water for recounting (1:5 dilution). Multiply the recovered volume by the swim-up concentration and then divide by the desired incubation concentration to yield the final desired volume. [Volume (ml) × conc. ($\times$ 10^6 cells/ml)]/ (5×10^6 cells/ml) = final volume (ml)).

All the "swim-up" samples are centrifuged for 5 min at 600 g followed by immediate aspiration to 0.1 ml and then resuspended to the desired volume with BWW-0.3% HSA. Two 50 μl droplets are placed in a small (35 × 10 mm, Falcon, #1008) culture dish (Figure 2G) and overlaid with 37°C silicon oil (Dow Corning 200 Fluid, 50cs viscosity) (Figure 2H).

The selection of motile sperm is beneficial for the patient who has poor semen quality, since the selection process separates the immotile sperm, white blood cells and extra cellular debris which interfere with assay outcome. Therefore, swim-up sperm eliminates debris interference as a source of false negative results for the oligospermic patient. However, selection of 100% motile sperm does not artificially enhance the SCI results. We have previously demonstrated that a good correlation ($r = 0.98$) exists between swim-up sperm and total sperm from various normospermic individuals when tested in the SPA.[7,16] The use of 100% motile cells permits accurate adjustment of the motile concentration of sperm in the sperm-ova incubation (5×10^6/ml ± 10%). This is important since we have previously shown that the SCI is correlated to the motile sperm concentration.[16] Thus, selection of 100% motile cells enhances assay accuracy as well as reproducibility.

4. Quality Control: The Frozen Standard
a. Freezing the Sperm Standard
Semen samples that contain over 200×10^6 motile sperm collected from high penetrating, as well as low penetrating individuals are diluted with an equal volume of TYB containing 8% glycerol (TYB-G).[13] The sample is divided into 0.5 ml french straws and both ends sealed with putty (Critoseal, Fisher Scientific Co.). The straws are placed horizontally in a 150 × 15 mm petri dish (Falcon, #1058) and incubated at −20°C for 10 min prior to freezing. The straws are rapidly transferred to liquid nitrogen vapor and frozen for 30 min prior to placing them in liquid nitrogen for long term storage. Using this method the sperm are frozen in suspension rather than settling to the bottom of the straw.

b. The Use of the Frozen Standard in the SPA
The straws containing the frozen semen for the standard are retrieved from the liquid nitrogen and immersed in a 4°C water bath. Optimal sperm recovery and capacitation of

SPA Frozen Standard Processing

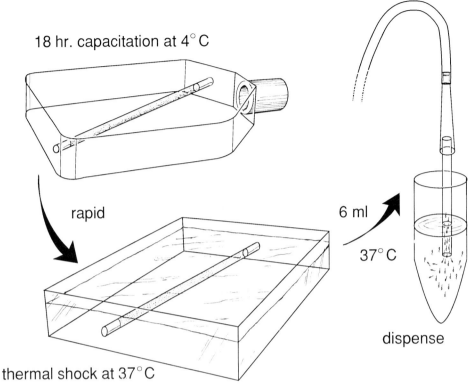

18 hr. capacitation at 4°C

rapid

6 ml

37°C

thermal shock at 37°C

dispense

FIGURE 3.   SPA frozen standard processing. The frozen straw containing semen and TYB-G is thawed and incubated in a 4°C water bath for 18 h. The straw is rapidly warmed to 37°C (thermal shock) and the end of the straw cut-off. The semen is washed from the straw using a tube with a pipette tip adaptor.

frozen sperm occur when the straws are submerged horizontally for 18 h at 4°C. We use a 250 ml flat tissue culture flask (Falcon, #3023) filled with 4°C water to hold the straws which is then placed in the refrigerator (Figure 3).

c. Thermal Shock of the Frozen Standard

After the overnight low temperature incubation of the frozen standard, the straw is quickly transferred to a 37°C water bath for 3 min (Figure 3). The straw is removed and one end cut off. This end is submerged in 6 ml of 37°C buffer in a 15 ml conical tube (Lux, #4106). The other end of the straw must be cut to allow the sperm to flow directly into the buffer. Using a tube fitted with a pipette tip, the straw can be flushed with buffer to insure total recovery of sperm. These sperm are subsequently processed as described in Section II.B.3. A high and low standard are run in *every* SPA assay.

d. Analysis of Quality Control Data

Figure 4 shows the Quality Control Plot from 11 different standard semen specimens with SCIs in the high, medium, and low ranges. Individual straws were assayed each week over an 8-month period and the SCI plotted over time. Our results from the SPA on the frozen standard are plotted on a Westgard multi-rule control chart,[15] with limits drawn at the X ±1, 2, and 3 standard deviations. The SCI is plotted on the y-axis vs. the time on the x-axis. However, for simplicity only the limits at 2-standard deviations are drawn in Figure 4.

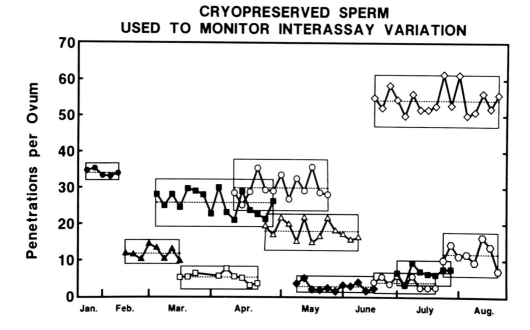

FIGURE 4. Quality control chart for the sperm penetration assay. The frozen semen from low, medium, and high penetrating individuals was assayed in each SPA over an 8-month period. The data was plotted using a control chart and is diagrammed with control limits drawn at ±2 standard deviations about the mean.[15]

The average coefficient of variation for the five specimens in the high and medium penetrating range was 8.4% compared with 28.3% for the six specimens in the low (SCI <12) range. In contrast, when two donors with 2 days abstinence were tested weekly for one year, the coefficients of variation were 41 and 50%, respectively, which reflects normal biologic variation. Frozen semen has proved to be a reliable standard for the SPA.

The Westgard Multi-Rule Control Chart uses a series of strict control rules for interpreting control data and the probability for error detection is improved over earlier methods. Only when all the rules are met, is an assay considered to be in control and the results are reported.[15]

C. OVA PREPARATION

1. Synchronization of Hamster Ovulation

Ova are obtained from Golden Syrian hamsters by supraovulating and inducing ovulation using a method similar to one originally described by Yanagimachi.[4-6] At 11:00 A.M. on day 1 of the assay period (or 70 h before ova harvest) each hamster is stimulated with 30 IU pregnant mare serum (PMS, Calbiochem, #367222).

Seven- to twelve-week-old hamsters are injected intraperitoneally with 0.3 ml of 100 IU/ ml PMS dissolved in sterile saline. The injection is made substernally with downward angulation using a syringe fitted with a 26 gauge ³/₈″ needle. A 30 IU dose of human chorionic gonadotropin (HCG, Sigma, #CG-10) is given at 3:30 on day 3 (or 17.5 h before ova harvest) in an identical volume and manner. Both PMS and HCG injection solutions can be aliquoted and stored in a −20°C freezer for a year. It is important to inject these solutions within 30 min after thawing to maximize ova yield. The assay requires that one hamster be injected for every two patients scheduled.

2. Hamster Ova Recovery

At 9:00 A.M. of the 4th day the hamsters are sacrificed in an atmosphere saturated with carbon dioxide. The oviducts are excised and placed in the first of three ice cold saline washes after which the oviducts are singularly transferred to a 35 × 10 mm culture dish containing iced saline on a dissecting scope. At 40× magnification the bulbous section of the duct is punctured with a 26 gauge needle to free the cumulus mass enclosing the ova into the cold saline. Once the entire mass has been teased free it is transferred by a pasteur pipette to a collection tube containing 0.5 ml ice cold solution of 1 mg/ml hyaluronidase (Sigma, H-2126) in BWW-0.3% HSA (BWW-0.3% HSA-0.1% HYL). The cumuli are collected and kept on ice.

In 28 consecutive assays using this regimen a total of 315 hamsters were stimulated. These animals were selected at random and not synchronized with respect to their ovulation cycles. However, the administration of pharmacological doses of gonadotropin successfully aligned ovulation. We recovered ova from an average 94.5% (range 78 to 100%) of the hamsters on any stimulation cycle. Of those, we recovered an average of 44.3 ± 6.6 SD (range 35 to 64) ova per hamster. Only 1.1% (range 0 to 4.6%) of the ova were not selected for use in the assay due to their small size. We have also examined ova recovered 13, 15, and 18 h after the HCG injection and found no differences in the peneterability of these ova.

3. Preparation of Ova for Incubation with Sperm

In order to synchronize the ova and sperm preparations, the cumuli are transferred to a culture dish containing a drop of room-temperature BWW-0.3% HSA-0.1% HYL at the time of harvest of the swim-up sperm. As the smaller cumulus cells are enzymatically detached from the ova it is necessary to remove them to prevent their interference with the subsequent trypsinization step. By stirring and allowing the ova to settle, the suspended cumulus cells in the supernatant and most of the buffer are easily removed with a pasteur pipette. The ova are then resuspended in fresh BWW-0.3% HSA and the less dense cumulus cells are again removed by aspiration. Repeating this step a third time produces a fairly clean group of ova. The ova can now be transferred using a flame drawn pasteur pipette (micropipette) connected to a mouth tube. The processing micropipettes should have an inner bore twice the diameter of the zona-intact ova. Skillful application of mouth suction and pressure can enable one to quickly harvest the ova while excluding remaining cellular debris. To remove the zona pellucida and the first polar body, ova are placed in a 200 μl droplet of BWW-0.3% HSA containing 0.5 mg/ml trypsin (ICN Pharmaceuticals, #103140). After 2 min the ova are washed free of trypsin by passage through three drops of BWW-0.3% HSA. The ova are now ready for incubation with sperm.

It is important to process the ova (up to 500) within 20 min from the time the cumulus mass is warmed to room temperature with BWW-0.3% HSA-0.1% HYL. We have demonstrated that zona-free and zona-intact ova lose their ability to be penetrated by human sperm with half-lives of 50 and 120 min, respectively.[14] However, by keeping the ova at low temperatures the penetration quality of fresh ova can be preserved for up to 24 h. For this reason, we store the oviducts and cumulus masses in iced buffer until needed. This also prevents ova recovered from animals sacrificed early from having a lower penetration rate than those harvested later.

We have also tested the effect of the cumulus size on subsequent ova penetration. Figure 5 shows that regardless of whether sperm were incubated with ova obtained from a hamster producing two large, medium, or small cumuli, nearly identical penetration rates were obtained. Figure 5 also demonstrates that the number of penetrations per ovum is directly dependent upon the number of sperm incubated with the ova.

D. SPERM AND OVA INCUBATION

To minimize interassay variation, the time after thermal shocking the sperm to the time the sperm and ova are incubated is kept between 2 and 2 $^1/_2$ h. The sperm and ova processing

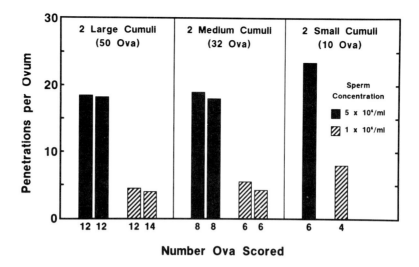

FIGURE 5. Effect of cumulus size on sperm penetration. Ova were isolated as described above from three different Golden Syrian hamsters. Both cumuli obtained varied in size (small, medium, and large) and in the number of ova they contained. The ova were incubated in duplicate with sperm at two different concentrations and the sperm capacitation index determined. Results are expressed as penetrations per ovum.

must be coordinated to finish simultaneously. Eight ova are placed in each twin 50 μl droplet containing 250,000 100% motile sperm. This dish should be kept on a 37°C heat block for *no more* than 5 min before adding the ova. The dishes are placed in a tissue culture incubator providing 95% humidity at 37°C for 3 $\frac{1}{2}$ h.

E. MOUNTING OVA

When the incubation is complete there are hundreds of unreacted excess sperm bound to the outer ovum membrane (oolema) which must be removed to provide an unobstructed view of those sperm that have penetrated. This is accomplished using a mounting micropipette with an inner bore the same diameter as the zone-free ova. Passing ova through three individual drops of buffer creates forces in the micropipette tip that shear off the loosely attached sperm. The ova are kept in buffer while a standard microscope slide is cleaned with ethanol. The cover slips (20 × 20 mm #1) are also prepared just prior to use by placing a very small amount of a paraffin-vaseline (1:1) mixture on all corners. The ova are retrieved so that a sufficient volume of buffer is drawn up into the micropipette after the last ovum. When the ova are placed on the slide a small droplet will be formed before the ova are expelled; this will prevent the rupturing of the fragile ova. The final droplet containing ova (1 to 2 μl) should be covered quickly with the coverslip to prevent any evaporation. Gentle pressure on one of the corners will cause the droplet to spread and gradually force the coverslip down expelling all the air. This process flattens the penetrated ova into one or two focal planes when viewed for scoring. The borders of the cover slip may now be sealed with nail polish. These slides can be kept for at least 3 days at 4°C before scoring even though a fixative is not used.

F. SCORING SLIDES

Since no stain is used, scoring must be performed using a phase-contrast microscope at 400× magnification. A penetrated sperm is indicated by the presence of a swollen head associated with a tail (Figure 6A). Using our assay, sperm penetrations are so numerous that the clear areas of the heads will often coalesce and appear somewhat indistinguishable (Figure 6B). In this case, it is necessary to count the tails without heads. It is extremely

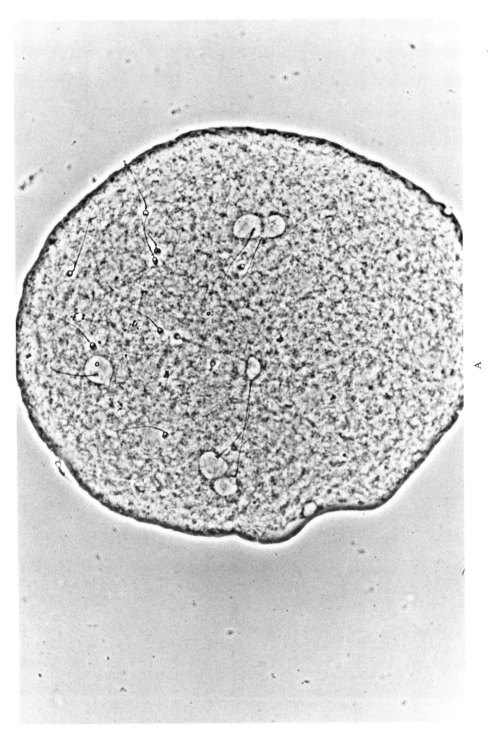

A

FIGURE 6.   Hamster ova penetrated by human sperm after mounting. After penetration the ova are washed and mounted for viewing by phase contrast microscopy at 400 × magnification. Panel A hamster ova with six human sperm penetrated which appear as clear areas (decondensed heads) with their tails. A number of unreacted sperm are attached to the outside of the ovum membrane. In Panel B the higher number of penetrations (28) demonstrate the importance of counting tails, since the clear areas of decondensed heads merge together.

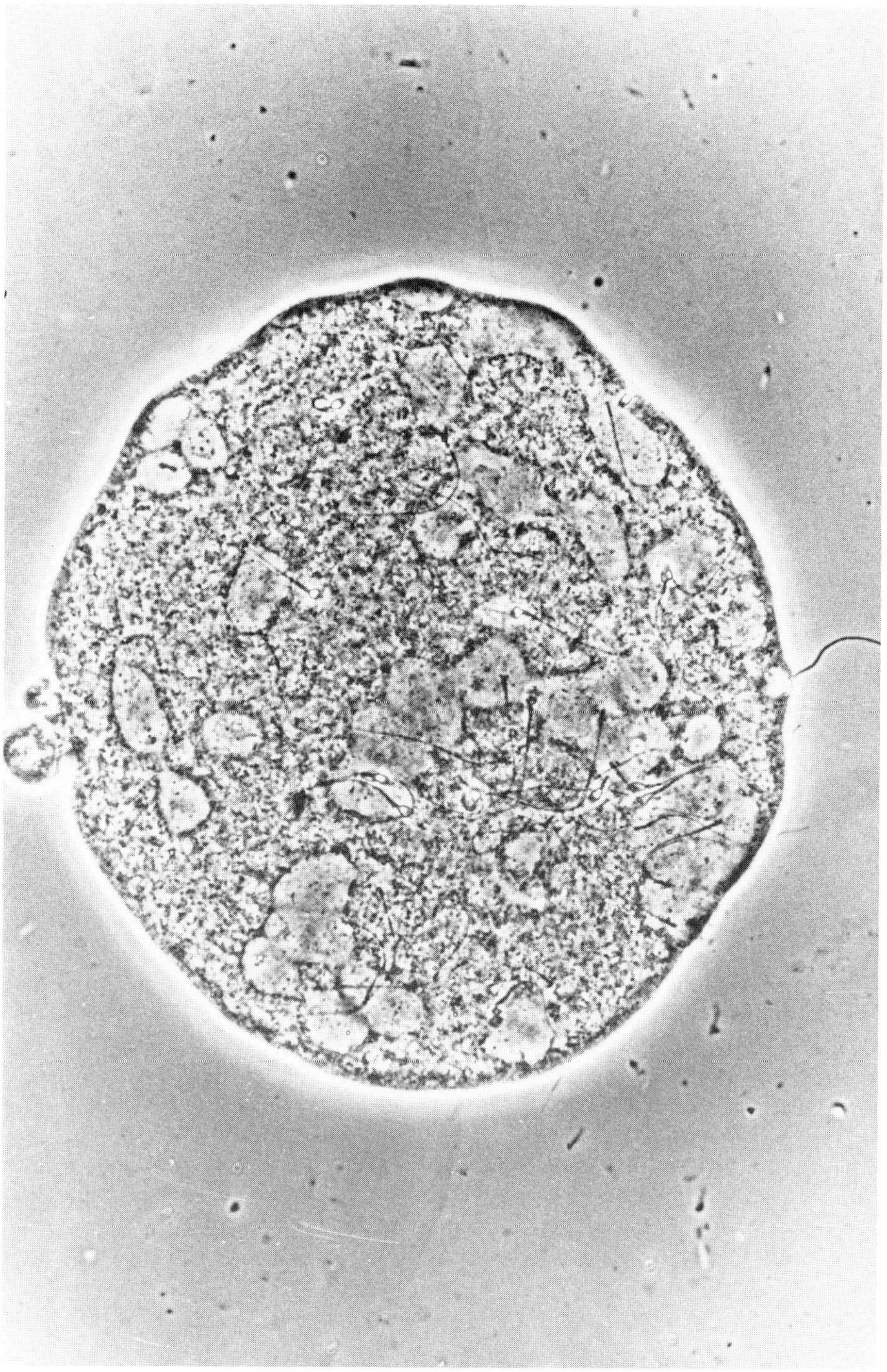

FIGURE 6B.

Penetrations per Hamster Ovum S.C.I.	Human Ova Fertilized I.V.F.			
	0	10–30	31–90	100%
68.0 to 5.1	2	3	64	42
5.0 to 0.1	9	6	7	2
0	3	0	0	0

FIGURE 7.   SCI and IVF correlation. The results obtained with our SPA were correlated with the percent of human ova fertilized by 138 couples participating in the Baylor IVF program. Individuals with an SCI of ≤5 have a lower probability of fertilizing human ova.

rare that an unpenetrated (unreacted) sperm bound to the outside of the ovum membrane will separate head from tail during mounting. The number of penetrated sperm in each ovum is recorded. The sperm capacitation index (SCI) is simply the average number of penetrations per ovum for *all* ova scored.

G. SPA CORRELATION WITH IVF

Figure 7 shows that a positive score in the SPA is highly predictive of a positive outcome in *in vitro* fertilization. With a SPA score >5, 95% of the patients fertilized 31% or more of the human ova. In contrast, of the individuals whose SPA score was ≤5, 44% of the patients did not fertilize any human ova and an additional 22% of these patients penetrated 30% or less of the human ova. It is important to note that the three patients receiving an SCI of zero also failed to fertilize a single ovum in IVF.

III. SUMMARY

Our laboratory has optimized the procedure for the SPA, resulting in greatly increased sensitivity. Although the conditions for the capacitation and penetration of the sperm are much different from the *in vivo* situation, the test nevertheless provides meaningful information concerning the ability of the sperm to capacitate and penetrate the ovum membrane. It must be emphasized that this test yields no information concerning the ability of the sperm to penetrate a cumulus mass and the zona pellucida, but affords information pertaining to the sperm-ovum membrane interaction.

Of utmost importance in a clinical bioassay of this nature are the optimization of assay conditions and the inclusion of adequate quality control. The test itself is rather labor-intensive and requires a *minimum* of two trained technicians for the most efficient operation if multiple samples are to be similarly processed. In our experience, in order for this assay to be cost effective we suggest that the SPA be established in a laboratory which would handle a minimum of 25 to 30 samples per week.

The optimized sperm penetration assay as described here has proven to be a valuable diagnostic tool for the infertile couple and provides an important supplement to the more traditional tests of semen quality.

REFERENCES

1. **Barros, C.,** *In vitro* capacitation of golden hamster spermatozoa with fallopian tube fluid of the mouse and rat, *J. Reprod. Fertil.,* 17, 203, 1968.
2. **Hanada, A. and Chang, M. C.,** Penetration of zona-free eggs by spermatozoa of different species, *Biol. Reprod.,* 6, 300, 1972.
3. **Barros, C. and Leal, J.,** *In vitro* fertilization and its use to study gamete interactions, in *In Vitro Fertilization and Embryo Transfer,* Hafez, E.S. E. and Semm, K., Eds., MTP Press, Lancaster, 1982, 37.
4. **Yanagimachi, R.,** Penetration of guinea pig spermatozoa into hamster eggs *in vitro, J. Reprod. Fertil.,* 28, 477, 1972.
5. **Yanagimachi, R.,** Mechanisms of fertilization in mammals, in *Fertilization and Embryonic Development In Vitro,* Mastroianni, L. and Biggers, J. D., Eds., Plenum Press, New York, 1981, 81.
6. **Yanagimachi, R., Yanagimachi, H., and Rogers, B. J.,** The use of zona-free animal ova a test system for the assessment of the fertilizing capacity of human spermatozoa, *Biol. Reprod.,* 15, 471, 1976.
7. **Smith, R. G., Johnson, A., Lamb, D. J., and Lipschultz, L. I.,** Functional tests of spermatozoa, in *The Urologic Clinics of North America: Male Infertility,* Vol. 14, #3, Lipshultz, L. I., Ed., W. B. Saunders, Philadelphia, August, 1987, 451.
8. **Perreault, S. D. and Rogers, B. J.,** Capacitation pattern of human spermatozoa, *Fertil. Steril.,* 38, 258, 1982.
9. **Overstreet, J. W., Yanagimachi, R., Katz, D. F., Hayashi, K., and Hanson, F. W.,** Penetration of human spermatozoa into the human zona pellucida and the zona-free hamster egg: a study of fertile donors and infertile patients, *Fertil. Steril.,* 33, 534, 1980.
10. **Wolf, D. P. and Sokoloski, J. E.,** Characterization of the sperm penetration bioassay, *J. Androl.,* 3, 445, 1982.
11. **Johnson, A. R., Syms, A. J., Lipschultz, L. I., and Smith, R. G.,** Conditions influencing human sperm capacitation and penetration of zona-free hamster ova, *Fertil. Steril.,* 42, 603,
12. **Johnson, A. R., Lipshultz, L. I., and Smith, R. G.,** Thermal shock (37°C) to spermatozoa stored at 4°C optimizes capacitation, *J. Urol.,* 133, 74, 1985.
13. **Johnson, A. R., Syms, A. J., Lipschultz, L. I., and Smith, R. G.,** Cryopreservation of sperm for use as a standard in the sperm penetration assay, *J. Androl.,* 6, 137, 1985.
14. **Syms, A. J., Johnson, A. R., Lipschultz, L. I., and Smith, R. G.,** Effect on aging and cold temperature storage of hamster ova as assessed in the sperm penetration assay, *Fertil. Steril.,* 43, 766, 1985.
15. **Westgard, J. I., Barry, P. L., and Hunt, M. R.,** A multi-rule Shewhart chart for quality control in clinical chemistry, *Clin. Chem.,* 27, 493, 1981.
16. **Johnson, A. R., Smith, R. G., et al.,** Group Discussion, in *The Zona-Free Hamster Oocyte Penetration Test and the Diagnosis of Male Fertility,* Aitken, R. J., Ed., *Int. J. Androl.,* Suppl. 6, 144, 1986.

Chapter 8

SPERM-CERVICAL MUCUS INTERACTION

Kamran S. Moghissi

TABLE OF CONTENTS

I. INTRODUCTION

The cervix represents the terminal portion of the uterus and plays a major role in human reproduction. From a functional point of view, the cervix acts as a biologic valve which, at certain periods during the reproductive cycle, allows the entry of sperm into the uterus and at other times bars their admission. Other properties of the cervix and its secretion include (1) protecting sperm from the hostile environment of the vagina and from being phagocytized; (2) supplementing the energy requirements of sperm; (3) filtering effect, that is discarding abnormal and unfit sperm and allowing the penetration only of vigorous normal sperm; and (4) acting as a sperm reservoir. An understanding of the physiology of the cervix, cervical mucus, and sperm transport is essential to interpret the usefulness and significance of various tests to evaluate the function of the cervix in infertile women.

II. INVESTIGATION OF THE CERVICAL FACTOR

The evaluation of sperm-cervical mucus interaction is an integral part of an infertility investigation. Abnormalities of the cervix and its secretion are reported to be responsible for failure to conceive in approximately 15 to 30% of infertile women; among properly investigated infertile couples, however, the true incidence of such abnormalities is probably not greater than 10%.

During coitus, 50 to 500 million spermatozoa are deposited on the cervix and posterior vaginal fornix. Human semen coagulates immediately after ejaculation and traps most sperm cells until proteolytic enzymes bring about liquefaction. The first portion of the ejaculate contains the highest concentration of spermatozoa (75% in humans), which, under favorable conditions, promptly penetrate cervical mucus.

Vaginal secretions are usually acid, with a pH of about 3 to 5. However, cervical secretions coat the upper part of the vagina and its fornices and considerably increase the pH of the vaginal milieu, providing a favorable medium for spermatozoa and apparently promoting their motility and longevity.

Seminal plasma, an alkaline fluid, also has a buffering effect upon the vaginal environment and alters the vaginal pH, thus smoothing the transition of sperm from the semen into the cervical mucus.

Human sperm are endowed with intrinsic motility, a property essential for penetrating cervical mucus and subsequent fertilization. There is no evidence that immotile or dead sperm can either pass through the human cervix or effect fertilization.

A stepwise plan for the evaluation of sperm-cervical mucus interaction in infertility is shown in Figure 1. Semen analysis and examination of cervical mucus should precede postcoital tests and more specific *in vitro* studies.

Substantial variance in all semen measures over an extended period in humans has been reported. The length of abstinence has implications for the study of variation in semen quality among and within subjects and should be recorded and standardized. A period of 2 to 3 days abstention before every test is recommended. It has been shown that three specimens spread at least 2 weeks apart are needed for the determination of a reliable measure of an individual's semen profile.[1]

A. EVALUATION OF CERVICAL MUCUS

The condition of cervical mucus greatly influences sperm receptivity; therefore, it should be evaluated accurately before a postcoital test is performed. Preovulatory mucus receptive to sperm penetration is profuse, thin, clear, acellular, and alkaline. It exhibits 4+ ferning (crystallization) and high spinnbarkeit. To evaluate objectively the properties of cervical mucus, a scoring system has been devised by Moghissi and endorsed by a Task Force of

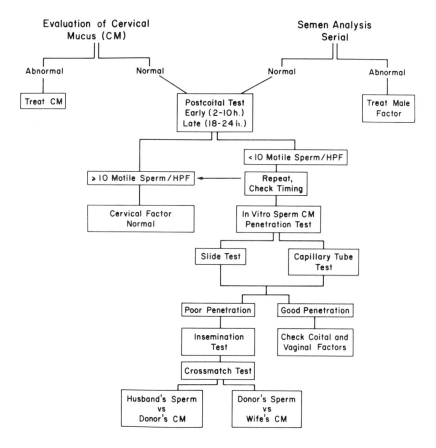

FIGURE 1. Steps in the evaluation of cervical factor infertility.

the World Health Organization.[2,3] This system takes into account five important properties of cervical mucus which are known to influence sperm penetration, survival, and migration: the amount, spinnbarkeit, ferning, viscosity, and cellularity. Each item receives a score of 0 to 3. A score of 3 represents the most optimal changes. A maximum score of 15 indicates preovulatory cervical mucus that is receptive to sperm penetration. A score of less than 10 is associated with relatively unfavorable cervical secretion, and a score of less than 5 represents hostile cervical mucus usually impenetrable by the sperm[4] (Figure 2). Insler and colleagues[5] have also devised a cervical scoring system aimed principally at monitoring the ovulation time. In this system, the quantity, spinnbarkeit, and ferning capacity of cervical mucus and the appearance of cervical os are assessed clinically. A 4-point score (0 to 3) is given to all variables except for the appearance of the external os, which is estimated by a 3-point score (0, 2, and 3). The sum of scores provides the total cervical score. Immediately prior to ovulation, a score of 10 to 12 is usually expected. The system is more suited to monitoring the response of the cervix to ovulation-inducing agents such as human menopausal gonadotropins rather than evaluation of sperm-cervical mucus interaction.

Several techniques for collecting cervical mucus have been described. The methods most commonly used include aspiration with a tuberculin syringe (without needle), pipette, or polyethylene tube; sampling with a mucus forceps is another method. Cervical mucus should be collected and studied as close to the time of ovulation as possible. Clinical examination of cervical mucus includes determination of amount, viscosity, cellularity, pH, ferning, spinnbarkeit, and, if infection is suspected, bacteriologic cultures. Ferning is performed by spreading cervical mucus on a glass slide and allowing it to dry (Figure 3). It is customarily

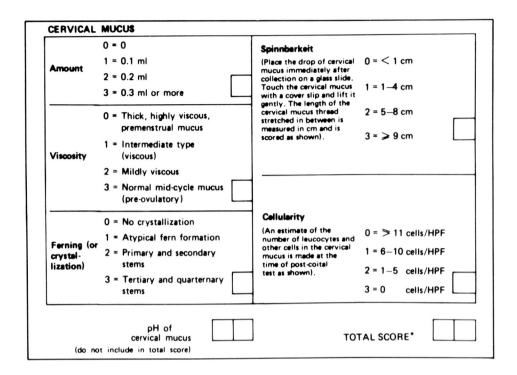

FIGURE 2. Cervical score for evaluation of preovulatory mucus. (From Moghissi, K. S., *Fertil. Steril.*, 17, 663, 1966. Reprinted with permission of the American Fertility Society.)

graded from 0 to 4 +, depending on the extent of crystal formation. Spinnbarkeit is measured by placing an adequate amount of cervical mucus on a microscope slide, covering it with a coverslip, and drawing the mucus between slide and coverslip. An estimate of spinnbarkeit (in centimeters) is made by measuring the length of the thread before it breaks (Figure 4). The pH of cervical mucus should be measured *in situ* or immediately following collection. Care should be taken to assay the pH of endocervical mucus correctly, since the pH of the exocervical mucus is always lower than that of the endocervical canal. In the laboratory, a pH meter may be used. In clinical practice, a pH paper with a range of 5 to 8 is commonly utilized.

III. POSTCOITAL TEST

The postcoital test, also known as the Sims-Huhner test or Huhner test, is an office procedure and should be performed in the early stages of the infertility investigation. Despite its popularity, there is a lack of standardization, and disagreement remains on how to interpret the test results.

A. TIMING

Postcoital test should be performed as near as possible to the time of ovulation as determined by the usual clinical or laboratory means (basal body temperature, cervical mucus changes, and hormonal assays). The couple is instructed to abstain from sexual intercourse for 2 days prior to the test, which is performed approximately 6 to 10 h after intercourse (standard test). If the initial test result is satisfactory, the test may be repeated at a longer interval of 18 to 24 h (delayed test) when infertility persists. The presence in the endocervix of an adequate number of motile spermatozoa at this stage suggests favorable mucus and adequate survival of sperm in the cervix. It excludes cervical factors as a cause of infertility.

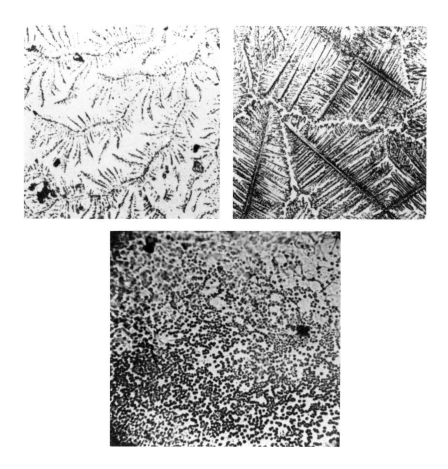

FIGURE 3. Ferning or crystallization of cervical mucus: (upper right) preovulatory ferning (4 +); (upper left) atypical ferning (1 +); (lower) absent ferning.

When the initial test yields poor results, the second test is planned 1 to 3 h after coitus (early test).

On the basis of cervical mucus examination following artificial insemination, it has been suggested that the most appropriate time to perform a postcoital test is 2.5 h after intercourse, since the largest sperm population in the mucus has been found at this time.[6] This timing does not allow for the adequate evaluation of sperm survival in the cervix. The purpose of a postcoital test is not only to determine whether there is a sufficient number of active spermatozoa in the cervical mucus, but also to evaluate sperm survival and behavior many hours after coitus (reservoir role). Therefore, 6 to 10 h after coitus is a balanced time to determine both sperm density and longevity. Earlier timing may be reserved for subjects who have negative or abnormal tests.

B. TECHNIQUE

An unlubricated speculum is inserted into the vagina and a sample of the posterior vaginal fornix pool is aspirated with a tuberculin syringe (without needle), mucus syringe, pipette, or polyethylene tube. With a different syringe, samples of cervical mucus are obtained from the endocervix and endocervical canal. These are placed on a separate glass slide, covered with a coverslip, and examined under a microscope at 200 and 400 × magnification. If exocervical mucus is covered with cells, debris, and vaginal content, the area should be wiped dry with cotton before the endocervical specimen is obtained. Whenever possible, the quality of the mucus should be evaluated immediately after collection.

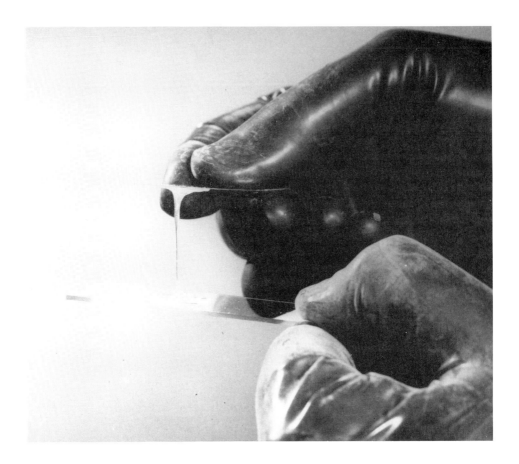

FIGURE 4.   Technique for determining spinnbarkeit (fibrosity) of cervical mucus.

C. INTERPRETATION

Interpreting the postcoital test requires an understanding of cervical function and sperm transport. Cervical mucus protects sperm from the hostile environment of the vagina and from phagocytosis.

Within seconds, ejaculated sperm enter midcycle mucus.[7] Subsequent migration through the cervical canal is accomplished principally by intrinsic motility. It may also be influenced by seminal plasma and the orientation of strands of cervical mucin. This last phenomenon may be responsible for the storage of sperm in the cervical crypts and their gradual release over an extended period into the uterus and oviducts.

The function of the cervix as a sperm reservoir is of considerable importance in fertility. Only occasionally does coitus occur at ovulation. In most instances, the union of gametes depends on a constant supply of sperm at the site of fertilization for some hours before and after ovulation. Following coitus, a gradient is established within the cervix which is entirely time-dependent. With increasing intervals between coitus and examination, there is an orderly progression of sperm from the lower to the upper part of the canal.[8]

With these facts in mind, postcoital tests may be interpreted on a rational basis as follows:

1. Vaginal pool sample: Spermatozoa are usually destroyed in the vagina within 2 to 4 h and lose their fertilizing ability within a few hours. The purpose of examining the vaginal pool sample, therefore, is to ensure that semen has actually been deposited in the vagina.

2. Exocervical sample: The number of sperm in the lower part of the cervical canal varies with time elapsed after coitus. Within 2 to 3 h after intercourse, there is a large accumulation of sperm in the lower part of the cervical canal. In a normal woman who has had coitus with a fertile man, more than 25 motile sperm (with $2+$ to $3+$ motility) per high-power field ($400\times$) are commonly observed in the exocervical specimen; 10 or more sperm per high-power field with a score of $3+$ motility is considered satisfactory.[3] Fewer than 5 sperm per high-power field, particularly when associated with sluggish or circular motion, is an indication of oligoasthenospermia or abnormality of cervical mucus.[9] Sperm motility in cervical mucus is graded from 0 to 3 as follows: 0, immotile; $1+$, *in situ* motility; $2+$, sluggish motility; $3+$, vigorous forward motility. Beginning approximately 4 h after coitus, the number of sperm in the exocervical pool gradually decreases. Thus, tests performed at intervals of 4 h or more following coitus may reveal fewer sperm in the mucus collected from the lower cervical canal.

3. Endocervical sample: After ejaculation, sperm rapidly reach the level of the internal os. Their number gradually increases and reaches a peak approximately 2 to 3 h later.[6] Thereafter, their number remains relatively constant for up to 24 h. At 6 to 10 h after intercourse, more than 10 sperm with adequate motility (score of $3+$) should normally be found per high-power field.[4] A similar number of sperm is usually detected on a delayed test (18 to 24 h after intercourse).

D. ABNORMAL POSTCOITAL TEST

One abnormal postcoital test has little clinical value and must be repeated. Controversy continues as to the significance of sperm found in cervical secretions several hours after coitus. Some investigators have suggested that they consist mainly of sperm populations of poor quality that have failed to pass into the uterus. This conclusion is not supported by animal and human studies.

A few older studies have compared the results of postcoital tests and endometrial aspirations and found that although motile sperm were present in the uteri of some patients, they could not be demonstrated in the cervical mucus.[10] An explanation of this finding may be that, in cases of oligospermia or when cervical mucus is relatively hostile, the more vigorous and healthier sperm penetrate the cervix and reach the uterine cavity shortly after coitus (rapid phase of transport). Other sperm, which are normally stored in cervical crypts and mucus, do not survive long enough to be detected (disturbed delayed phase of transport).

Most investigators believe that persistently negative postcoital tests indicate either an abnormality of the mucus or oligoasthenospermia.

E. SIGNIFICANCE OF THE POSTCOITAL TEST

Semen analysis fails to evaluate two important properties of sperm, namely, the ability to penetrate cervical mucus and fertilizing capacity. Although spermatozoa from an ejaculate with adequate sperm concentration, motility, and morphology are expected to penetrate the normal cervical mucus readily, this does not occur in all cases. The principal function of the postcoital test of *in vitro* sperm penetration studies is to assess sperm-cervical mucus interaction and the ability of sperm to negotiate the cervical barrier and eventually reach the distal portion of the oviducts.

Although widely practiced as a clinical test, the PCT has not been adequately standardized with respect to methodology and interpretation, and remains highly subjective. A task force of the World Health Organization has attempted to standardize PCT and *in vitro* tests of sperm-cervical mucus interaction,[2] but many clinicians and investigators continue to use their own technique or, at times, no acceptable technique. Because of lack of standardization and other variables affecting human fertility, it is difficult to correlate the results of PCT with conception rate. When variables are better controlled, as in a donor artificial insemination process, a positive correlation can be demonstrated between conception and sperm survival in the cervix.[11]

Soon after ejaculation, spermatozoa are transferred from seminal plasma to female genital fluid, in which they are suspended. Migration, survival, and fertilizing potential of spermatozoa depend to a large extent on how well they adapt to this new environment. The postcoital test provides valuable information on the adaptation of sperm to this environment.

A survey of published reports on postcoital tests indicates much controversy. Most investigators believe that the postcoital tests correlate well with sperm concentration, morphology, and motility in the semen as well as with *in vitro* studies.[12] Motile sperm have been observed in samples of cervical mucus obtained from the cervical os and canal 1.5 to 3 min after ejaculation.[7] Under normal conditions, the percentage of motile and morphologically normal spermatozoa is usually higher in cervical mucus than in semen.[13]

Serial postcoital tests have shown that the increased ferning and spinnbarkeit of preovulatory cervical mucus coincides with a greater number of motile sperm being observed in mucus samples.[14] After ovulation, the mucus becomes thick, and few, if any, live sperm cells are found in it. Combined postcoital tests and endometrial aspirations have demonstrated that the greatest numbers of sperm in the endometrial cavity are found at or near the time of ovulation. Very few are present in the uterus during the luteal or early follicular phases of the cycle.[15]

A direct relationship between the numbers of artificially inseminated motile sperm and those recovered from the cervical mucus has been demonstrated.[16] The ratio of cervical mucus sperm to inseminated sperm was fairly constant 15 min to 24 h after insemination. By 48 h, the number of sperm in cervical mucus was negligible.

In studies reported by Ahlgren and colleagues,[17] the number of sperm in cervical mucus and the uterine cavity correlated well with the number in the oviducts and pouch of Douglas. Most progressively motile sperm in these locations were observed in the presence of a mature follicle in the ovaries. A significant decrease in motile sperm population has been seen when the ovaries contained corpora lutea. Once the sperm reached the uterine cavity, however, their further progression to the oviduct was not influenced by the stage of ovarian cycle. The presence of sperm in the uterus correlated directly with high sperm density of the cervical mucus approximately 25 to 41 h after coitus.

Several investigators have reported a lack of correlation between the results of sperm recovery from the peritoneal cavity following artificial insemination and the results of postcoital testing.[18-20] It should be recognized, however, that the two procedures assess sperm transport in different segments of the reproductive tract. Postcoital testing evaluates sperm-cervical mucus interaction, whereas sperm recovery from the pelvic cavity evaluates sperm transport through the entire reproductive tract. Also, it is conceivable that the rapid sperm transport may provide for the presence of some sperm in pelvic cavity, but a disturbance in the delayed transport mechanism causes absence of sperm in cervical mucus some hours after coitus. Finally, it is known that the spermatozoa can survive within the reproductive tract of the female for up to 7 days.[21] Therefore, sperm recovered from the peritoneal cavity (cul-de-sac), particularly those without motility, may have been the result of coital activities that have occurred several days before testing.

F. RELATIONSHIP BETWEEN PCT AND FERTILITY

The postcoital test has also been correlated with occurrence of pregnancy. If the cervical mucus is good and an adequate number of active motile sperm are found at the time of the postcoital test, the pregnancy rate is significantly greater than if sperm migration is poor in the context of good cervical mucus.[22]

In a series of 555 infertile women reported by Jette and Glass,[23] the pregnancy rate was significantly higher in the presence of favorable cervical mucus and when there were more than 20 sperm per high-power field in the mucus as demonstrated on postcoital testing. These results were confirmed by Moghissi,[4] who performed a fractional postcoital test as a part of a complete infertility survey in 208 infertile women. Results of the best postcoital tests of 58 women who became pregnant were compared with the test results of 143 women who did not become pregnant. Excluded from the study were all women who had a definite impediment to fertility that could not be corrected and tests that were not timed to coincide with ovulation. Cervical scores were not significantly different in the two groups. Significantly more sperm were found on postcoital testing of women who achieved pregnancy than on postcoital testing of women who remained infertile. Since cervical scores in the two groups were comparable, the data indicated that a high number of sperm in cervical mucus is associated with a greater chance of pregnancy.

In another study, Hanson and Overstreet[24] analyzed the relationship of the number of motile sperm seen in cervical mucus 48 h after artificial insemination with a donor (AID) with subsequent fertility. They demonstrated a significant association between conception after AID and sperm survival for 48 h in the cervical mucus. Examination of their data suggested that when spermatozoa were consistently present in the mucus, there was a significantly higher probability of conception in that insemination cycle.

The lack of correlation of postcoital test results with the occurrence of pregnancy has also been documented in some studies. For example, Harrison,[25] in a study of 423 couples, found that the postcoital test was not a good indicator of fertility potential, since 24.5% of 98 women who had persistently negative postcoital test results achieved pregnancy.

In a more recent report, Collins and associates[26] evaluated the result of cervical mucus characteristics and postcoital test results with subsequent pregnancies. They found that cervical mucus characteristics has a significant association with postcoital sperm motility but not with pregnancy. Also, postcoital sperm motility in cervical mucus was strongly associated with total sperm count per ejaculate.

Other similar reports have appeared from time to time[27] in various publications and have created a certain degree of controversy and confusion relative to the validity and significance of postcoital tests. To assess these contradictory reports objectively, several facts need to be emphasized.

First, in humans, it is biologically impossible for spermatozoa to reach the site of fertilization without penetrating the cervical mucus and traversing the cervical canal. Second, without exception, all *in vitro* and adequately designed *in vivo* studies indicate that sperm are unable to penetrate viscous and hostile cervical mucus. Third, it is now well recognized that the sperm concentration and quality of most men are subject to considerable changes when serial semen analyses are performed.[1] These alterations are reflected in the results of postcoital or *in vitro* sperm-cervical mucus tests. Fourth, timing of the tests, technical differences, subjective interpretation, experience of the physician, and other variables may affect the test results. Finally, it should be realized that pregnancy results only when various factors involved in the reproductive process, in addition to sperm-cervical mucus interaction, are optimal. The mere presence of sperm in the cervical mucus cannot be equated with successful resolution of infertility. It remains to be determined whether sperm found in the mucus are capable of reaching the oviducts and fertilizing ovum.

IV. *IN VITRO* STUDIES

Negative or abnormal postcoital test results are indications for *in vitro* cervical mucus-sperm penetration tests. Three different techniques have been used for *in vitro* investigation of sperm penetration of cervical mucus; (1) the slide method, (2) the sperm-cervical mucus contact test, and (3) the capillary tube test.

The first two techniques are simple to perform and provide useful information. The capillary tube test is a more sophisticated form of analysis which provides a semi-quantitative measure of the level of sperm penetration into the mucus.

When performing tests *in vitro*, fresh semen not older than 1 h after ejaculation should be used.

A. THE SLIDE TEST

A drop of cervical mucus is placed on a slide and flattened by a coverslip (25 × 40 mm). A drop of semen is deposited at each side and in contact with the edge of the coverslip so that the semen moves under the coverslip by capillary force. In this way a clear interface is obtained between the cervical mucus and semen.

At the interface, finger-like projections or phalanges of seminal fluid develop within a few minutes and penetrate into the mucus. Most spermatozoa penetrate the phalangeal canal before entering the mucus. In many instances, a single spermatozoon appears to lead a column of sperm into the mucus. Once in the cervical mucus the spermatozoa fan out and move at random. Some return to the seminal plasma layer, while most migrate deep into the cervical mucus until they meet with resistance from cellular debris of leukocytes. In interpreting the tests, the number of spermatozoa per HPF from the interface are counted. The sperm within the phalanges should not be included in the result. Only those spermatozoa which are clearly within the substance of cervical mucus must be considered as having penetrated. To quantify the test,[28] the first microscopic field from the interface, called F_1, is counted (400× magnification) 5 and 15 min after the initiation of the test. The magnification used must be recorded with each test. In order to study the depth of penetration, the second microscopic field adjacent to the first one (F_2), and the third (F_3) can also be evaluated and the number of spermatozoa in these fields recorded (see Figure 5).

1. Interpretation
The results are evaluated as follows:

(a) Excellent: $\geq$ 25 sperm/HPF in F_1; $\geq$25 sperm/HPF in F_2
(b) Good: 15 sperm/HPF in F_1; 10 sperm/HPF in F_2
(c) Poor: 5 sperm /HPF in F_1; 0 to 1 sperm/HPF in F_2
(d) Negative: no penetration in F_1 or in F_2

When the purpose of the test is to compare the quality of various cervical mucus specimens, a single sample of semen with optimal count, motility and morphology should be used. On the other hand, when the interest is to evaluate the quality of several semen specimens, the same sample of cervical mucus should be used to assess the ability of spermatozoa to penetrate into it.

B. THE SPERM-CERVICAL MUCUS CONTACT (SCMC) TEST

The purpose of this test is to detect the presence of anti-sperm antibodies in cervical mucus and/or sperm.[29]

The SCMC test is performed by placing a small amount (e.g., about 10 to 50 µl) of preovulatory cervical mucus and an approximately equal amount of fresh semen on one end of a microscopic slide. The two materials are thoroughly mixed. Another drop of the same semen sample is placed on the other end of the slide. The semen-mucus mixture and the semen drop are covered with coverslips. The preparation is stored in a moist Petri dish at room temperature. After 30 min the percentage of motile spermatozoa that are rapidly shaking is determined. The semen alone served as a control for sperm activity. Immotile and slowly shaking spermatozoa are ignored. Spermatozoa shaking but moving slowly forward and shaking spermatozoa with intermittent forward movements are considered to belong to the shaking fraction.[2]

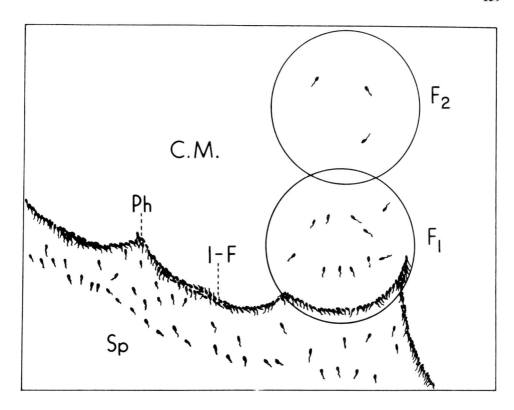

FIGURE 5. Schematic representation of the *in vitro* sperm-cervical mucus penetration (slide) test. CM, cervical mucus; SP, spermatozoa; IF, interface; Ph, phalanges; F_1, first microscopic field; F_2, second microscopic field adjacent to F_1 (From Moghissi, K., *Int. J. Fertil.*, 15, 43, 1970. With permission.)

1. Interpretation

The results are classified as follows:

(a) Negative: 0 to 25% shaking
(b) Weakly positive: 26 to 50% shaking (the result should be repeated)
(c) Positive: 51 to 75% shaking
(d) Strongly positive: 76 to 100% shaking

When a positive SCMC test is obtained using the husband's semen and the wife's mucus, crossover testing using donor semen and donor cervical mucus should be performed to identify whether the antibodies concerned are present in the semen or in the cervical mucus.

Although a high percentage of shaking is very specific for the present of anti-sperm antibodies, false-positive reactions can occur. The false-positive reactions are almost always due to cervical mucus factors.

C. THE CAPILLARY TUBE TEST

The test was originally designed by Kremer[30] and modified in 1980.[31] It measures the ability of spermatozoa to penetrate a column of cervical mucus in a capillary tube. Various types of capillary tubes have been used but those with a rectangular cross-section are recommended.

The Kremer sperm penetration meter (Figure 6) may be constructed in the laboratory as follows:

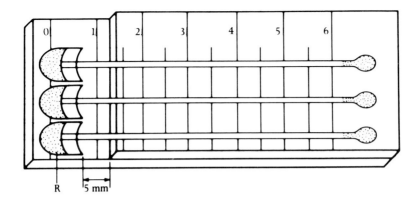

FIGURE 6.   The Kremer sperm penetration meter for capillary tube test of sperm-cervical mucus penetration.[2] (From World Health Organization, *Laboratory Manual for Examination of Human Semen and Semen-Cervical Mucus Interaction,* Cambridge University Press, Cambridge, 1987.)

1.   Glue onto a glass slide three reservoirs (R) with a semi-circular cross-section (radius about 3.5 mm).
2.   A second glass slide is then glued onto the first. The second slide is 1.5 cm shorter and is positioned at a distance of 5 mm from the reservoirs. This construction prevents creeping of the seminal fluid between the capillary tube and the glass slide. A centimeter scale is present on the second slide.

The glass capillary tubes may be obtained from Vitro Dynamics, U.S. They are rectangular in cross-section and are available in a variety of sizes. A depth of 300 or 400 μm and a length of 6 cm is appropriate for the capillary tube test.

1. Method
Fresh semen, not older than 1 h after ejaculation, should be used. Cervical mucus is aspirated into a capillary tube, making sure that no air bubbles are introduced. One end of the tube is sealed with plasticine or modeling clay. Application of the sealer forces a drop of mucus to protrude from the tube. The open end of the capillary tube is then placed on a slide so that it projects about 0.5 cm into the reservoir containing the semen sample. During the process of sperm penetration, the slide should be placed in a covered Petri dish with a damp sponge on the sides, to maintain humidity and prevent drying of the semen and mucus. The measurements are carried out preferably in a chamber with an ambient temperature of 37°C.

2. Assessment of the Test
After 2 h, the migration distance, penetration density, migration reduction, and presence of spermatozoa with forward motility are read.
The capillary tubes may be inspected again after 24 h for the presence of forward moving spermatozoa only.
Variables to be assessed after 2 h are defined as follows.

a. Migration Distance
The distance from the semen reservoir to the foremost spermatozoon in the capillary tube.

b. Penetration Distance
This is determined at distances of 1 and 4.5 cm from the semen reservoir. At each

TABLE 1
Order of Classes of Penetration
Density

Penetration density class	Rank order
0	1
0—5	2
6—10	3
11—20	4
21—50	5
51—100	6
>100	7

distance the mean number of spermatozoa per low power field (LPF; 10×10) is determined. The mean number is obtained from estimations of five adjacent low-power fields. The mean of the estimations is expressed in one of the penetration density classes (see Table 1). For the classification of the test, the highest penetration density class is recorded.

c. Migration Reduction

This indicates the decrease in penetration density at 4.5 cm compared to the penetration density at 1 cm. It is expressed as the difference in rank order number.

d. Examples

1. Penetration density at 1 cm is 51 to 100 and at 4.5 cm is 6 to 10. The migration reduction value is 3 (rank order 6 to rank order 3; Table 1).
2. Penetration density at 1 cm is 21 to 50 and 4.5 cm 51 to 100. The migration reduction value is zero because there is no decrease in penetration density.

Duration of the progressive movements—The presence in the cervical mucus of spermatozoa with forward motility may be determined after 2 and 24 h. The results are classified according to Table 2.

V. CORRELATION BETWEEN *IN VITRO* AND *IN VIVO* TESTS

A good correlation has been found between the results obtained by slide tests and capillary tube test techniques.[32] The results of *in vitro* sperm-cervical mucus penetration tests also correlate with sperm concentration, motility, percent morphology in semen samples, and the amplitude of the lateral head displacement about the axis of progression of the progressive spermatozoa.[33] Finally, there is a significant correlation among the results of postcoital tests, *in vitro* tests, and semen analysis findings.[34]

When both *in vivo* and *in vitro* tests are negative, normal donor sperm may be tested *in vitro* against the woman's cervical mucus, and preovulatory mucus obtained from a fertile donor should be tested with the man's sperm. This cross-match test will determine whether the sperm or the cervical mucus is responsible for abnormal results (Figure 1).

VI. INSEMINATION TEST

When postcoital tests are consistently negative but *in vitro* tests show adequate sperm penetration in cervical mucus obtained from the woman, an insemination test may be considered. In this test, the couple is instructed to abstain from intercourse for 2 days and to report at the time of anticipated ovulation. The ejaculate is allowed to liquefy and the woman

TABLE 2
Classification of the Test Results

Migration distance (cm)		Penetration density (spermatozoa LPF[a])		Migration reduction from 1 to 4.5 cm (Decrease in rank order number)		Duration of the progressive movements in cervical mucus (h)	Classification
1		0		—		—	Negative
<3	or	<10	or	>3	or	<2	Poor
All combinations of test results that cannot be classified as: negative, poor or good							Fair
4.5	and	>50	and	<3	and	>24	Good

[a] LPF = low power field (10 × 10).

is artificially inseminated with this sample, using the intracervical technique of insemination. Approximately 1 to 2 h later, samples of mucus from exocervix and endocervix are obtained and the concentration and quality of sperm are observed and recorded, using the technique described for postcoital test. If large semen volume, oligospermia, or liquefaction defects have previously been observed on semen analysis, the first portion (or better portion) of a split ejaculate may be used.

The results of postinsemination tests are interpreted in the same way as those of postcoital tests. If the postinsemination test shows 10 or more vigorously motile sperm per high-power field, one should suspect the presence of vaginal factor(s) or alterations of buffering capacity of seminal plasma and/or cervical mucus as contributing to early destruction of sperm in the vagina. This situation may be encountered particularly when the volume of the ejaculate is small and cervical mucus is scanty.

The results of postinsemination tests may also be used as a guide to management of the patient. If the test result is favorable, there is a good prognosis for attaining pregnancy with the use of homologous artificial insemination.

VII. USE OF BOVINE ESTRUS CERVICAL MUCUS AND SYNTHETIC MUCUS FOR *IN VITRO* TESTS

Bovine estrus cervical mucus may be used as a substitute for human mid-cycle mucus.[35,36] Bovine estrus cervical mucus is biochemically and functionally similar to human mucus. Human spermatozoa can enter bovine cervical mucus (BCM) readily *in vitro* and maintain good motility and viability for several hours.[37] The pattern and depth of sperm penetration in human cervical mucus (HCM) and BCM are very similar. Human sperm migrate somewhat more slowly in BCM than in HCM. A highly significant correlation between BCM penetration distance and sperm count, motility, velocity, motile density, and percent normal morphology has been demonstrated.[38] Similarly, the depth of sperm penetration in preovulatory HCM correlates significantly with that of BCM.[35]

The results of *in vitro* sperm penetration tests in HCM and BCM have also been compared with postcoital tests.[34] Postcoital test results correlate significantly with those from *in vitro* sperm penetration.

Commercially prepared capillary tubes containing standarized samples of bovine mucus are now available (PeneTrak Kit, Serono, Norwell, MA). The use of BCM can considerably facilitate testing of the ability of spermatozoa from a given man to penetrate normal cervical mucus and will provide a new means to evaluate the cause of an abnormal sperm-cervical mucus interaction. However, these tests are not meant to replace more specific *in vivo* or *in vitro* evaluation of couples sperm-cervical mucus interaction.

Urry et al. have also described the use of a synthetic or artificial cervical mucus (ACM) made of polyacrylamide gel for use as a substitute for cervical mucus in sperm migration tests. ACM was found to have characteristics similar to those of BCM. Penetration distance of the vanguard sperm was significantly greater in BCM than ACM, whereas sperm concentration at 5 and 10 mm distance in capillary tube testing was not different for either BCM or ACM.[39]

VIII. CORRELATION OF SPERM FERTILIZING ABILITY AND SPERM-CERVICAL MUCUS INTERACTION

Fertilization of zona-free hamster egg or sperm penetration assay (SPA) has been used to evaluate the ability of sperm to initiate fertilization. Comparisons have been made between SPA results and postcoital tests, HCM penetration, and BCM penetration. The correlation was significant between the postcoital test and SPA in a retrospective study of 79 infertile couples.[40] *In vitro* sperm penetration in HCM correlated more significantly with SPA. Similarly, a significant correlation between SPA and BCM penetration was found. When known fertile and infertile groups were tested, the mucus test predicted 74% correctly and the SPA predicted 90% correctly.[41]

Postcoital test results have also been compared with the results of *in vitro* fertilization. The findings indicated that spermatozoa that were unable to penetrate preovulatory cervical mucus were generally also unable to fertilize the human oocytes.[42]

IV. CONCLUSION

Evaluation of cervical factor and sperm-cervical mucus interaction must be an integral part of the studies performed on infertile couples and should be initiated before more invasive procedures are contemplated. The postcoital test determines the adequacy of sperm and receptivity of cervical mucus. It is the only test that evaluates the interaction between the sperm and the female genital tract fluids. Since cervical mucus accurately reflects the ovarian cycle, the postcoital test is also a useful indicator of endocrine preparation of the female reproductive tract. Finally, postcoital tests and sperm penetration studies assess an important functional aspect of spermatozoa which is not readily available from the results of semen analysis. When the postcoital test is abnormal, *in vitro* sperm-cervical mucus tests should assist the clinician in determining whether the sperm or the cervical mucus is responsible for abnormal results.

REFERENCES

1. **Poland, M. L., Moghissi, K. S., Giblin, P. T., Ager, J. W., and Olson, J. W.,** Variation of semen measures within normal men, *Fertil. Steril.,* 44, 396, 1985.
2. World Health Organization, *Laboratory Manual for Examination of Human Semen and Semen-Cervical Mucus Interaction,* Cambridge University Press, Cambridge, 1987.
3. **Moghissi, K. S.,** The cervix in infertility, *Clin. Obstet. Gynecol.,* 22, 27, 1979.
4. **Moghissi, K. S.,** Significance and prognostic value of postcoital test, in *The Uterine Cervix in Reproduction,* Insler, V. and Bettendorf, G., Eds., Georg Thieme, Stuttgart, 1977, 231.
5. **Insler, V., Melmed, H., Eichenbrenner, I., Serr, D. M., and Lunenfeld, B.,** The cervical score: a simple semiquantitative method for monitoring of the menstrual cycle, *Int. J. Gynaecol. Obstet.,* 10, 223, 1972.
6. **Tredway, D. R., Settlage, D. S. F., Nakamura R. M., Motoshima, M., Umezaki, C. U., and Mishell, R. R., Jr.,** Significance of timing for the postcoital evaluation of cervical mucus, *Am. J. Obstet. Gynecol.,* 121, 387, 1975.
7. **Sobrero, A. J. and Macleod, J.,** The immediate postcoital test, *Fertil. Steril.,* 13, 184, 1962.
8. **Moghissi, K. S.,** The function of the cervix in human reproduction, *Curr. Prob. Obstet. Gynecol.,* 7, 1, 1984.
9. **Davajan, V.,** Cervical factor, in *Reproductive Endocrinology, Infertility and Contraception,* Mishell, D. and Davajan, V., Eds., Davis Co., Philadelphia, 1979, 339.
10. **Grant, A.,** Cervical hostility, *Fertil. Steril.,* 9, 321, 1958.
11. **Hanson, F. W., Overstreet, J. W., and Katz, D. F.,** A study of the relationship of motile sperm numbers in cervical mucus 48 hours after artificial insemination with subsequent fertility, *Am. J. Obstet. Gynecol.,* 143, 85, 1982.
12. **Davajan, V. and Kunitake, G.,** Fractional in vivo and in vitro examination of postcoital cervical mucus in the human, *Fertil. Steril.,* 20, 197, 1969.
13. **Fredricsson, B. and Bjork, G.,** Morphology of postcoital spermatozoa in the cervical secretion and its clinical significance, *Fertil. Steril.,* 28, 841, 1977.
14. **Sujan, S., Danezis, J., and Sobrero, A. J.,** Sperm migration and cervical mucus studies in individual cycles, *J. Reprod. Fertil.,* 6, 87, 1963.
15. **Frenkel, D. A.,** Sperm migration and survival in the endometrial cavity, *Int. J. Fertil.,* 6, 285, 1961.

16. **Settlage, D. S. F., Matoshima, M., and Tredway, D.,** Sperm transport from the vagina to the fallopian tubes in women, in *Biology of Spermatozoa Transport, Survival and Fertilizing Ability,* Hafez, E. S. E. and Thibault, C. G., Eds., S. Karger, Basel, 1975.

17. **Ahlgren, M., Bostrom, K., and Malmqvist, R.,** Sperm transport and survival in women with special reference to the fallopian tube, in *Biology of Spermatozoa Transport, Survival and Fertilizing Ability,* Hafez, E. S. E. and Thibault, C. G., Eds., S. Karger, Basel, 1975.

18. **Templeton, A. A. and Mortimer, D.,** Laparoscopic sperm recovery in infertile women, *Br. J. Obstet. Gynaecol.,* 87, 1128, 1980.

19. **Asch, R. H.,** Sperm recovery in peritoneal aspirate after negative Sims-Huhner test, *Int. J. Fertil.,* 23, 57, 1978.

20. **Stone, S. C.,** Peritoneal recovery of sperm in patients with fertility associated with inadequate cervical mucus, *Fertil. Steril.,* 40, 802, 1983.

21. **Perloff, W. H. and Steinberger, E.,** In vivo survival of spermatozoa in cervical mucus, *Am. J. Obstet. Gynecol.,* 88, 439, 1964.

22. **Buxton, C. L. and Southam, A. L.,** Cervical physiology, in *Human Infertility,* PB Hoeber, New York, 1958.

23. **Jette, N. T. and Glass, R. H.,** Prognostic value of the postcoital test, *Fertil. Steril.,* 23, 29, 1972.

24. **Hanson, F. W. and Overstreet, J. W.,** The interaction of human spermatozoa with cervical mucus in vivo, *Am. J. Obstet. Gynecol.,* 140, 173, 1981.

25. **Harrison, R.,** The diagnostic and therapeutic potential of the postcoital test, *Fertil. Steril.,* 36, 71, 1981.

26. **Collins, J. A., So, Y., Wilson, E. H., Wrixon, W., and Casper, R. F.,** The postcoital test as a predictor of pregnancy among 355 infertile couples, *Fertil. Steril.,* 41, 703, 1984.

27. **Giner, J., Merino, G., Luna, J., and Aznar, R.,** Evaluation of the Sims-Huhner postcoital test in fertile couples, *Fertil. Steril.,* 25, 145, 1974.

28. **Moghissi, K. S.,** Cyclic changes of cervical mucus in normal and progestin treated women, *Fertil. Steril.,* 17, 663, 1966.

29. **Kremer, J. and Jager, S.,** The sperm-cervical mucus contact test: a preliminary report, *Fertil. Steril.,* 27, 335, 1976.

30. **Kremer, J.,** A simple sperm penetration test, *Int. J. Fertil.,* 10, 209, 1965.

31. **Kremer, J.,** In vitro sperm penetration in cervical mucus and AIH, in *Homologous Artificial Insemination (AIH),* Emperaire, J. C., Audobert, A., and Hafez, E. S. E., Martinus, Nijhoff, The Hague.

32. **Kremer, J., Jagers, S., and Kuiken, J.,** The meaning of cervical mucus in couples with antisperm antibodies, in *The Uterine Cervix in Reproduction,* Insler, V. and Bettendorf, G., Eds., George Thieme, Stuttgart, 1977.

33. **Mortimer, D., Pandya, I. J., and Sawers, R. D.,** Relationship between human sperm motility characteristics and sperm penetration into the human cervical mucus in vitro, *J. Reprod. Fertil.,* 78, 93, 1986.

34. **Hayes, M. F., Segal, S., Moghissi, K. S., Magyar, D. M., and Agronow, S.,** Comparison of the in vitro sperm penetration test using human cervical mucus and bovine estrus cervical mucus with the postcoital test, *Int. J. Fertil.,* 29, 133, 1984.

35. **Moghissi, K. S., Segal, S., Meinhold, D., and Agronow, S. J.,** In vitro sperm cervical mucus penetration: studies in human and bovine cervical mucus, *Fertil. Steril.,* 37, 823, 1982.

36. **Amit, A., Bergman, A., Yedwab, G., David, M., Homannai, T., and Paz, G.,** Penetration of human ejaculated spermatozoa into human and bovine cervical mucus. II. Pattern and velocity of penetration, *Int. J. Fertil.,* 27, 160, 1982.

37. **Gaddam-Rosse, P., Blandau, R. J., and Lee, W. I.,** Sperm penetration into cervical mucus in vitro: human spermatozoa in bovine cervical mucus, *Fertil. Steril.,* 33, 644, 1980.

38. **Keel, B. A. and Webster, B. W.,** Correlation of human sperm motility characteristics with an in vitro cervical mucus penetration test, *Fertil. Steril.,* 49, 138, 1988.

39. **Urry, R. L., Middleton, R. C., and Mayo, D.,** A comparison of the penetration of human sperm into bovine and artificial cervical mucus, *Fertil. Steril.,* 45, 135, 1986.

40. **Rogers, B. J.,** The sperm penetration assay: its usefulness reevaluated, *Fertil. Steril.,* 43, 821, 1985.

41. **Aitkin, R. J., Warner, P. E., and Reid, C.,** Factors influencing the success of sperm-cervical mucus interaction in patients exhibiting unexplained infertility, *J. Androl.,* 7, 3, 1986.

42. **Hull, M. G. R., McLeod, F. N., Joyce, D. N., et al.,** Human in vitro fertilization, in vivo sperm penetration of cervical mucus and unexplained infertility, *Lancet,* 2, 245, 1984.

Chapter 9

DETECTION OF AGGLUTINATING AND IMMOBILIZING ANTISPERM ANTIBODIES

Mary K. Korte and Alan C. Menge

TABLE OF CONTENTS

I. INTRODUCTION

The diagnosis of infertility has progressed considerably in recent years as witnessed by the numerous techniques described in this book. The role of immunologic infertility has become more defined as a greater number of laboratories have become involved in assaying for antisperm antibodies in response to the demands of human *in vitro* fertilization and intrauterine insemination procedures and the infertile patient's persistence at overcoming the condition.

As with many other causative factors, immunologic infertility due to sperm antibodies still lacks complete delineation in terms of etiology and treatment, however, diagnosis has progressed to the stage of fairly well characterized assays and repeatibility of results. Two assays that we have found to be reliable and rather easy to perform and interpret are the agglutination and complement-dependent immobilization of sperm cells. These can be applied not only to serum samples but also to genital tract secretions.

II. MEASUREMENT OF ANTISPERM AGGLUTINATING ANTIBODIES

Serum agglutinating antisperm antibodies are detected in infertility patients by the Kibrick macroscopic gelatin agglutination test (GAT);[1] the Franklin and Dukes microscopic tube-slide agglutination test (TSAT);[2] and the Friberg tray agglutination test (TAT).[3]

Friberg's tray agglutination test offers the following advantages over the gelatin agglutination and tube-slide agglutination tests: allows a large number of tests to be performed using a single donor sperm sample; allows differentiation between types of sperm agglutination (head-to-head, H-H; tail-to-tail, T-T; and head-to tail or mixed, H-T) and titrations are easily performed.[4] In a comparison between TAT and GAT, similar titers for T-T and H-T sperm agglutinins were found. The TAT, however, was found to be more sensitive (i.e., had higher titers) with respect to H-H sperm agglutinins.

As the Friberg TAT methodology was implemented in our laboratory certain drawbacks became apparent. The disposable microchambers (Møller-Coates AS, Moss, Norway) used were sometimes toxic to the sperm and often the sperm-serum mixture became displaced from the bottom surface of the plate. Much of the difficulty with obtaining consistent results seemed to be associated with the surface of the microchambers. In order to circumvent the problems which accompanied the use of these chambers, our laboratory adapted the use of a disposable 96 well Costar tissue culture cluster (#3696) to perform the TAT. Extensive comparisons using the TAT were made between the Møller-Coates disposable microchamber and the Costar tissue culture cluster. The modified method was also standardized with positive and negative serum agglutinating controls in order to evaluate the results obtained on the 96-well Costar tissue culture cluster. We concluded that the results obtained on the Costar tissue culture cluster were reliable and could be consistently reproduced. The microadaptation of the Friberg TAT is presented below in the clinical laboratory procedures section.

A. CLINICAL LABORATORY PROCEDURES
1. Materials

- 0.01 M phosphate-buffered saline (PBS)—pH 7.4
    $NaH_2PO_4 \cdot H_2O$ (MW 137.99)   1.9 mM
    $Na_2HPO_4 \cdot 7H_2O$ (MW 268.07)   8.1 mM
    NaCl (MW 58.45)   0.145 M
- Dextrose—0.01% in PBS
- Costar tissue culture clusters (catalog #3696)

- Hamilton micro-syringe model 1705 50 μl gas-tight (Hamilton Micro-Syringe Co., Anaheim, CA)
- Hamilton repeating dispenser model PB6001; dispenses 1/50 of syringes capacity
- Inverted microscope

2. Serum Specimen Collection

A 15 ml red or pink top tube of blood should be drawn from each patient. The sample may be drawn at any time from males. However, it is recommended that the sample be drawn during the interval between the cessation of menses and prior to the temperature rise at ovulation in females. Human serum at low dilution has been shown to contain a nonimmune globulin which causes agglutination similar to antisperm antibodies.[5] The serum factor is present in women more commonly in the luteal phase of the menstrual cycle, during pregnancy, and when taking oral contraceptives. It has been identified as a β lipoprotein-steroid conjugate. After the blood has clotted, serum should be drawn off and stored at $-20°C$ until tested.

3. Sperm Donor Criteria

Since the TAT involves the use of motile spermatozoa to detect the presence of antisperm antibodies. It is therefore necessary that the donor specimen used in the test system be of consistently good quality. The specimen should meet the following criteria: volume 3 to 5 ml, complete liquifaction within 30 min, ≥70% initial motility and 60% after 2 to 3 h, 3—4 forward progression, and ≥70% normal forms. The specimen should also be free from spontaneous agglutinates, debris, and other cell types such as white blood cells, red blood cells, and epithelial cells. Raw and diluted semen specimens should be protected from sudden changes in temperature and prolonged exposures to intense natural or artificial light. Specimens with low motility or poor forward progression may decrease the sensitivity of the test. Use of a single reference donor has the added advantage of reducing interassay variation.

Semen samples with a high concentration of sperm will be diluted further than samples with a lower concentration. This will aid in reducing the concentration of seminal plasma which may contain some competing cross-reacting antigens and anticomplement activity.

4. Methodology for Modified Friberg Tray Agglutination Test (TAT)

Sixteen test specimens may be screened on one tray at dilutions of 1:16, 1:32, and 1:64. The controls comprise 12 wells on the tray. Four hours should be allowed to complete the testing procedure.

1.   Patient serum samples to be tested are quick-thawed in a 37°C waterbath and heat-inactivated at 56°C in a waterbath for 45 min.
2.   Serial dilutions are made with PBS-Dextrose at 1:16, 1:32, and 1:64. Solutions should be prepared fresh before each assay.
3.   Thirty microliters of each diluted serum sample are transferred onto a 96-well Costar tissue culture cluster. The outer 36 wells of the tray are not used as the evaporation rate tends to be higher in the outer wells. It is also more convenient to set up a protocol using the inner 60 wells.
4.   Three microliters of filtered donor semen, adjusted to 40×10^6 sperm/ml in PBS-dextrose, are added to each well with a Hamilton repeating dispenser syringe. Raw donor semen is filtered through glass wool to removed debris and gelatinous clumps. A few drops of PBS-dextrose are used to wet the glass wool column[6] before the semen is added.
5.   The trays are then incubated for 2 h at 37°C in an air incubator. A humid chamber may be used to prevent evaporation.

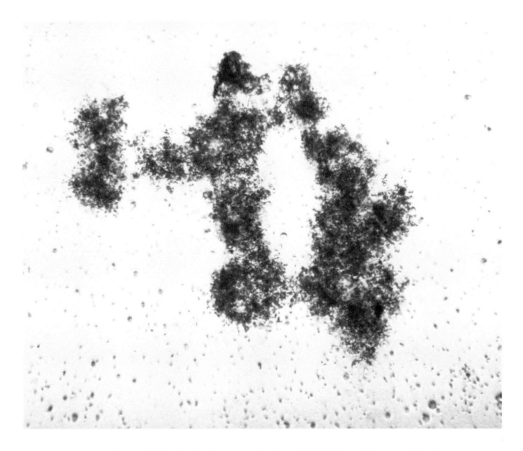

FIGURE 1.   Positive head-tail agglutination as seen in the modified TAT (original magnification was ×58).

6.   Results are read on an inverted microscope. The degree of agglutination is observed at low power magnification (×40 and ×100). High power magnification is used to assess the type of agglutination (×200).

The test serum is read as positive if an obvious agglutination of donor sperm is noted (Figure 1). The test results are scored negative when no agglutination of sperm is observed (Figure 2).

If the majority of sperm are agglutinated (≥75%), the test result is scored as 3 +. Large agglutinates together with free spermatozoa (≥50% and ≤75%) are scored as 2 +. Scattered but still apparent aggregates of agglutinated sperm (≤50%) are scored as 1 +. A patient's serum is considered positive for serum agglutinating antibodies if the sperm agglutination activity is observed in at least two dilutions, 1:16 and 1:32. If sperm agglutinating activity is observed at a dilution of 1:16 but not at 1:32, the patient's serum sample is retested at dilutions of 1:8, 1:16, and 1:32. When agglutinating activity is observed at 1:64, the patient serum is retested and titered at dilutions of 1:16, 1:32, 1:64, 1:256, 1:1024, and 1:4096. Patient serum is scored positive at the highest dilution in which 1 + agglutinating activity is observed. The type of agglutination is discerned using a high power objective (×200) (Figures 3 and 4).

5. Quality Control
A media control, PBS-dextrose used to make the serial dilutions, and a known negative control serum that has been tested as negative, are incorporated into the protocol to stand-

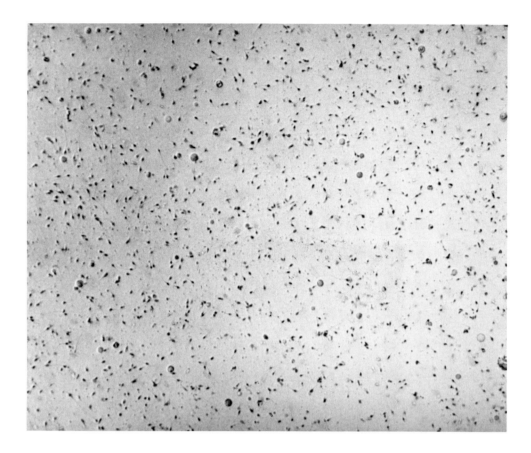

FIGURE 2.   Negative sperm agglutination as seen in the modified TAT (original magnification was ×58).

ardize and ensure validity of the test results. If there is agglutination in the media or negative control, the results are not considered valid and the test must be repeated. A known positive titered control is also included with the serum samples and titered to ensure the sensitivity and validity of the results. There should be agglutination of sperm to within one dilution of the serum observed. If there is no agglutination in the positive control or a difference of more than two dilutions, the results are not considered valid and the test should be repeated. Controls are stored at −70°C in 100 μl aliquots and thawed as needed.

In the event that a new control must be employed, it must meet the above criteria and titered with the old controls. Test serum specimens are initially screened at three dilutions 1:16, 1:32, and 1:64. A serum sample is considered negative if there is no agglutination at any dilution. Serum samples are recorded as positive when agglutination is observed in at least two dilutions. Serum samples positive at 1:64 are retested and titered i.e., 1:16, 1:32, 1:64, 1:256, 1:1024, and 1:4096.

6. Troubleshooting

Differences in serum titers may appear when samples are tested with another donor sperm sample. This is usually attributed to a variation in the quality of the donor specimen. To standardize the test and reduce interassay variation, its preferable that a single reference donor be used.

Occasionally nonspecific sperm clumping may be observed at lower dilutions of 1:16 and 1:32. This may be attributed to nonantibody factors in the serum, the donor semen quality, and in some cases the quality of test serum specimens. At high power, sperm

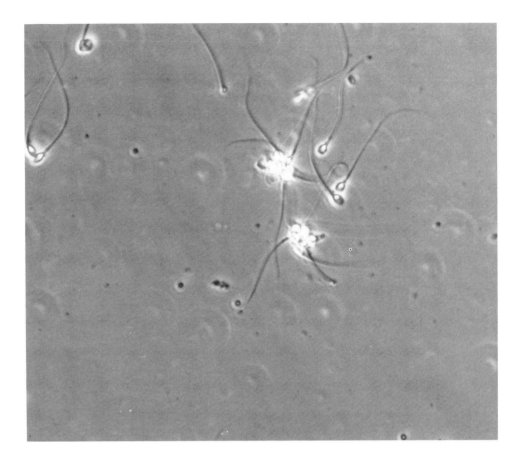

FIGURE 3.   Head-head agglutination of serum antisperm antibodies (original magnification was × 125, phase contrast).

clumping on debris or clumping of dead sperm may become visible. If not, it is recommended that the serum be retested at a dilution of 1:8.

In the event that sperm agglutination is observed in the PBS-dextrose control and/or the negative control the assay should be repeated. The donor reference sample should be checked for spontaneous agglutinates and new PBS-dextrose used. Agglutination can be caused by bacteria and some nonimmunoglobulin proteins in serum that may give false positive results especially at low dilutions.

III. MEASUREMENT OF SPERM CYTOTOXIC ANTIBODIES

The clinical evaluation of antisperm antibodies in the infertile patient should also include a method for the detection of sperm antibodies that are complement dependent. These complement-dependent antibodies may be of the IgM and IgG classes. In order for the complement to be fixed, antibody must form a complex with the antigen. The fixation or activation of complement results in an observable immobilization of the sperm cell or an uptake of dye. Isojima et al.[7] and Husted and Hjort[8] have published methods of detecting sperm immobilizing antibodies. A micotray modification of the Isojima sperm immobilization test is presented below in the Clinical Laboratory section.

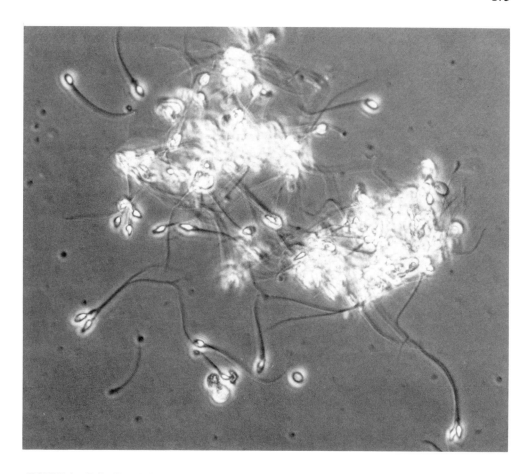

FIGURE 4.   Tail-tail agglutination of sperm by serum antisperm antibodies (original magnification was ×125, phase contrast).

A. CLINICAL LABORATORY PROCEDURES
1. Materials

- 0.01 M phosphate-buffered saline (PBS)—pH 7.4

$NaH_2PO_4 \cdot H_2O$) (MW 137.99)	1.9 mM
$Na_2HPO_4 \cdot 7H_2O$ (MW 268.07)	8.1 mM
NaCl (MW 58.45)	0.145 M

- Dextrose—0.01% in PBS
- Bovine serum albumin (BSA—0.5%) in PBS dextrose, used in the semen overlay technique
- Rabbit complement, Pel freeze Biologicals
- Lightweight mineral oil
- Lux tissue culture 60-well HL-A plates with a 0.01 ml working volume (catalog #5260)
- Hamilton micro-syringe model 1705 50 μl gas-tight (Hamilton Micro-Syringe Co., Anaheim, CA)
- Hamilton repeating dispenser model PB6001; dispenses 1/50 of syringes capacity
- Inverted microscope

2. Serum Specimen Collection
The serum specimen collection is the same as described above for the TAT.

3. Sperm Donor Criteria

The sperm donor criteria is the same as described above for the TAT.

4. Methodology for Sperm Immobilization Test (SIT)

Eight test specimens may be screened at dilutions of 1:4, 1:8, and 1:16 on one plate. The controls comprise 24 adjacent wells. Approximately 2 h should be allowed to complete the testing procedure.

1. Patient serum samples to be tested are quick-thawed in a 37°C waterbath and heat-inactivated at 56°C in a waterbath for 45 min.
2. Serial dilutions are made with PBS-dextrose (0.01%) at 1:4, 1:8, and 1:16.
3. Ten microliters of diluted serum test sample are transferred onto two adjacent wells of a Lux tissue culture 60-well HL-A plate.
4. One microliter of swim-up sperm (see below) at a concentration of 10×10^6 sperm/ml is added to each well with the Hamilton repeating dispenser.
5. One microliter of heat inactivated rabbit complement is added to the even numbered wells with the Hamilton syringe.
6. One microliter of pretested rabbit complement (see below) is added to the odd numbered wells.
7. Lightweight mineral oil is gently poured over the trays to cover the wells.
8. The trays are then covered and incubated at 37°C for 1 h.
9. Results are read using an inverted microscope at high power ($\times 100$).

The test serum is considered positive if the sperm immobilizing value of the sample is greater than two. The sperm immobilizing value (SIV) is calculated by observing motility for the sample with active and inactivated rabbit complement at the same serum dilution.

$$SIV = \frac{\text{\% motility of sample with inactivated complement}}{\text{\% motility of sample with active complement}}$$

Motility is observed using an inverted microscope under $\times 100$ objective and is judged as the percentage of sperm cells showing progressive movement.

Test results are scored negative if the SIV is less than two.

5. Quality Control

A serum overlay technique is used to insure high initial sperm motility. It also helps to alleviate the influence of seminal plasma. 0.5 to 1.0 ml of semen is layered under $\times 2$ the volume of PBS-dextrose buffer with BSA using a pasteur pipette.

The test tube is then incubated on a horizontal slant for 30 min at 37°C. After the incubation period the test tube is carefully withdrawn and allowed to settle for a couple of minutes, care being used to preserve the interface. The top layer which contains the highly motile sperm is withdrawn, counted and diluted to 10×10^6 sperm/ml.

Rabbit complement is used at a dilution that immobilizes the sperm 90 to 95% in the presence of antibody and that has no immobilizing activity in a control serum without antibody. The rabbit complement is assayed for activity using a checkerboard titration. Dilutions of the active rabbit complement, 1, 1:2, 1:3, 1:4, etc., are tested against known positive and negative controls.

A media control (PBS-dextrose buffer), a negative control, and a known titered positive control is tested with the patient serum sample. If known controls do not give the expected values then the assay is not considered valid and must be repeated.

Controls and complement are stored at -70°C in 100 μl aliquots and are thawed as used. In the event that new controls must be implemented, they are standardized against the old control and meet the above criteria.

Three serum dilutions are prepared with each sample, 1:4, 1:8, and 1:16. A serum sample is considered negative if the SIV is less than two at each dilution.

Each serum dilution with complement is standardized with a dilution without complement. Motility is compared between the two.

6. Troubleshooting

As seminal plasma contains anti-complement activity, the processing of the raw sample becomes important in standardizing the sperm immobilization test and obtaining consistent results. It is therefore preferable that a single reference donor be used when working with a lot of rabbit complement. It may be necessary to restandardize the complement with different donor sperm. When drawing off the top layer of motile sperm it is also important to avoid interrupting the raw sample-media interface and to avoid drawing up seminal plasma with the motile sperm. An increase concentration of seminal plasma may decrease the activity of the complement and thus decrease the sensitivity of the test.

Rabbit complement is heat labile and must be stored and processed with care. Complement is thawed in 37°C waterbath until a frozen sliver remains about one hour before use. Aliquots are stored at −70°C.

The TAT and SIT may also be used to measure seminal plasma agglutinating and cervical mucus immobilizing antisperm antibodies with minor modifications (see Chapter 10 for details on preparation of seminal plasma and cervical mucus).

REFERENCES

1. **Kibrick, S., Belding, D. L., and Merill, B.,** Methods for detection of antibodies against mammalian spermatozoa. II. A gelatin agglutination test, *Fertil. Steril.,* 3, 430, 1952.
2. **Franklin, R. R. and Dukes, C. D.,** Antispermatozoal antibody and unexplained infertility, *Am. J. Obstet. Gynecol.,* 89, 6, 1964.
3. **Friberg, J.,** A simple and sensitive micro-method for demonstration of sperm-agglutinating activity in serum from infertile men and women, *Acta Obstet. Gynecol. Scand. (Suppl.),* 36, 21, 1974.
4. **Friberg, J.,** Clinical and immunological studies on sperm-agglutinating antibodies in serum and seminal fluid, *Acta Obstet. Gynecol. Scand. (Suppl.),* 36, 21, 1974.
5. **Boettcher, B., Hay, J., Kay, D. J., Baldo, B. A., and Roberts, T. K.,** Sperm agglutinating activity in some human sera, *Int. J. Fertil.,* 15, 143, 1970.
6. **Paulson, J. D. and Polakoski, K. L.,** A glass wool column procedure for removing extraneous material from the human ejaculate, *Fertil. Steril.,* 28, 179, 1977.
7. **Isojima, S., Li, T. S., and Ashitaka, Y.,** Immunologic analysis of sperm-immobilizing factor found in sera of women with unexplained sterility, *Am. J. Obstet. Gynecol.,* 101, 677, 1968.
8. **Husted, S. and Hjort, T.,** Microtechnique for simultaneous determination of immobilizing and cytotoxic sperm antibodies, *Clin. Exp. Immunol.,* 22, 256, 1975.

Chapter 10

DETECTION OF ANTISPERM ANTIBODIES USING IMMUNOBEADS

Gary N. Clarke

TABLE OF CONTENTS

I. BACKGROUND

Since there are many reviews which discuss sperm antibodies and their role in infertility,[1-5] I need only make some brief points and observations by way of introduction to this chapter. First, there is considerable evidence that sperm antibodies impair fertility,[6-10] Secondly, sperm antibodies are detectable in either male or female partner in a significant (approximately 10%) proportion of couples presenting with infertility problems.[11,12] It is therefore essential that all couples being investigated for infertility should be adequately screened for sperm antibodies. The immunobead test (IBT) is a simple, sensitive and specific test for routine sperm antibody screening of semen,[11] cervical mucus,[12] serum,[13] or follicular fluid.[14] Research on the IBT for sperm antibodies was initiated in our laboratory in 1979 and descriptions of our initial work were published in 1982.[15,16] A slightly different version of this assay was developed independently by Bronson et al. (1982).[17] The IBT has since been widely accepted as a reliable screening test for sperm antibodies.[18-22]

The IBT is a technically simple assay for sperm-bound antibodies which in essence involves microscopic observation of bead/sperm mixtures to determine if the marker beads have bound to motile sperm (Figure 1). The immunobeads are microscopic polyacrylamide spheres (approximately 2 to 10 μm) which carry covalently bound rabbit antibodies directed against human immunoglobulins. Immunobeads are commercially available and are directed against whole human immunoglobulin (Ig) or against individual immunoglobulin classes (IgG, IgA, IgM). The IBT has distinct advantages over conventional tests for sperm antibodies because it can identify the immunoglobulin class(es) of the antibody, it provides information on the regional distribution of antibodies on the sperm surface and simultaneously allows determination of the proportion of antibody coated motile spermatozoa.

A major advantage of the IBT is that it allows the direct detection of antibodies bound to a patient's spermatozoa. This is important because sperm antibodies are unlikely to impair fertility unless they bind to the sperm surface. There is also good evidence indicating that locally produced antibodies of IgA class (? secretory IgA) are the main inhibitors of sperm function. [23-26] The IBT can be used for the detection of antibodies in serum or other fluids and can be semi-quantitated using titration procedures.[27] An IBT titer can be very useful for monitoring a patient's response to corticosteroid treatment.

Sperm antibodies may impair fertility by blocking cervical mucus penetration by spermatozoa,[25] by inhibiting fertilization,[28] or possibly by exerting an embryotoxic effect. The extent to which some of these effects are expressed is related to the antibody level, immunoglobulin class and regional specificity of the antibodies concerned. For example, tail-tip antibodies do not significantly affect cervical mucus penetration[29] or fertilization[30] and often occur in fertile individuals.[31-33] There is evidence that sperm-bound antibodies of IgA class are more effective at blocking *in vitro* fertilization (IVF) than those of IgG class.[30] There is also evidence that antibody titer is correlated directly with the severity of sperm functional impairment[34] and inversely with fecundability.[6]

The preliminary investigation of the male partner from an infertile couple should include an IBT to screen for sperm-bound antibodies. A positive result should be followed up with a repeat test and mucus penetration testing (see Chapter 8) to make a preliminary assessment of the functional significance of the antibodies. Selected men can be treated with corticosteroids to reduce their sperm antibody levels and to concomitantly improve sperm function.[35] The female partner should initially be tested for circulating antibodies. High levels of circulating antibodies may severely reduce the chances of successful treatment by IVF or donor insemination. Assessment of *in vitro* sperm-mucus interaction by means of the capillary (Kremer) test and/or the semen-cervical mucus contact test (SCMCT) may suggest the likely presence of sperm antibodies in CM even though circulating antibodies may have been weak or undetectable. The presence of antibodies in CM should be confirmed by indirect IBT on

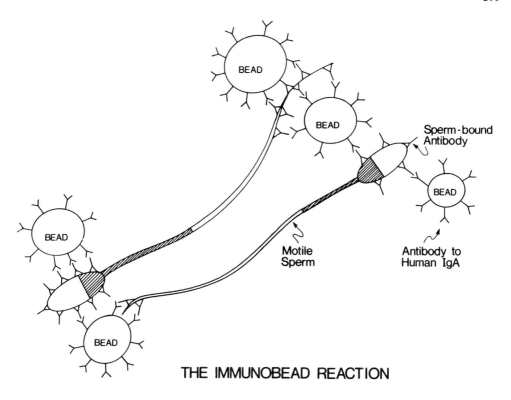

THE IMMUNOBEAD REACTION

FIGURE 1.   Diagrammatic representation of the interactions between immunobeads and motile spermatozoa in a positive IBT.

liquefied CM.[12] The presence of high cervical antibody levels and associated negative/weak circulating antibodies gives a good prognosis for treatment of the couple by intrauterine artificial insemination using husband's semen (AIH). On the other hand, the presence of high antibody levels both locally and systemically gives a poor prognosis.

This laboratory is now concentrating on the development of assays which will allow objective quantitation of sperm antibodies. Our aim is to use an objective assay to complement the IBT, rather than to supplant it. Thus, all our initial sperm antibody screening will still be performed by IBT, followed by quantitation of positive activity using a radioimmuno-binding assay (RIBA) or a modified enzyme-linked immunosorbent assay (ELISA). An objective assay will allow more accurate monitoring of antibody levels in patients' undergoing treatment, and enable us to investigate the relationship between antibody density on the sperm surface, and sperm function. Our preliminary work in this area is encouraging.[36] However, the first step for all semen laboratories is to establish a relatively simple assay such as the IBT before proceeding to objective (but in some ways less informative) assays such as the RIBA.

II. DETAILED PROCEDURES

A. EQUIPMENT

1.   Waterbath (56°C)
2.   Incubator (37°C)
3.   Autopipettes (2—10 μl, 10—50 μl, 40—200 μl, 200—1000 μl
4.   Microscope (phase-contrast optics, magnification ×200 and ×400)
5.   Centrifuge (to 1000 g)

TABLE 1
Composition of Tyrode Solution

Chemical	Formula	mg/100 ml
Sodium chloride	NaCl	800
Potassium chloride	KCl	20
Calcium chloride (fused)	$CaCl_2$	20
Magnesium chloride	$MgCl_2 \cdot 6H_2O$	10
Sodium dihydrogen orthophosphate	$NaH_2PO_4 \cdot 2H_2O$	6.4
Glucose	D-Glucose	100
Sodium bicarbonate	$NaHCO_3$	100

TABLE 2
Composition of Dulbecco's Phosphate Buffered Saline

Chemical	Formula	mg/100 ml
Sodium chloride	NaCl	800
Potassium chloride	KCl	20
Disodium hydrogen orthophosphate (anhydrous)	Na_2HPO_4	115
Calcium chloride (fused)	$CaCl_2$	10
Magnesium sulfate	$MgSO_4 \cdot 7H_2O$	12

6.   Conical centrifuge tubes, graduated to 10 ml
7.   Disposable 0.45 and 0.8 μm membrane filters
8.   Hemacytometer or Makler sperm counting chamber
9.   Freezer ($-30°C$ or below but preferably $-70°C$ for long-term storage of sera)

B. REAGENTS
1. Buffer
Tyrode solution or Dulbecco's phosphate buffered saline can be used as the buffer medium for the IBT. Both are available commercially from Commonwealth Serum Laboratories (CSL), Melbourne, Australia or from Gibco, Grand Island, New York, U.S. Alternatively, the buffers can be prepared in the laboratory. Only analytical reagent (AR) grade chemicals should be used in preparing the buffered solution (Tables 1 and 2). In order to prevent precipitation, it is important to dissolve calcium chloride separately in cold distilled water, then add this to the solution containing the other dissolved components. If not used within 24 h, the solution should be autoclaved or filtered to sterilize it.

2. Bovine Serum Albumin (BSA)
The source or purity of the BSA are unlikely to affect the performance of the IBT. However, it is important to obtain the BSA in dried or powder form without preservatives and to filter the dissolved BSA before use, as explained below. Preservatives such as sodium azide can affect sperm viability and some bacterial contaminants of crude BSA products can cause false positive interactions between immunobeads and spermatozoa. In this laboratory we have always used dried, unsterile BSA from the same company (CSL, catalog no.7441301).

3. Tyrode Solution Containing 0.3% BSA (TBSA)
TBSA is prepared on the day of use. For example, to prepared 300 ml of TBSA, weigh out 0.9 g of BSA, dissolve this in approximately 20 ml of Tyrode solution, then filter (0.45 μm Millipore) the solution into a conical flask and make up to 300 ml with Tyrode solution. Warm the mixture to 30 to 37°C before use.

4. Tyrode Solution Containing 5% BSA (TBSA-5)

TBSA-5 is prepared occasionally, aliquoted in 2 to 5 ml volumes and stored frozen (below $-30°C$). The BSA (5 g/100 ml) is weighed out, dissolved in Tyrode solution, filtered through a 0.45 μm Millipore filter, then aliquoted. A vial is removed from the freezer when required, thawed and warmed to 30 to 37°C before use.

5. Immunobeads

Immunobeads are obtained from Biorad Laboratories and consist of polyacrylamide beads of 2 to 10 μm diameter with covalently bound rabbit antibodies directed against human immunoglobulin classes (IgG Cat. No. 170-5100; IgA Cat. No. 170-5114). The beads are initially in dry form and are reconstituted by adding 10 ml of plain Tyrode solution (pre-filtered, 0.45 μm) to a bottle containing 50 mg of beads (i.e., 5 mg/ml working solution). After reconstitution, the beads can be used for up to 2 months if kept at 4°C. Because the beads contain sodium azide as preservative they must be washed once in TBSA immediately prior to use. This can usually be done at the same time as the second sperm wash.

6. Bromelain (Calbiochem Cat. No. 20376)

Bromelain is prepared occasionally and stored frozen at $-70°C$ in the freezer. Bromelain powder is weighed out and dissolved in Tyrode solution at a concentration of 2 mg/ml then aliquoted in 2 ml volumes before freezing. Bromelain is used to dissolve cervical mucus prior to testing.

C. DIRECT IMMUNOBEAD TEST (FIGURE 2) [11,16]

Application—To detect sperm-bound immunoglobulins of IgG or IgA immunoglobulin classes in a patient's semen sample. The direct IBT should be applicable to most semen samples with $> 2 \times 10^6$ sperm/ml and motile sperm present, assuming that the sample is of normal volume.

Positive control—Sera which are strongly positive ($\geq 90\%$) for IBT-IgG and IBT-IgA in the indirect IBT (see Section II. D) are occasionally pooled, aliquoted (100 μl) into 10 ml centrifuge tubes and stored frozen until used. On the day of use a tube is thawed, 50 μl of semen (best available on the day) is added and the mixture is preincubated at 37°C for 15 to 30 min.

Negative control—Transfer 50 μl of the positive control mixture to a separate tube, do not wash this tube. The free serum-derived immunoglobulins will inhibit any specific sperm-bead binding.

Procedure

1. Dispense an aliquot of the semen to be tested into a 10 ml plastic conical centrifuge tube. The volume of semen dispensed is determined by the sperm count and motility. The aliquot should preferably contain $5—10 \times 10^6$ motile spermatozoa.
2. The volume is then made up to 10 ml with TBSA. The TBSA should be prewarmed to 30 to 37°C and checked using thermometer.
3. The tube is centrifuged at $600 g$ (2000 rpm) for 5 min. The supernatant is then aspirated down to approximately 0.2 ml and the pellet is resuspended and made up to 10 ml again with TBSA. Aliquots (e.g., 0.2 ml) of the appropriate immunobead reagents can be washed at the same time as the second sperm wash.
4. Repeat centrifugation and finally resuspend the sperm and immunobead pellets in 0.2 ml TBSA-5. If the density of motile sperm is too low to obtain an accurate reading, then centrifuge again (*without* adding washing buffer), remove 150 μl of the supernatant, and set up the slide preparations again. If this fails then request a second semen sample to perform and indirect IBT on seminal plasma.

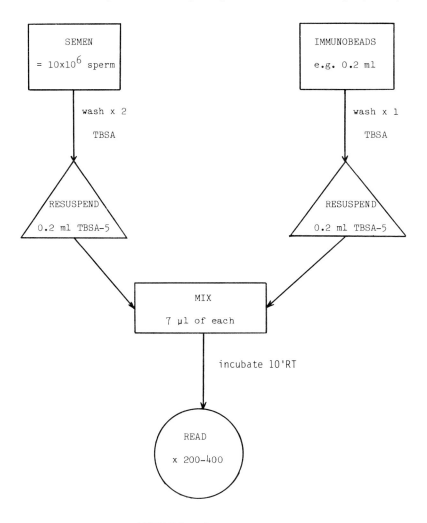

FIGURE 2.   Direct IBT protocol.

5.   The test is performed by mixing 7 μl of washed sperm with 7 μl of the appropriate immunobead reagent on a slide and covering with a standard (22 × 22 mm) coverslip. The slide is incubated at room temperature in a moist chamber for 10 minutes before reading under phase-contrast optics (×200 to 400). Set up slides for both IgG and IgA.

6.   A test is positive if ≥50% of the motile sperm have ≥2 attached beads. The percentage of motile sperm bound to beads is recorded and also the pattern of binding, i.e., head (H), tail mainpiece (M), tail endpiece (E) or all (A). Examples of positive and negative IBT reactions are shown in Figure 3.

D. INDIRECT IMMUNOBEAD TEST (FIGURE 4)

Application—indirect test is used to detect sperm antibodies in seminal plasma,[11] serum,[13] follicular fluid,[14] or cervical mucus.[12] In the past we have recommended preliminary screening of sera using immunobeads directed against whole human immunoglobulin (IBT-GAM), followed by secondary testing of positives by IBT-IgG, -IgA, and -IgM.[27] However, our experience over the last few years has led us to conclude that it is much more cost effective to simply screen for IgG and IgA class antibodies only. This is because sera are rarely positive for IgM class antibodies alone, and we do not believe that IgM class antibodies are of clinical significance.

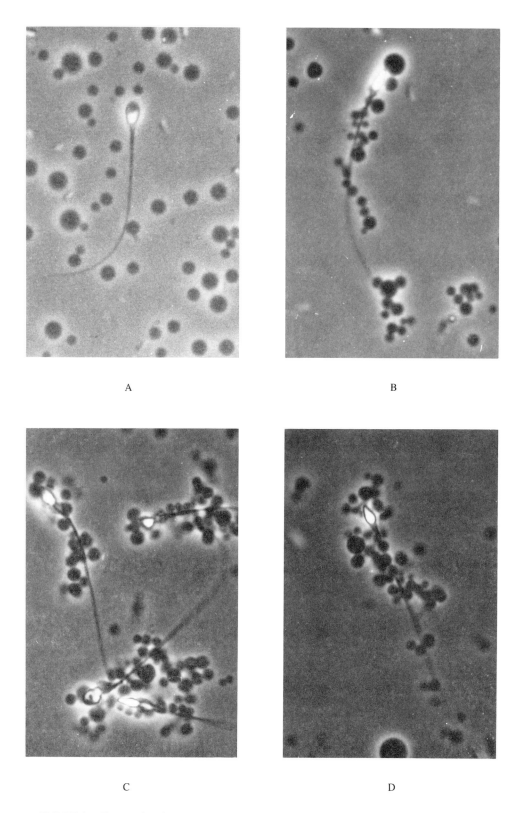

A

B

C

D

FIGURE 3. Photographs of negative (A) and positive (B—D) IBT reactions (magnification × 1200).

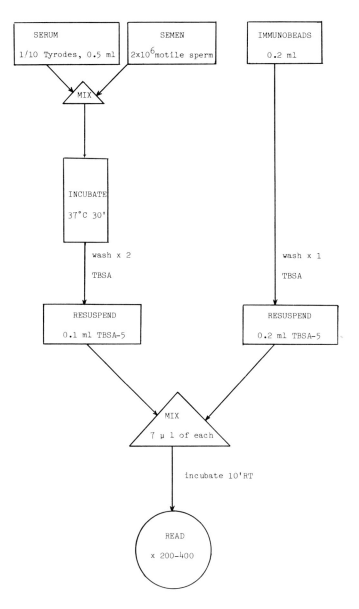

FIGURE 4.   Indirect IBT protocol.

Positive control—Sera which are strongly positive for IBT-IgG, and/or IBT-IgA, in the indirect IBT are occasionally pooled, passed through a 0.45 μm disposable Millipore filter, diluted 1/10 in Tyrode solution, aliquoted (500 μl) and frozen (− 70°C) until used. On the day of use a tube is thawed and processed with the batch of sera to be tested.

Negative control—Sera which are negative for IBT-IgG and IBT-IgA are pooled and processed as above.

E. SAMPLE PREPARATION
1. Seminal Plasma

An indirect IBT is performed on seminal plasma if there are not enough motile sperm to perform a direct test. Seminal plasma is prepared by filtering the semen through a 0.45 μm or 0.8 μm Millipore filter (disposable). Semen with increased viscosity must be syringed (see Chapter 3) before filtering. Seminal plasma can be tested without inactivation of complement. Dilute 0.25 ml seminal plasma with an equal volume of Tyrode solution to test. Store at $-70°C$ until tested.

2. Cervical Mucus

Cervical mucus is prepared by adding an equal volume of Tyrode solution containing 2 mg/ml of Bromelain and incubating the mixture at room temperature for 10 to 15 min with frequent shaking. Check the viscosity by dropping the solution from a pasteur pipette— if the drop hangs on at all then syringe the mixture several times. The mixture is then centrifuged at 600 g (2000 rpm) for 5 min to remove debris, and inactivated at 5°C for 30 min prior to testing. If not tested on the same day, then freeze at $-70°C$.

3. Serum or Follicular Fluid

Inactivate at 56°C for 30 min. Store at $-70°C$ until tested. The initial screening test is performed on sera diluted 1/10 in TBSA:

$$1/10 \ = \ 50 \ \mu l \ serum \ + \ 450 \ \mu l \ TBSA$$

Samples which are strongly positive (i.e., $\geqslant 80\%$ of sperm with attached beads for IgG, or IgA classes) at 1/10 dilution can then be titrated in tenfold steps and retested immediately:

- $1/100 \ = \ 50 \ \mu l \ of \ 1/10 \ dilution \ + \ 450 \ \mu l \ TBSA$
- $1/1000 \ = \ 50 \ \mu l \ of \ 1/100 \ dilution \ + \ 450 \ \mu l \ TBSA$

Procedure

Add 20 to 50 μl (approximately 2×10^6 motile sperm) of semen, previously found negative ($< 5\%$ of sperm coated) by direct IBT, to 0.5 ml of the fluid to be tested. Mix and then incubate the mixture at 37°C for 30 min. At the completion of incubation perform steps C2-C6 as described for the Direct Test except that final sperm resuspension is in 80 μl of TBSA-5. The Indirect Test can be semiquantitated as a titer by preparing tenfold dilutions of the fluid to be tested, then processing, as described above.

III. QUALITY CONTROL PROCEDURES

A. POSITIVE AND NEGATIVE CONTROLS

The procedures for generating positive and negative controls have been described in Section II. Pooled serum containing sperm antibodies is used to produce a positive control for the direct IBT. This is necessary because of the logistic problem of obtaining natural positive semen on a day to day basis. The negative control is generated by inhibiting specific immunobead binding with serum-derived immunoglobulins. Alternatively it might be feasible for some laboratories to use fresh or cryopreserved semen from an individual previously found to be negative by direct IBT. This would provide a 'true' negative control which would be preferable to the artificially generated control. In any case it is important to include a negative control with each test batch in order to determine if significant nonspecific bead-sperm binding may be occurring. The positive control demonstrates that the immunobead preparation is functionally intact—this controls against deterioration during storage or the possible introduction of extraneous factors, for example, if the technician accidentally used a buffer containing human serum the positive control would give a weak or negative result.

In the event of a weak positive control result, the following should be investigated:

1. The date of reconstitution of the immunobead preparation. If the immunobeads have

been reconstituted and stored at 4°C for more than 8 weeks, it would be advisable to discard them and open a new bottle. If the laboratory is testing small numbers of samples it would prove more economical to weigh out perhaps 10 mg of the lyophilized immunobeads instead of reconstituting the full 50 mg.

2. Examine the immunobead stock for fungal or bacterial contamination. Discard immunobead stock if contaminated.
3. Was the negative rather than a positive control tube mistakenly used?
4. Could the TBSA have been contaminated with human serum?
5. Was the incorrect buffer used by mistake?

In the event of positive results occurring in the negative control, the following should be investigated:

1. Bacterial contamination of immunobeads—discard stock if contaminated.
2. Bacterial contamination of TBSA—was the BSA filtered? Is the TBSA more than 24 h old or has it been maintained at 37°C for many hours? Prepared fresh TBSA if indicated.
3. Mix-up of control tubes?
4. Mix-up of slide preparations?
5. Was the semen sample heavily contaminated with bacteria? If so, repeat the IBT on a fresh semen sample.

Fortunately these problems are rare occurrences in a reasonably competent laboratory, but it is wise to be aware of the possibilities.

B. CROSSED-INHIBITION TEST[12,13]

This procedure may be useful for troubleshooting or as an extra proof that a positive IBT result is due to immunologically specific binding between immunobeads and sperm-bound antibodies. The inhibition test is performed as follows:

1. Add an equal volume of pure IgG or IgA (Calbiochem or Sigma, 2 mg/ml) to an aliquot of the appropriate immunobead preparation (e.g., anti-IgG immunobeads).
2. Incubate the immunoglobulin/bead mixture for 30 min at 37°C to allow binding between the rabbit anti-human IgG antibodies attached to the beads and the pure immnoglobulins added.
3. Retest the sperm preparation which was positive for sperm-bound antibodies of IgG class, but using the beads preincubated with pure immunoglobulin. A specific positive result for IgG should be inhibited by purified IgG, but not by IgA. Similarly, a specific positive for IgA class antibodies should be inhibited by pure IgA, but not by IgG. A dose-response curve depicting the inhibition of positive cervical mucus IgA-IBT reactions by purified human IgA is presented in Figure 5.

C. CROSS-REFERENCING

It is important for the scientist or technician performing the IBT to note if there are other indications of the presence of sperm antibodies, rather than relying entirely on a single test result. Did the patient have pronounced sperm-agglutination in his semen? Has he had a vasectomy reversal (vasovasostomy) operation performed? Did his sperm penetrate normal cervical mucus? Did they show the shaking phenomenon in the semen-cervical-mucus contact test (SCMCT)? Have any tests for circulating sperm antibodies been performed? Have the couple had negative postcoital tests (PCT)? Have they had unexplained poor fertilization results in IVF? Similar points need to be noted for a positive IBT for sperm antibodies in

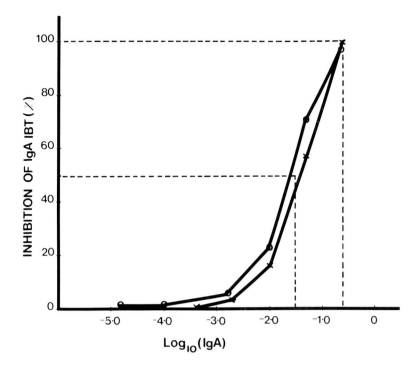

FIGURE 5. Inhibition of positive cervical mucus IgA-IBT reactions using purified human IgA. The curves represent the results of two experiments using mucus samples from two women with strongly positive IBT results.

cervical mucus. It is important to note that there is not an exact relationship between these variables and IBT results. Cross-referencing is a useful exercise however, particularly when establishing the IBT in your laboratory, because it will give confidence that the test is detecting sperm antibodies of clinical relevance, particularly when strong IBT results are obtained.

IV. INTERPRETATION OF RESULTS

Many clinicians seem to hold incongruously unsophisticated opinions regarding the relevance of sperm antibodies to infertility. They say something to the effect that "a patient with a positive sperm antibody results achieved a pregnancy, therefore sperm antibodies must be irrelevant". I have come to the conclusion that this may be largely due to the tendency of laboratories to test insufficiently diluted serum and to generally report weak results as positive. For example, many laboratories test undiluted or 1/4 diluted serum, when it is arguable that 1/10 should be the minimum serum dilution tested in order to minimize nonspecific factors, detection of natural antibodies and possible pro-zone phenomena. We consider 50% sperm-coating at 1/10 serum dilution to be the *minimum* indirect IBT result likely to have any clinical significance. This criterion will no doubt require modification as knowledge accumulates. I think that this is a conservative criterion, considering the sensitivity of the IBT. It is possible that 1/100 may be a more appropriate serum dilution to use. This may also vary with the immunoglobulin class of the antibody detected or being tested for.

With respect to the direct IBT, because of several considerations we think that a *minimum* of 50% of *motile* spermatozoa must be antibody coated for the IBT result to have any likely clinical significance. Firstly, from a statistical point of view, it is unlikely that sperm function will be significantly impaired if less than 50% of the motile are coated with antibodies. This opinion was confirmed by comparison of IBT results with IVF, cervical mucus penetration,

PCT and conception rates. In certain circumstances, even >90% sperm coating may not necessarily give a poor prognosis for fertility. This is particularly so if the sperm antibodies are predominantly restricted to the sperm tail-tip. Careful inspection of the slide preparation using phase-contrast optics ($\times 400$) often reveals that there is only one bead-sperm binding event at the tail-tip (clumps of beads are ignored unless more than once bead actually appears bound to the sperm). We therefore use the criterion of ≥ 2 beads bound to $\geq 50\%$ of sperm as the criterion of positivity which is likely to have clinical significance. However, this criterion alone is not sufficient to conclude that a patient has 'immunoinfertility' or 'sperm autoimmunity'. We restrict the use of these terms for cases where both sperm antibodies have been unequivocally detected, *and* there is evidence of poor cervical mucus penetration by spermatozoa and/or repeated negative PCT, suggesting functional impairment consistent with infertility or subfertility.

What is the appropriate course of action after sperm antibodies have been detected in either husband or wife, or both? If the antibody test was initially performed on the patient's serum, then the following steps should be followed:

1.   Repeat the indirect IBT on serum, including 1/100 and 1/1000 serum dilutions.
2.   Perform an IBT on semen or cervical mucus.
3.   If not already done, test for sperm/cervical mucus penetration.

If, *as is preferable,* tests for local antibodies have been performed first, then proceed as follows:

1.   Test for sperm/cervical mucus penetration.
2.   Repeat IBT tests on semen and/or cervical mucus.
3.   Test sera by indirect IBT.

How should the various results be interpreted in order to advise and treat the couple for their infertility problem? If a man has a positive direct IBT associated with a poor capillary (Kremer) test result (<3) cm penetration in 2 h), then the patient can be treated with corticosteroids such as prednisolone.[35] However, before proceeding it is imperative that the female partner is thoroughly evaluated to ascertain whether she is ovulating, has patent fallopian tubes and does not have endometriosis. If indicated, she may require prior or concomitant treatment to ensure optimal chances for a successful outcome. The man must be thoroughly screened and counseled regarding the possible side effects of corticosteroid treatment. Any evidence of a peptic ulcer, high blood pressure, tuberculosis, diabetes, or any serious illness is a contraindication for corticosteroid treatment.

What course should be followed if the female partner has sperm antibodies? If the patient has a positive indirect IBT for IgA class antibodies in cervical mucus, associated with poor cervical mucus penetration results, but relatively low titer (<1/100) circulating antibodies, then the patient has a reasonable chance of conceiving by intrauterine insemination of husband's semen or washed spermatozoa (assuming essentially normal semen quality). High titer antibodies (>1/1000) give a generally poor prognosis.

V. FUTURE DIRECTIONS

A. DIAGNOSTIC PROCEDURES

The IBT is a sensitive and specific test for detection of sperm antibodies in serum or reproductive tract secretions. It detects only those antibodies which react with native (i.e., unfixed) surface antigens on motile sperm. This is a crucial requirement for diagnostic sperm

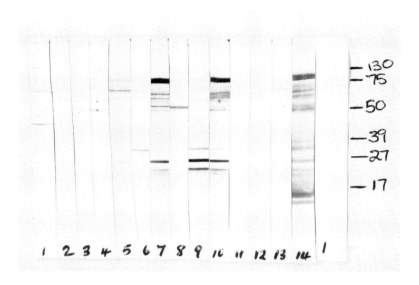

FIGURE 6. Comparison of western blotting and IBT. IBT negative sera were used for lanes 1,2,5,6, and 7, and high titer (>1/1000) positive sera for lanes 3,4,8,9, and 10. The other lanes were controls. The positions of molecular weight markers are indicated down the right side.

antibody screening assays. Assays which use extracted or fixed antigens will often detect antibodies reacting with subsurface or sequestered determinants.[37] which are not accessible in the spermatozoa *in vivo* and therefore are of no diagnostic significance. Thus, a number of laboratories have reported extremely poor correlation between 'fixed antigen' and 'live antigen' assays.[37-39] We have observed complete lack of correlation between a commercially available ELISA kit (ZER, Israel) and the IBT[39] Preliminary experiments have also demonstrated poor correlation between standard Western blotting procedures and IBT. Sera which are negative for surface reacting antibodies by IBT often give positive results by Western blotting (Figure 6). It is of course feasible that antibodies to some internal antigens (? inner acrosomal membrane or acrosomal enzymes) may play a role in immunofertility and this area should be investigated further. However, for the moment I believe it is safer to use live sperm assays for diagnostic screening purposes.

Although the IBT is an excellent screening test, it does not allow objective quantitation of antibodies bound to the spermatozoa. Titration using a tenfold dilution series gives a valuable indication of antibody levels in serum or other fluids, but it lacks sensitivity for patient monitoring. We have therefore developed the protein G assay (PGA)[36] which allows objective and specific quantitation of IgG class antibodies by using [^{125}I]-protein G as the radioligand. The PGA correlates well with the IBT titers in serum, suggesting that these assays are detecting the same antibodies. Current investigations are aimed at improving the PGA and development of a similar assay for IgA class antibodies. Parslow et al.[24] have reported a double layer antibody procedure which allows quantitation of IgA on the sperm surface. Using this procedure they found an inverse relationship between the amount of IgA and secretory piece on sperm and cervical mucus penetration. The drawback of their procedure is that it requires multiple centrifugation/washing cycles which will prohibit its routine use. We are therefore trying to develop a quantitative IgA assay which is faster and less tedious, and therefore more amenable to routine application. The availability of more sophisticated diagnostic procedures is essential for increasing our understanding of immunoinfertility.

B. TREATMENT

The traditional treatment for sperm autoimmunity has involved the use of immunosuppressive doses of corticosteroids such as prednisolone taken continuously[35] or intermittently.[40] This therapy is successful in helping approximately 25% of men with definite immunoinfertility to impregnate their partners. However, this treatment is only suitable for men who are in good health. Unpleasant side-effects lead some men to discontinue treatment and it is not advisable to continue treatment for extended periods. It would be preferable if *in vitro* procedures could be developed for treating the patients' semen to overcome their infertility. Initial attempts using ejaculation directly into a physiological buffer looked promising,[41] but more recent results are discouraging (Dr. David Kay, personal communication).

Several other approaches have significant potential for therapeutic use in this area. Bronson's laboratory has been investigating enzymatic treatment to remove sperm-bound antibodies.[42] Treatment with IgA-protease, which is specific for IgA class immunoglobulins, removes IgA antibodies as assessed by IBT, and allows improved cervical mucus penetration by the treated spermatozoa.[42] Further investigation is required to assess the fertilizing capacity of antibody-coated sperm before and after enzyme treatment. This approach could be used to treat sperm prior to their use in IVF or artificial insemination, especially if highly purified gene-cloned enzyme becomes available. This is likely since four different laboratories have now cloned the IgA-protease gene.[43]

Another possible *in vitro* procedure involves the application of immunoaffinity chromatography to selectively remove spermatozoa which are heavily antibody coated, thereby enriching the unbound population of less heavily coated sperm.[44] This approach relies on the veracity of the assumption that there is heterogeneity in antibody density on the surface of different sperm. Our observations with immunobead labeling suggest that this assumption is reasonable. Initial experiments using an anti-IgA affinity column have shown some promise. We will publish a detailed report on this work shortly.

VI. SUMMARY

Sperm antibodies are detected in one or both partners in approximately 10% of couples presenting with infertility/subfertility. It is therefore essential that routine sperm antibody screening be performed during initial investigations of infertile couples. The IBT provides a rapid, robust, specific and sensitive procedure which is applicable to routine screening of these patients. The IBT can be used for detection of sperm-bound antibodies in a patient's serum, or for detection of free sperm antibodies in semen, cervical mucus, follicular fluid or seminal plasma. We are now attempting to develop assays which will allow quantitation of sperm antibodies initially detected by IBT screening. These assays may allow more refined assessment of patients and better monitoring ability during treatment protocols.

REFERENCES

1. **Menge, A. C.,** Clinical immunologic infertility: diagnostic measures, incidence of antisperm antibodies, fertility and mechanisms, in *Immunological Aspects of Infertility and Fertility Regulation,* Dhindsa, D. S. and Schumacher, G. F. B., Eds., Elsevier– North Holland, 1980, 205.
2. **Bronson, R., Cooper, G., and Rosenfeld, D.,** Sperm antibodies: their role in infertility, *Fertil. Steril.,* 42, 171, 1984.
3. **Shulman, S.,** Autoimmune aspects of human reproduction, *Conc. Immunopathol.,* 2, 189, 1985.
4. **Haas, G. G. and Beer, A. E.,** Immunologic influences on reproductive biology: sperm gametogenesis and maturation in the male and female tracts, *Fertil. Steril.,* 46, 753, 1986.
5. **Alexander, N. J. and Anderson, D. J.,** Immunology of semen, *Fertil. Steril.,* 47, 192, 1987.

6. **Rumke, P., Amstel, N. V., Messer, E. N., and Bezemer, P. D.,** Prognosis of fertility of men with sperm agglutinins in the serum, *Fertil. Steril.,* 25, 393, 1974.

7. **Menge, A. C., Medley, N. E., Mangione, C. M., and Dietrich, J. W.,** The incidence and influence of antisperm antibodies in infertile human couples on sperm-cervical mucus interactions and subsequent fertility, *Fertil. Steril.,* 38, 439, 1982.

8. **Rumke, P., Renckens, C. N. M., Bezemer, P. D., and Amstel, N. V.,** Prognosis of fertility in women with unexplained infertility and sperm agglutinins in the serum, *Fertil. Steril.,* 42, 561, 1984.

9. **Ayvaliotis, B., Bronson, R., Rosenfeld, D., and Cooper, G.,** Conception rates in couples where autoimmunity to sperm is detected, *Fertil. Steril.,* 43, 739, 1985.

10. **Witkin, S. S. and David, S. S.,** Effect of sperm antibodies on pregnancy outcome in a subfertile population, *Am. J. Obstet. Gynecol.,* 158, 59, 1988.

11. **Clarke, G. N., Elliott, P. J., and Smaila, C.,** Detection of sperm antibodies in semen suing the immunobead test: a survey of 813 consecutive patients, *Am. J. Reprod. Immunol. Microbiol.,* 7, 118, 1985.

12. **Clarke, G. N., Stojanoff, A., Cauchi, M. N., McBain, J. C., Speirs, A. L., and Johnston, W. I. H.,** Detection of antispermatozoal antibodies of IgA class in cervical mucus, *Am. J. Reprod. Immunol.,* 5, 61, 1984.

13. **Clarke, G. N., Stojanoff, A., Cauchi, M. N., and Johnston, W. I. H.,** The immunoglobulin class of antispermatozoal antibodies in serum, *Am. J. Reprod. Immunol. Microbiol.,* 7, 143, 1985.

14. **Clarke, G. N., Hsieh, C., Koh, S. H., and Cauchi, M. N.,** Sperm antibodies, immunoglobulins and complement in human follicular fluid, *Am. J. Reprod. Immunol. Microbiol.,* 5, 179, 1984.

15. **Clarke, G. N. and Baker, H. W. G.,** Treatment of sperm antibodies in infertile men: sperm antibody coating and mucus penetration, in *Proc. Int. Symp. Immunology of Reproduction,* Bratanov, K., Ed., Bulgarian Academy of Sciences Press, Bulgaria, 1982, 337.

16. **Clarke, G. N., Stojanoff, A., and Cauchi, M. N.,** Immunoglobulin class of sperm-bound antibodies in semen, in *Proc. Int. Symp. Immunology of Reproduction,* Bratanov, K., Ed., Bulgarian Academy of Sciences Press, Bulgaria, 1982, 482.

17. **Bronson, R. A., Cooper, G. W., and Rosenfeld, D. L.,** Correlation between regional specificity of antisperm antibodies to the spermatozoan surface and complement-mediated sperm immobilization, *Am. J. Reprod. Immunol. Microbiol.,* 2, 222, 1982.

18. **Pretorius, E., Franken, D. R., Shulman, S., and Gloeb, J.,** Sperm cervical mucus contact test and immunobead test for sperm antibodies, *Arch. Androl.,* 16, 199, 1986.

19. **Jennings, M. G., McGowan, M. P., and Baker, H. W. G.,** Immunoglobulins on human sperm: validation of a screening test for sperm autoimmunity, *Clin. Reprod. Fertil.,* 3, 335, 1985.

20. **Junk, S. M., Matson, P. L., O'Halloran, F., and Yovich, J. L.,** Use of immunobeads to detect human antispermatozoal antibodies, *Clin. Reprod. Fertil.,* 4, 199, 1986.

21. **Adeghe, J. A., Cohen, J., and Sawers, S. R.,** Relationship between local and systemic autoantibodies to sperm, and evaluation of immunobead test for sperm surface antibodies, *Acta Eur. Fertil.,* 17, 99, 1986.

22. **Pattinson, H. A. and Mortimer, D.,** Prevalence of sperm surface antibodies in the male partners of infertile couples as determined by immunobead screening, *Fertil. Steril.,* 48, 466, 1987.

23. **Jager, S., Kremer, J., Kuiken, J., and Van Stochteren-Dradisma, T.,** Immunoglobulin class of antispermatozoal antibodies from infertile men and inhibition of in vitro sperm penetration into cervical mucus, *Int. J. Androl.,* 3, 1, 1980.

24. **Parslow, J. M., Poulton, T. A., Besser, G. M., and Hendry, W. F.,** The clinical relevance of classes of immunoglobulins on spermatozoa from infertile and vasovasostomized males, *Fertil. Steril.,* 43, 621, 1985.

25. **Clarke, G. N.,** Immunoglobulin class and regional specificity of antispermatozoal antibodies blocking cervical mucus penetration by human spermatozoa, *Am. J. Reprod. Immunol. Microbiol.,* 16, 135, 1988.

26. **Hjort, T.,** Immune subfertility caused by anti-sperm antibodies: an IgA mediated disease?, *Res. Reprod.,* 10, 1, 1988.

27. **Clarke, G. N.,** An improved immunobead test procedure for detecting sperm antibodies in serum, *Am. J. Reprod. Immunol. Microbiol.,* 13, 1, 1987.

28. **Clarke, G. N., Hyne, R. V., Du Plessis, Y., and Johnston, W. I. H.,** Sperm antibodies and human in vitro fertilization, *Fertil. Steril.,* 49, 1018, 1988.

29. **Wang, C., Baker, H. W. G., Jennings, M. G., Burger, H. G., and Lutjen, P.,** Interaction between human cervical mucus and sperm surface antibodies, *Fertil. Steril.,* 44, 484, 1985.

30. **Clarke, G,. N., Lopata, A., McBain, J. C., Baker, H. W. G., and Johnston, W. I. H.,** Effect of sperm antibodies in males on human in vitro fertilization (IVF), *Am. J. Reprod. Immunol.,* 8, 62, 1985.

31. **Hammitt, D. G., Muench, M. M., and Williamson, R. A.,** Antibody binding to greater than 50% of sperm at the tail tip does not impair male fertility, *Fertil. Steril.,* 49, 174, 1988.

32. **Jager, S., Rumke, P., and Kremer, J.,** A fertile man with a high sperm agglutination titer in the seminal plasma: a case report, *Am. J. Reprod. Immunol. Microbiol.,* 15, 29, 1987.

33. **Clarke, G. N.,** Sperm antibodies in normal men: association with a history of nongonococcal urethritis (NGU), *Am. J. Reprod. Immunol. Microbiol.,* 12, 31, 1986.

34. **Fjallbrant, B.,** Interrelation between high levels of sperm antibodies, reduced penetration of cervical mucus by spermatozoa and sterility in men, *Acta Obstet. Gynecol. Scand.,* 47, 102, 1968.

35. **Baker, H. W. G., Clarke, G. N., Hudson, B., McBain, J. C., McGowan, M. P., and Pepperell, R. J.,** Treatment of sperm autoimmunity in men, *Clin. Reprod. Fertil.,* 2, 55, 1983.

36. **Clarke, G. N.,** A simple radioimmunobinding assay for quantitation of sperm antibodies of IgG immunoglobulin class, *Am. J. Reprod. Immunol. Microbiol.,* 18, 1, 1988.

37. **Haas, G. G., DeBault, L. E., D'Cruz, O., and Shuey, R.,** The effect of fixatives and/or air-drying on the plasma and acrosomal membranes of human sperm, *Fertil. Steril.,* 50, 487, 1988.

38. **Stredonska-Clark, J., Clark, D. A., and Hendry, W. F.,** Antisperm antibodies detected by ZER enzyme-linked immunosorbent assay kit are not those detected by tray agglutination test, *Am. J. Reprod. Immunol. Microbiol.,* 13, 76, 1987.

39. **Clarke, G. N.,** Lack of correlation between the immunobead test (IBT) and the enzyme-linked immunosorbent assay (ELISA) for sperm antibody detection, *Am. J. Reprod. Immunol. Microbiol.,* 18, 2, 1988.

40. **Hendry, W. F., Treehuba, K., Hughes, L., Stredonska, J., Parslow, J. M., Wass, J. A. H., and Besser, G. M.,** Cyclic prednisolone therapy for male infertility associated with autoantibodies to spermatozoa, *Fertil. Steril.,* 45, 249, 1986.

41. **Boettcher, B., Kay, D. J., and Fitchett, S. B.,** Successful treatment of male infertility caused by antispermatozoal antibodies, *Med. J. Aust.,* 2, 471, 1982.

42. **Bronson, R. A., Cooper, G. W., Rosenfeld, D. L., Gilbert, J. V., and Plaut, A. G.,** The effect of IgA$_1$ protease on immunoglobulins bound to the sperm surface and sperm cervical penetrating ability, *Fertil. Steril.,* 47, 985, 1987.

43. **Pohlner, J., Halter, R., Beyreuther, K., and Meyer, T. F.,** Gene structure and extracellular secretion of *Neisseria gonorrheae* IgA protease, *Nature,* 325, 458, 1987.

44. **Kiser, G. C., Alexander, N. J., Fuchs, E. F., and Fulgham, D. L.,** In vitro immune absorption of antisperm antibodies with immunobead-rise, immunomagnetic, and immunocolumn separation techniques, *Fertil. Steril.,* 47, 466, 1987.

Chapter 11

SPERMATOZOA WASHING AND CONCENTRATION TECHNIQUES

David L. Fulgham and Nancy J. Alexander

TABLE OF CONTENTS

I. INTRODUCTION

The semen analysis is one of the first and the least expensive diagnostic procedure that can be performed on the husband of a couple presenting for an infertility work-up. Unless the sample is azoospermic or severely oligozoospermic, the results often are not adequate to discern the presence of male factor problems. Since systemic approaches to treatment of males are of limited value, therapeutic procedures often involve sperm manipulation and artificial insemination (vaginal, intracervical, intrauterine, intraperitoneal), gamete intrafallopian transfer (GIFT), *in vitro* fertilization (IVF) and embryo transfer (ET), or sperm microinjection into the egg.

The focus of this chapter is to describe laboratory techniques of sperm processing in order to improve various parameters (i.e., concentration, motility) or to select particular sperm subsets (i.e., X-Y separation, antibody-free sperm from antibody-bound sperm, capacitated sperm from acrosome-reacted sperm). Although these procedures usually improve sperm quality (e.g., increasing the percentage with progressive motility), the fertility potential of the treated sperm is not necessarily increased. In fact, processing of sperm may decrease fertility potentials. For example, sperm longevity is reduced after repeated centrifugation. Furthermore, processing for a technique may differ from that for IVF. The ability of sperm to capacitate, acrosome react, bind to the oocyte plasma membrane, penetrate, and finally to undergo nuclear decondensation can be assessed in the hamster egg penetration test (refer to Chapter 7). However, the clinician performing *in vitro* fertilization does not generally process sperm in the same manner as for the hamster egg penetration assay.

This chapter describes the processing of semen for artificial insemination, methods for concentrating sperm recovery of sperm from retrograde ejaculates, and the selection of X- or Y-bearing sperm for gender preselection. Efforts have been made to cross-reference the procedures so that this chapter can be used at the bench top.

II. PREPARATION OF SPERMATOZOA FOR ARTIFICIAL INSEMINATION

Before performing manipulation of a semen sample, previous semen analysis results must be available so that the expected ejaculate quality can be anticipated. Before collection, usually 2 to 3 days of abstinence is requested. The sample is provided by masturbation and, whenever possible, on site so that the sperm can be processed immediately. A clean glass or sterile plastic container with a lid is used to collect the ejaculate. The container should be of sufficient volume and size for ease of collection. If necessary, non spermicidal condoms may be used to obtain postcoital semen sample (Silastic Seminal Fluid Collection Device, HD corporation, Mountain View, CA). Since postcoital semen samples may be superior to those collected by masturbation,[1,2] a patient with a sample of marginal quality might produce a better sample through the use of these condoms.

Semen is not a sterile fluid and both aerobic and anaerobic bacteria are common[3] (refer to Chapter 14). In addition, other cell types are usually present in ejaculate including macrophages and lymphocytes.[4,5] Extracellular debris and/or sloughed (epithelial) cells may be found in semen samples. It is not, however, common to find fungi or red blood cells.

Soon after ejaculation, the seminal fluid coagulates and then usually liquefies within 30 min at 37°C. The physiological state of human sperm obtained at ejaculation is asynchronous; sperm of different states of maturation, i.e., pre-capacitated, capacitated, or acrosome-reacted[6] will be found. The longer sperm reside in seminal plasma, the less fertile they become relative to certain procedures.[7] Whether decapacitation factor(s) in seminal plasma play a role is not clear. While capacitation is reversible, the acrosome reaction results in the fusion of the plasma membrane and outer acrosomal membrane and is irreversible.

Sperm motility is a function of temperature[8] and requires an energy source (fructose or glucose). Serum-free media may be used for short term sperm incubation, but for lengthy incubations, serum is required as well as sperm concentrations not exceeding 10^6/ml. The requirement of serum is especially important when sperm are incubated under tissue culture conditions (i.e., 5% CO_2 in air at 37°C).

A plethora of buffers and media have been used in sperm processing and generally, substitution of one for another is feasible. However, human sperm that have swum-up into Baker's buffer[9] without serum will spontaneously head-to-head agglutinate, so Ham's F-10 or BWW is recommended (see below). The use of Tyrode's (for Y-bearing sperm enrichment) or Locke's solution (for X-bearing sperm enrichment) must not be substituted (see below).

Sperm are hardy cells and retain their motility after processing. Even so, there may be subtle changes (i.e., loss of membrane integrity) due to harsh treatment. Because of this, sperm should not be centrifuged at higher than $400 \times g$. Use of a swinging bucket centrifuge is recommended as a fixed-angle centrifuge will often pellet the sperm along the sides of a centrifuge tube rather than at the bottom. Because of the viscous nature of seminal plasma, diluting the ejaculate with an appropriate buffer or medium facilitates centrifugation by decreasing the time required to pellet the sperm.

The length of time necessary to pellet sperm by centrifugation is a function of the volume of the diluted semen sample. A sample of 10 ml will take 20 min in a normal 15 ml conical graduated centrifuge tube (see Materials and Methods, below) whereas a sample of 2 to 3 ml will require half that time. If the duration of sperm exposure to seminal plasma is a concern, aliquoting the semen sample into 2 to 3 ml fractions will decrease both the centrifugation and exposure time.

To minimize injury, sperm are resuspended from the pellet with gentle aspiration with a glass or nonspermicidal plastic pipette. The precise effect of vortexing on sperm membranes is unknown, though vortexed sperm in the anti-sperm antibody gel agglutination assay seem to remain viable during the test period.

Sperm are affected by osmolarity. In fact, a test has been described to ascertain membrane integrity by exposure to a hypo-osmotic solution.[10] In this test, the sperm that have suffered membrane damage retain a normal appearance, when evaluated microscopically, whereas sperm with intact membranes develop coiled tails.

The quality of a sperm sample that contains a large proportion of cellular debris can be improved by filtration (see below),[11] a procedure performed before washing by centrifugation. Washing of sperm does not change the cellular components of an ejaculate (dead/live sperm ratio, the number of white blood cells, etc.) but it will reduce the bacterial count[12] because the sperm pellet to the test tube bottom while the smaller bacteria stay in suspension. If the semen sample is thought to have a higher than normal bacterial contamination, then a sperm wash step should be performed and treatment with an antibiotic regime prior to use of the ejaculate is recommended.

On the following pages, three variations of the sperm rise technique are described. All three will result in an improvement of the percentage of motile sperm. The sperm pellet-then-rise procedure has an advantage in that it frees the sperm from seminal plasma more quickly than the other two methods do. With all three procedures the semen may be overlaid with medium or deposited under the medium with a pipette (although with the sperm-pellet-then-rise method, the sperm are resuspended in a small volume before being put under the medium). All three procedures allow isolation of the motile sperm cells from the white blood cells. A variation, the sperm swim-down procedure, is described under the methods for Y-bearing sperm enrichment method.

Since ejaculated sperm do not undergo capacitation in seminal plasma, the three sperm-rise and swim-down procedures are preliminary steps that allow sperm capacitation. Capacitation is a physiological maturation of spermatozoa in the presence of calcium ions without accompanying morphological changes.[13,14] A synchronous sperm preparation can be prepared through the use of a calcium free medium. During sperm maturation there are cholesterol shifts and a loss of disulfide groups.[15] Most specimens generally exhibit maximum sperm attachment and binding to zona pellucidae by 4 to 6 h post-sperm-rise (see Chapter 7). Although rapid sperm transport through the female tract has been described,[17] it is generally thought that sperm do not immediately reach the site of fertilization. It is important that sperm reach the egg when they are at a proper stage to fertilize. Therefore, artificial insemination in the vagina (or perhaps the cervical canal) with incubated sperm-rise samples may not be the best method to optimize pregnancy. Sperm-rise samples may be most effective in intrauterine or *in vitro* fertilization procedures. Sperm that have undergone capacitation will bind and attach to zona pellucidae, whereupon they undergo the acrosome reactions.[18] In fact, solubilized zona pellucidae can induce the acrosome reaction of capacitated sperm.[19-21] Since acrosome-reacted sperm will not bind and attach to zona pellucidae, fertility of the sample may be compromised if sperm processing promotes the acrosome reaction.

The best medium for sperm capacitation has not been defined. Only recently has a test been developed which can discern capacitated human sperm from pre- or post-capacitated human sperm (HZA, see Chapter 12). Use of the hemizona assay or a similar technique may allow definition of the optimal variables needed for capacitation.

III. PROCEDURES FOR THE PREPARATION OF SPERMATOZOA FOR ARTIFICIAL INSEMINATION

A. SPERM FILTRATION

When a semen sample is found to have large amounts of cellular debris or portions of the ejaculate that have not liquefied, sperm filtration can be used to clarify the sample. A filtration cone is made from two Kimwipes folded over on each other and placed in a glass funnel mounted over a test tube. The Kimwipe is moistened with media. Semen is pipetted onto the filter and the filtrate is collected. If the sperm sample is not clarified, diluting it 1:1 with buffer and allowing the sample to settle in a 15 ml graduated test tube for 20 min will allow the large particles to fall out.

B. SPERM WASH

The sperm cell can be washed and resuspended many times with no apparent immediate damage. Washed sample, however, may have somewhat reduced longevity. Sperm are sensitive to centrifugal force so they should not be pelleted by more than $400 \times g$. If cryopreserved sperm are being washed, then washes in media with less and less cryopreservative prevents possible osmotic shock (e.g., do not go from 10% glycerol solution straight to a 0% glycerol solution.)

When washing sperm remove the supernatant from the sperm pellet soon after centrifugation as the sperm will swim free from the pellet. As with any centrifugation procedure, the volume being centrifuged dictates the centrifugation time. Viscous seminal plasma will require a longer centrifugation time.

Diluting the semen sample 1:4 with buffer before washing (0.5 ml semen:1.5 ml buffer) is recommended. This should result in a sperm pellet after 10 minutes centrifugation at $300 \times g$ at room temperature. For seminal plasma-free sperm, wash the sperm three times. After the first wash, to conserve material, sperm may be pooled together (or split into two centrifuge tubes).

C. SPERM RISE

A — About 0.5 ml of semen is deposited into the bottom of a 15 ml graduated centrifuge tube. As many tubes as necessary should be used. The semen is then overlayed with 2 ml buffer (BWW or Ham's F-10; Baker's buffer should not be used as human sperm tend to spontaneously head-to-head agglutinate). The samples are then incubated at 37°C in a vertical position for 90 min. The supernatant buffer layer is removed with a Pasteur pipette taking care not to remove any of the semen layer. The buffer layers are pooled together and the sperm density and motility recorded. The sperm are then centrifuged in a 6 ml volume in 15 ml centrifuge tubes for 20 min at room temperature and the sperm pellets resuspended to the desired concentration in the appropriate buffer. For long-term incubation, such as for capacitation procedures, do not incubate the sperm at a concentration higher than 1×10^7 motile sperm/ml.

B — This procedure is similar to the above except that the sperm are incubated in tubes that are at an inclined orientation.[22] For every 0.5 ml of semen, prepare a 15 ml graduated centrifuge tube. Place 0.5 ml semen in the bottom of a centrifuge tube and overlay the semen with 3 ml buffer (note that 1 ml more buffer is used here). Incubate the semen at 37°C with the centrifuge tube inclined at a 30° angle for 60 min (the incubation time is shorter than for the above described method). The tubes are then gently and slowly placed back into an upright position and then the upper 1.5 ml of the buffer layer is removed and the buffer samples are pooled together (the amount of buffer layer taken is much more conservative than the above described procedure).

C — This sperm rise procedure has an advantage over the other two described procedures in that the sperm are removed quickly from the seminal plasma with a washing step done prior to the rise.[23] This procedure does not seem to isolate the sperm from microorganisms any better than does a simple washing procedure.[12] A one-step sperm wash method is combined with the first sperm rise method. For every 0.5 ml of semen, add 1.5 ml buffer and centrifuge the 2 ml volumes for 10 min at room temperature at $300 \times g$. Remove the supernatant from the sperm pellet as soon as the centrifugation has finished. Add 1 ml fresh buffer over the sperm pellets and incubate at 37°C for 1 h in the vertical position. Remove the upper 0.5 ml of buffer and pool the sample. Note the sperm density and motility. The sperm sample is then centrifuged again and resuspended to the desired concentration.

IV. ANTISPERM ANTIBODY PROCESSING G-200

Vasectomy is a popular method for permanent male contraception. Microsurgical reversal (vasovasostomy) is often successful although men with high levels of antisperm antibodies (both IgA and IgG) often seem less fertile.[24,25] The procedures used for detection of antisperm antibodies are described in Chapters 9 and 10. Immunoglobulin, one of the components in the ejaculate, is thought to be contributed by transudation from the prostate. However, there is also evidence that sperm antibodies may be present and bind to sperm within the epididymis.

Based on the assumption that a large percentage of antisperm antibodies bind at or after ejaculation, procedures have been developed for ejaculation into buffer containing sonicated sperm. These disrupted sperm could absorb the immunoglobins with the idea that more living sperm might remain antibody free. Sometimes the samples seem improved after this procedure. Given below is the ASAP G200 procedure that we have developed which was the easiest, simplest, and cheapest of the methods that we investigated.[26]

Although we were able to greatly improve the semen samples in terms of sperm motility, longevity, and ability to penetrate hamster eggs, we did not always observe a lower percentage of sperm with antisperm antibodies on their surface. These results suggest that an antisperm reaction may occur in the reproductive tract before ejaculation. Even though the percentage of immunobead-positive samples often remained unchanged post-treatment, there was a significant decrease of sperm agglutination. Possibly the sperm-antibody reaction that occurs in the reproductive tract does not promote cross linkage (resulting in sperm agglutination), and the ASAP G-200 procedure isolates the sperm from the additional antibodies to which they would be exposed upon ejaculation.

This procedure quickly isolates sperm from an ejaculate that contains anti-sperm antibodies. The sperm sample is collected by masturbation into 30 ml medium (Ham's F-10 or complete BWW). Within 5 to 10 min of collection, the semen-rich medium is separated from the ejaculate coagulum. The sperm are concentrated by centrifugation and then passed over a Sephadex G-200 column; those sperm which fall though the column are used for insemination. A variation involves a column constructed with gel conjugated with anti-antibody to separate sperm that are coated with antisperm antibody from sperm that are not.

A. REAGENTS
1. Sephadex G-200 (Pharmacia—do not use the "fine" or "super fine"); commercially available as a dry powder; 17-0080-01
2. Complete BWW media
    0.55 g NaCl
    0.036 g KCl
    0.02 g $CaCl_2$ (anhydrous) or 0.03 g $CaCl_2 \cdot 2H_2O$
    0.02 g KH_2PO_4
    0.03 g $MgSO_4 \cdot 7H_2O$

Dissolve in 50 ml ddH_2O* and bring to 100 ml. To 50 ml of above salt solution add the following:

- 0.003 g pyruvic acid, sodium salt (Calbiochem)
- 0.1 g glucose
- 0.35 g albumin (Fraction V)
- 0.21 g $NaHCO_3$
- 0.05 ml 0.5% phenol red
- 0.37 ml 60% *dl* lactic acid syrup (Sigma)
- **● 1.0 ml pen/strep at 100,000 U/ml (GIBCO)

Dissolve the above components and pH to 7.4 with no more than 2 ml 2 *M* HEPES; bring volume to 100 ml with more stock salt solution; sterilize through 0.22 μm filter.

*ddH_2O is abbreviation for double distilled tissue culture quality water; ddH_2O 1 is type one water (18 megaOhm resistant, filter sterilized and pyrogen free).
**Pen/strep is abbreviation for penicillin and streptomycin.

3. 5.0 ml disposable graduated pipette, glass bead and tubing with clamp
4. 70% ethanol; 70 ml 95% ethanol; bring to 100 ml with ddH_2O
5. Semen collection vial with lid able to hold 150 ml liquid (American Scientific Products, C8827-4)
6. Laboratory bench ring stand with test tube holder clamp
7. Swing-bucket centrifuge calibrated to 300 $\times g$
8. 16 $\times$ 125 mm test tube (about 10)
9. Two 15 ml graduated conical centrifuge test tubes
10. Pasteur pipettes

B. METHOD
Two days before the procedure, BWW medium is made and 1.5 g of Sephadex G-200 is weighed. The dry powder is placed in a glass flask and 50 ml of BWW added. The gel is swirled to disperse clumps and then degassed under vacuum for 4 h while the mixture is swirled from time to time. A stock solution of gel may be stored with 0.01% sodium azide

added as a preservative. The sodium azide, however, must be washed out of the gel matrix before sperm are added.

Three hours before the ASAP G-200 procedure, a graduated pipette is etched with a diamond pencil at the 2 ml mark (from the top) and the glass broken at this site. The end is flame-polished so that it is not sharp. Tubing is attached to the pipette end and a glass bead placed inside. The column is attached by means of a test tube clamp to a ring stand and orientated so that it is perpendicular with the base and level. The column is washed with 100 ml 70% ethanol (to aid in column sterilization) and then rinsed with BWW. At this time the flow of the column can be checked. If the glass bead is too tightly sealed in the column, the flow may be too slow. Generally, the column cannot run too fast at this stage. The flow rate will slow when the column is packed. The column is then filled with BWW until there is about 1 ml medium left in the column, and the tubing is clamped off. The column is filled with a slurry of G-200 and the gel is allowed to settle for 20 min. Excess BWW is removed from the top, and the column is refilled with more G-200 slurry, and again allowed to settle. Repeat until the settled gel is 5 mm from the top. The tubing clamp is opened and the flow is started slowly by holding the tubing above the column tip and letting the end of the tubing go below the tip as the gel packs. Too fast of an initial outflow may cause the gel to pack unevenly in the lower portion of the column and result in reduced flow rate. The gel is packed by washing 30 ml BWW through the column. (Do not let the gel matrix dry out.) Just before the patient is to arrive, excess BWW medium is removed from the surface of the gel. Labeled test tubes are placed in a rack and the column tubing end is placed in the first tube. Thirty milliliters BWW is put into the collection jar and kept at 37°C until the sperm donor arrives. As soon as possible after the sperm sample has been given, the collection jar is swirled gently and then inclined at an angle. A Pasteur pipette is used to collect the excess BWW medium from the coagulum. The sperm-rich medium is divided into two equal volumes and then placed into 15 ml graduated centrifuge tubes. The sample is centrifuged at $300 \times g$ for 20 min at room temperature, the supernatant is removed, 0.4 ml of BWW added to the sperm pellet, and the pellet is gently dispersed. The BWW and sperm mixture is removed and used to disperse the sperm pellet in the second centrifuge tube.

One half milliliter of the sperm is loaded onto the G-200 column and one half milliliter fractions are collected. Sperm appear in the outflow by tube 3, this tube is pooled with the next two (tubes 4 and 5), centrifuged for 5 min at $300 \times g$, and the supernatant is discarded. The sperm pellet is dispersed into 1 ml BWW and inseminated. Intracervical insemination is recommended.

The resulting sperm sample should not exhibit any motility loss or agglutination that is often seen in patients with antisperm antibodies. However, these samples often retain a high percentage of sperm with antibody on their surface. These antibodies do not seem to interfere with fertilization (hamster egg penetration tests results are significantly improved), but whether they reduce fertility in women is not clear. Some laboratories report success after artificial insemination, whereas others do not.

V. ASAP AFFINITY CHROMATOGRAPHY

For *in vitro* insemination procedures, sperm with antibodies on their surface may still be able to fertilize as long as there is no agglutination and the sperm can capacitate, attach and bind to the zona pellucidae, etc. However, for *in vivo* insemination procedures, quick removal of opsonized sperm (antibodies on their surface) by macrophages could be a problem. The affinity ASAP G200 procedure is a simple and effective method for separating antibody-bound sperm from antibody-free sperm. We recommend that before an affinity ASAP G200 procedure is considered, an immunobead antisperm antibody assay be performed. Since sperm that have antibodies on their surface will be eliminated by the procedure, the resultant count may be too low for subsequent insemination if a high percentage of the sperm are immunobead positive.

The principle of this procedure is essentially that described above except that IgG anti-human antibody conjugated beads are dispersed within the gel. Antibody-bound sperm will be separated from the population of sperm that are free of antisperm antibody.

A. REAGENTS

1. 1.0 mM HCl: pH 2—3
   8.3 µl 12 M HCl
   100 ml ddH$_2$O
2. 0.5 M NaCl
   13.86 g NaCl
   500 ml ddH$_2$O
3. 0.1 M Tris buffer. pH 8.0
   2.42 g Tris base (MW = 121.1)
   Dissolve in 100 ml ddH$_2$O
   pH to 8.0 with 6 N HCl
   Raise volume to 200 ml with ddH$_2$O
4. 0.2 M glycine
   1.5 g glycine
   100 ml 0.1 M Tris buffer
5. 0.1 M NaHCO$_3$ buffer, pH 9
   1.68 g NaHCO$_3$ (MW = 84.0)
   200 ml 0.5 M NaCl
6. **Acetate buffer**—Prepare a 0.1 M acetic acid solution by adding 0.50 ml glacial acetic acid to 100 ml 0.5 M NaCl. Then dissolve 0.82 g sodium acetate (MW = 82.0) in 50 ml 0.5 M NaCl and pH to 4.0 with 0.1 M acetic acid solution; raise volume to 100 ml with 0.5 M NaCl.
7. **CNBr-activated Sepharose 4B (Pharmacia) 117-04030-01**—commercially available
8. **Affinity purified IgG anti-human IgG and anti-IgA**—(if there is an indication that there may be IgM antisperm antibodies involved then these antibodies should be included) These reagents are commercially available.

B. METHOD

One gram freeze dried CNBr-4B gel is weighed and 10 ml 1 mM HCl solution is added. The beads are allowed to swell for 1 h at room temperature while swirling the mixture to disperse the gel. The mixture is then degassed under vacuum for 1 h with occasional swirling.

The gel is poured into a column and washed with 100 ml 1 mM HCl solution. The washed gel is removed from the column using 0.1 M NaHCO$_3$ buffer and placed into a screw cap test tube capable of holding 10 ml volumes. To the CNBr beads add 15 mg of the affinity purified anti-antibodies and bring the volume to 5 ml with more 0.1 M NaHCO$_3$. The test tube is sealed and placed on a test tube rocker for 18 h at 4°C.

The conjugated gel is washed from the test tube into a column using 0.2 M Tris buffer. The gel matrix is then washed with 50 ml volumes with the following solutions in sequence:

> NaHCO$_3$ buffer > Tris buffer > Tris buffer > Acetate buffer >
> Tris buffer > Acetate buffer > Glycine solution > Acetate buffer >
> Tris buffer

The gel is washed out from the column with complete BWW and the volume is recorded.

To this volume (about 3 ml) is added an equal volume of G-200 slurry. This gel mixture is then loaded upon a column as described above for the ASAP G-200 column procedure.

The affinity gel is dispersed into the G-200 gel so that sperm that bind to the affinity beads will not plug the column. A column is used for washing the gel matrix in order to process the beads in a gentle but thorough manner. Often it is best to have both an ASAP G-200 column and an affinity ASAP G-200 column prepared for the patient. After receiving the semen sample and performing the first wash of the sperm, run a sperm mixed agglutinatin reaction (sperm MAR) assay to determine the percentage of sperm with antibody on their surface. Depending on the sperm density and the insemination procedure to be used, one may elect not to do the affinity treatment as too low a sperm count may result if more than 60% of the sperm are sperm Mar positive.

In all chromatography procedures, the fractions are subsequently pooled to eliminate possible selection of X- or Y-bearing sperm. With all procedures, the percentage of sperm with progressive motility will be improved. The ASAP G200 method can be used as an alternative to sperm rise procedure, since many sperm from vasovasostomized men with antisperm antibodies often do not swim-up well. Glass bead columns seem to offer nearly the same advantages as the ASAP G200 columns; the latter will also separate the sperm by molecular exclusion from any free antisperm antibodies.

VI. ZONA MANIPULATION

Since some men have sperm samples that do not undergo an acrosome reaction, mechanical methods to circumvent penetration of the zona pellucidae have been developed. Zona drilling and microinjection techniques have been described.[26-29] A dilemma of these techniques is how to select the single sperm to be used. What is even more important is how to select a sperm that is acrosome-reacted, since other sperm cannot fertilize or undergo nuclear decondensation. By changing the antibody component of the affinity ASAP G200 to an anticapacitated sperm-only antibody, only acrosome-reacted motile sperm are excluded from the column. In a like manner, by substituting the antibody directed to the inner acrosome components, one could enrich for capacitate sperm and eliminate the acrosome-reacted sperm. When antibodies become available, such a procedure might be useful with GIFT or intraperitoneal insemination.

VII. RECOVERY OF SPERMATOZOA FROM RETROGRADE EJACULATIONS

Retrograde ejaculation is a condition in which the sperm are not expelled through the ureter during ejaculation but, because of an incompetent bladder neck, reflux back into the bladder. Reasons for this problem include organic (diabetes) or pharmacological (alpha adrenergic blocker use for hypertension) mechanisms. The general approach is to neutralize the urine pH and to normalize the osmolarity to 300 to 500 mOsm/l and then to have the patient void postejaculation. The sample is subsequently washed and used for insemination.

The incidence of men who experience retrograde ejaculation into the bladder at the time of orgasm is not known. There is some evidence that there may be some efflux of semen into the bladder under apparently normal circumstances.[30] The exposure of sperm to urine is usually detrimental. Sperm have a relatively wide range of sensitivity to environmental pH and osmolarity[31] and are more sensitive to osmotic shock (especially hypotonic) than to pH shock.[32]

A man suspected of experiencing retrograde ejaculation should provide a postejaculatory urine specimen to be examined for sperm. Culture of a midstream urine sample will provide information on the possibility of a bladder infection. The patient must be informed of the requirement to urinate and to produce an ejaculate on demand. His urine should be evaluated for pH and osmolarity post treatment. In addition, the quality of the recovered sperm can then be evaluated.

On the morning of the procedure, the patient should drink a solution containing 3 to 5 g of sodium bicarbonate in 250 ml water. Within 2 to 3 h the patient should provide a urine sample which is evaluated for pH and osmolarity. The patient should be instructed to try and withhold a small portion of his urine at this time. If the urine sample pH is 7.6 to 8.1 and the osmolarity is between 300 and 500 mOsm/l, he is instructed to masturbate into a vial with 30 ml buffered medium and then urinate into another vial with 30 ml buffered medium. The urine sample is aliquoted into 5 ml volumes and centrifuged for 10 min at $300 \times g$ at room temperature. The supernatant is removed and the sperm pellets are pooled together and washed one more time in buffered medium.

If after the first visit the urine sample pH or osmolarity are not appropriate, on the next visit, the amount of sodium bicarbonate is increased from 3 to 5 g to 5 to 10 g (1 or 2 tablespoons). The osmolarity of the urine can be decreased by having the patient present with a half-full bladder and then drink 250 ml water. The patient is asked to urinate 30 to 60 min later while still retaining some residual in his bladder. Again, if the pH and the osmolarity are within the proper range, he is instructed to ejaculate and subsequently urinate into a vial with buffered medium. Process the sample as described above.

Instruct the patient that it is important that he not change any habits (i.e., kind of breakfast) so that his urine is more likely to be consistent with that found on the insemination day.

The kind of buffer used for the dilution of the urine does not seem to be important but the pH should be adjusted slightly higher (7.6 to 8.1, rather than 7.2 to 7.4 for normal tissue culture) and that the osmolarity should be adjusted to be around 300 mOsm/l (rather than the lower osmolarity of most media prepared for tissue culture, i.e., IVF). The use of albumin or HEPES will strengthen the buffering ability of the media. The use of antibiotics is recommended.

VIII. SEX SELECTION PROCEDURES

The concept of sexual pre-selection has been a common element of man's endeavors since antiquity. The Bible teaches that woman was derived from the rib of man. It is now known that it is the sperm, not the rib, that determines the sex of the offspring. Usually half of infants born are male and half female. Even so, a statistic predictive for a population is of little value for the individual. Since nearly half the time the desired sex is achieved without manipulation, many procedures which seem to improve the possibility of gender selection are met with acceptance. There are popular omens, douches, and potions and even timing for the pre-selection of gender.[33]

The most reasonable approaches to sex selection rely on the premise that there is a difference in weight or size between sperm that contain the Y (male) chromosome and those that contain the X (female). Y-bearing sperm differences include: its slightly lighter mass (the Y-bearing sperm has less chromatin and is thus 1% lighter),[34] the charge of its smaller surface area, its dynamic swimming abilities, and possible expression of a male-specific antigen.[35] Given sperm with equal motility, those with a smaller cross section and less drag would be expected ot obtain a higher velocity. However, those that win the race may not win the event. Apparently, no mechanism of fertilization favors one gender over another. The finding of sperm appearing high in the female reproductive tract within minutes of ejaculation would not favor gender based on swimming speed.[17]

A statistical shift in favor of one gender or the other may be possible by two methods. The Y selection protocol sample size of patients is far larger than that for the X selection protocol.

The precautions for the chromatography methods already noted above are also applicable to the X-bearing sperm enrichment method. Three methods are described in the Y-bearing sperm enrichment section but the first two are sperm swim-down protocols (with no claim to Y selection), whereas the third procedure is the method for Y sperm selection.

IX. ENRICHMENT OF X-BEARING SPERMATOZOA

This is a modification of the protocol described by Quinlivan et al.[36] The procedure is to prepare a Sephadex G-50 column (1 × 12 cm) and to collect 1 ml fractions of sperm from the column. Sperm should be completely excluded from the column due to their size, although there seems to be some retention possibly because of an interaction of the sperm surface with the sugar moieties of the Sephadex material. After the column void volume has passed (usually 1 to 2 ml), the first fraction of sperm are collected, enriched for X-bearing sperm, and used for insemination.

A. REAGENTS AND EQUIPMENT
1. Sephadex G 50 (Pharmacia, 17-0044-01)
2. Locke's Solution; 8.50 g sodium chloride; 0.42 g potassium chloride; 0.20 g sodium bicarbonate; 0.24 g calcium dichloride

The ingredients are combined into 500 ml tissue culture grade distilled water. After the salts have gone into solution, the final volume is brought to 1000 ml with more tissue culture grade water; pH of the solution should have a pH of 7.2 and then be filter sterilized by passing through a 22 μm filter. The water is degassed for 2 h under vacuum while stirring and then the solution is stored in 100 ml aliquots at 4°C. Locke's solution can be stored for at least 4 months. A fresh solution is prepared on each day.

3. Human serum albumin solution (intravenous grade; usually comes as 25% sterile solution)
4. Disposable glass 10 ml graduated pipette
5. A glass bead (5.0 mm diameter, approximately round, Thomas Scientific, New Jersey, U.S., 5663-L25)
6. Tygone tubing (Fisher Scientific Company, Pennsylvania, U.S., 14-169-1C, 3/32 I.D., 5/32 O.D. and 1/32 wall)
7. Hemostat or other clamping device to turn on and off the column
8. Glass Pasture pipettes and glass test tubes
9. Calibrated swinging bucket centrifuge

B. METHOD
Two days before the procedure is to be conducted, the Sephadex G-50 must be swollen and degassed. Ten grams of dry Sephadex G-50 is weighed and placed in a 500 ml side arm vacuum flask. Between 150 to 200 ml of Locke's solution is added to the gel in the vacuum flask and swirled together. A magnetic stir bar or other mechanical device should not be used to stir the ingredients. The use of mechanical stirring devices can cause damage to the Sephadex bead particles. A rotary table or another such device will work. After 2 h of swirling the mixture, the solution is degassed under vacuum for another 2 h. The G-50 is stored at 4°C (for long-term storage of the gel the addition of sodium azide to a final concentration of 0.01% is recommended). Sodium azide will preserve the gel for long period of time, but 2 days before the gel to be used, it should be viewed with light microscopy for possible bacterial contamination. Bacteria can reside within the gel beads as well as outside the beads. In general, this is a good practice for gels that have been stored for any

length of time. Be sure to view your gel with enough time before the anticipated need, such that more could be prepared if necessary (48 h before need).

Using a diamond pencil or a triangle file, etch a 10 ml glass pipette below the mouth piece and break at the etched mark. The broken pipette is flame polished. Tubing is attached to the end of the glass pipette and a glass bead placed inside. The column is gas sterilized and allowed to degas for at least 2 weeks before using. Alternatively, the column can be sterilized by washing the outside and the inside of the column with 70% ethanol in water.

The column is prepared at least 2 h before use. Once the column has been poured, it should not be moved excessively as movement of the glass bead may result in Sephadex gel particles being freed from the column and possibly contaminating the sperm sample. Glass wool should never be used to support the G-50 gel matrix as it is virtually impossible to prevent the glass wool fiber from shedding into the column eluate. The column is mounted vertically in a ring stand and leveled. The G-50 and an aliquot of Locke's solution are allowed to come to room temperature. The G-50 gel (15 ml) is degassed for 10 min. Approximately 10 ml Locke's solution is added to the empty pipette column with the glass bead seated in the bottom. The tubing is clamped off after 8 ml of Locke's solution has passed through the column, leaving 2 ml in the column. (This allows a check to be sure that the glass bead has not seated too well in the column, restricting the flow too much; if the flow is too slow, another less perfect glass bead should be selected). Washing the column with an aliquot of Locke's solution allows removal of air bubbles from around the glass bead and provides a bed on which to add the G-50 slurry. The G-50 is made into a thick suspension (slurry) by swirling the gel gently in a minimum volume of Locke's solution. The column is filled with G-50 slurry and allowed to settle for 10 min. Excess Locke's solution is removed from the top of the gel, and another layer of G-50 slurry placed on top. This procedure is repeated until the column is filled. After the column has settled and no more than 1 ml excess Locke's solution is at the top, the column is slowly opened and washed with Locke's solution. NEVER LET THE COLUMN RUN OUT OF LIQUID, AS IT WILL CRACK THE GEL BED AND REQUIRE REPACKING. The column is packed by running 20 ml of Locke's solution through the column and removing excess gel until there is a distance of 12 cm between the glass bead and the top of the gel bed. It is very important to prewash the column with excessive amounts of Locke's solution (60 ml) if the gel was stored with sodium azide; otherwise, a total of 35 to 40 ml of Locke's solution is adequate for washing the gel before the procedure. Finally, Locke's solution is allowed to enter the gel bed with only 0.5 ml liquid remaining over the bed and the column clamped off.

A fresh human sperm sample is collected and allowed to liquefy for 30 min at 37°C. The semen sample is diluted two- to threefold with Locke's solution. The diluted semen sample is centrifuged at room temperature at $300 \times g$ for 20 min and the supernatant is discarded. The pellet is resuspended to 1 ml with fresh Locke's solution.

The column is loaded with the 1.5 ml washed sperm. The sperm solution enters the bed of the column after the tubing is unclamped. Then the column is reclamped, and 1 ml of fresh Locke's solution is loaded. The column is then unclamped again and 1 ml fractions are collected. The separation is continued until 5 ml have been collected. The first 2 ml are discarded and the next three fractions are pooled and centrifuged at $300 \times g$ for 10 min. The supernatant is discarded and the sperm resuspended in 0.5 ml with 3% HSA and Locke's solution. This preparation is used for insemination.

The principle for the enrichment of X-bearing sperm by G-50 chromatography is not understood. The gel matrix must not be separated on the basis of size, since both Y-bearing and X-bearing sperm are too large for the exclusion abilities of G-50 to differentiate. In addition, it would seem that the flow rate of the column would negate any differences in swimming velocity between the two populations of sperm. Possibly the Y-bearing sperm interact with the gel matrix more than do the X-bearing sperm, or there is a sub-population of X-bearing sperm which do not interact with the gel matrix as extensively as do the other sperm.

X. ENRICHMENT OF Y-BEARING SPERMATOZOA

This procedure is a modification of the protocol described by Ericsson.[37] The method has been patented and consists of exposing sperm to various albumin gradients, resulting in the collection of the sperm which have exhibited a higher degree of linear swimming velocity. The assay is to set up a race between the two populations; the winners are collected at the end.

The procedure is performed employing two different discontinuous albumin gradients. The first gradient allows the sperm to separate upon a 7.5% gradient. Sperm which enter the gradient are placed upon a second gradient of 12.5% albumin overlaid on a 20% albumin gradient. Sperm within the last gradient are used for insemination.

There is a significant loss of sperm in this procedure (as is also true for the X-bearing sperm enrichment protocol). The initial quality of the semen sample undergoing the procedure must be taken into account.

A. REAGENTS AND EQUIPMENT

1. Tyrode's solution—The following are $10 \times$ concentrates of the stock salt solutions. The salts are prepared separately and combined in the order given.
    a. 80 g sodium chloride
       100 ml tissue culture grade water
    b. 1.95 g potassium chloride
       1000 ml tissue culture grade water
    c. 2.13 g magnesium chloride—6 waters ($MgCl_2.6\ H_2O$)
       1000 ml tissue culture grade water
    d. 10.15 g sodium bicarbonate
       1000 ml tissue culture grade water
    e. 1.554 g calcium dichloride (anhydrous)
       1000 ml tissue culture grade water

On the day of the procedure, 20 ml of each stock salt solution are combined; 0.2 g glucose is dissolved and brought to a final volume to 200 ml with tissue culture grade water.

2. A 25% solution of liquid human serum albumin, salt poor.
3. Glass Pasteur pipettes, 5 $^3/_4$ in. long

B. METHOD

The albumin gradients are prepared for separation and then loaded into Pasteur pipettes, the ends of which are heat-sealed taper. Alternatively, appropriate glass tubes may be purchased from Arrow Glass Co., South Vineland, NJ. A fresh human semen sample is allowed to liquefy at 37°C for 30 min. The sample is mixed 1:1 with Tyrode's solution and the volume is determined. Make a 7.5% albumin solution from the stock albumin solution using Tyrode's (0.3 ml 25% stock albumin + 0.7 milliliter Tyrode's). For every milliliter of the diluted semen sample prepared, two 7.5% albumin gradients are prepared. That is, if the diluted semen sample volume is 6 ml, then twelve 7.5% albumin gradient columns are prepared. For each milliliter of the diluted semen sample, a glass tube is placed into a 37°C water bath in a vertical position. Albumin (1.0 ml) is put into each glass tube. The albumin gradient is gently overlaid with 0.5 ml of the diluted semen, and the sample is incubated for 1 h.

The diluted semen sample is removed from the albumin layer (taking a small amount of albumin under the layer to assure that the sperm used in the subsequent portions of the procedure are from the albumin layer and not contaminated with sperm from the diluted semen layer). The diluted semen layer material is discarded. The 7.5% albumin fractions are pooled and the sperm density determined. The albumin pool is centrifuged in 4 ml aliquots for 10 min at $300 \times g$, and the supernatants are discarded. The sperm pellets are brought to 60×10^6 sperm/ml with Tyrode's solution. In other words, if the sperm density in 12 ml of the 7.5% albumin pool was 12×10^6 sperm/ml, then the pellets would be resuspended in a total volume of 2 ml Tyrode's.

For each ml of semen at the appropriate density, prepare two two-layer albumin gradient tubes as described above for the 7.5% gradients. Each of the gradient tubes is filled at the bottom with 0.5 ml 20% albumin (0.8 ml 25% albumin + 0.2 ml Tyrode's). Onto this layer is placed 1 ml 12.5% albumin (0.5 ml 25% albumin + 0.5 ml Tyrode's). Onto each of these tubes is placed 0.5 ml of the appropriately diluted sperm. The sample is incubated for 1 h. The 12.5% gradient is removed from the 20% gradient. The 12.5% fractions are discarded and the 20% albumin fractions are pooled. The 20% albumin pool is centrifuged at $300 \times g$ for 10 min and the pellet is resuspended in 0.5 ml Tyrode's solution. This sample is used for insemination.

As an alternative to layering sample onto the gradients, one can underlay it. The only change in the protocol is the order of placement. In the 7.5% columns, rather than loading 1 ml of the albumin solution first into the tubes, 0.5 ml of diluted semen is first placed into the tubes. Then 1 ml of 7.5% albumin solution is delivered under the sample with a Pasteur pipette. This procedure may also be an easier way of removing samples.

XI. HISTOCHEMICAL STAINING FOR THE Y-BEARING SPERMATOZOA

The visualization of the Y body [38,39] of the stained sperm requires fluorescent microscopy analysis at $1000\times$ magnification and the viewing of at least 200 cells. Since there can be variance in reading the slides, it is often advisable for the analysis to be performed by two individuals. The stained chromatin of the sperm will fluoresce with a mild yellow-green color. The basal one third of the sperm head will show a concentrated or denser spot of fluorescence when the Y chromosome is present. However, this pattern is often difficult to distinguish and is complicated by the fact that fluorescence is quenched rather quickly. Usually 45 to 50% of the sperm in a normal sample are stained. Doing a sperm rise before staining does not alter this percentage.

A. REAGENTS AND EQUIPMENT
1. Quinacrine mustard dihydrochloride (QMD) (Sigma Chemical Co., St. Louis, MO; Q-2000). Store the reagent under dessication and hold at 4°C.
2. McIlvane's buffer, prepare the following stock solutions:
    (a) **0.1 *M* citric acid anhydrous**—19.212 g citric acid anhydrous bring to 1000 ml with tissue culture grade water
    (b) **0.2 *M* disodium phosphate**—28.396 g disodium phosphate bring to 1000 ml with tissue culture grade water

    Prepare buffer

Volume	Citric acid	Disodium PO$_4$
20 ml	3.53 ml	16.47 ml
100	17.65	82.47
500	88.25	411.75

all solutions should be at pH 7.0

3. Sucrose mounting solution
    Dissolve 6 g sucrose into 10 ml tissue culture grade water and heat until the sucrose goes into solution.
4. Baker's Buffer (9)
    0.20 g sodium chloride
    3.00 g glucose
    0.354 g sodium phosphate, dibasic (anhydrous)
    0.03 g potassium phosphate, monobasic
    Bring all to 100.0 ml with tissue culture grade water; pH of the buffer will be 7.7; pH to 7.0 with HCl.
5. Methanol/acetic acid fixing solution mix one part absolute methanol with one part glacial acetic acid.
6. Fluorescent microscope equipped with a mercury lamp, exciter filter, barrier filter, dark field condenser, a 100× objective and immersion oil (if the objective requires).

B. METHOD

Dissolve 2.5 mg of QMD in 10 ml tissue culture water; further dilute with 40 ml McIlvane's buffer (final concentration 50 μg of QMD/ml). Protect the QMD solution from light AT ALL TIMES. Store in a dark, foil-wrapped bottle at 4°C for no more than 2 weeks. The fresher the QMD solution, the better the staining.

If a fresh semen sample is being evaluated, wash the sample twice in Baker's buffer at 300 × g. If the sperm are derived from one of the sex selection procedures, no prewashing is needed. Prepare a sperm cell smear. Let the slide air dry for 10 min. Dip the sperm slide into methanol/acetic acid fixing solution for 2 min. Air-dry the slides. Wash slides in McIlvane's buffer for 5 min. While protecting the slide from light, stain it with QMD solution for 10 min if the stain is fresh or for 20 min if the stain is up to two weeks old. While protecting the slide from exposure to light, wash twice in McIlvane's buffer for 5 min each. Air-dry the slide in the dark. Coverslip the slide with the sucrose mounting medium. Read the slide at a magnification of 1000×. Report the number of sperm seen with and without fluorescent spot. There is still a great deal of scepticism associated with X and Y separation techniques. Chromosomal evaluation by means of the hamster egg tests has not supported a shift in the percentage of treated sperm.[40]

C. MATERIALS

The observance of good laboratory practice procedures is needed for nearly all of the procedures used in this chapter. Water baths, slide warmers, refrigerators, freezers, incubators must have their temperatures, water and gas levels or mixtures and cleanliness monitored and recorded on a daily basis. Attaching daily record sheets and having a technician be responsible may aid in record keeping. In addition, periodic check of the accuracy of pipettes, pH meters, osmometers, microscopes, centrifuges, etc. will aid in maintaining a consistent laboratory environment for the routine processing of very sensitive cells *in vitro*.

Centrifuge—As was mentioned above, a swing bucket model tends to centrifuge cells more easily to the bottom of the test tube than does a fixed angle centrifuge. By the same token, a centrifuge with variable speed ability is more versatile than is a fixed speed centrifuge. In any case, the centrifuge needs to have its rotations (or revolutions) per minute (rpm) calibrated to the speed scale indicator. This is most easily and accurately performed by using a stroboscope. Finally, one needs to calculate the *g* force that is developed at the various settings (relative centrifugal field (xg $= 1118 \times R \times (\text{rpm}^2) \times 10^8$; where R is average radius in cm, and rpm is revolutions per minute). Sperm cells should not be centrifuged harder than $400 \times g$.

Incubator—The incubator gas must be monitored daily so that replacement tanks can be obtained without difficulty (many laboratories have a spare tank already attached to the incubator and reorder a replacement tank when the attached tank runs out and the spare is turned onto the system). Almost all incubators are water jacketed to aid in holding the temperature constant. Nevertheless, having a thermometer inside the incubator offers assurance to the temperature readings. No media, buffers or other reagents should be put into the incubator to warm up as nonsterile liquid will condense upon the outside of the vials and may run down into the incubator. Possible bacterial or fungi contamination may result. Some laboratories even wipe the outside of their vials and trays with 70% alcohol prior to placing them into the incubator to further aid control of bacteria or fungi contamination.

Hood—A laminar flow hood is an ideal aid in tissue culture, but is not necessary for normal sperm culture techniques. A ''clean'' area with no air drafts and little people traffic is usually enough. The hood must be kept clean and spills immediately wiped up.

Ejaculate specimen vials—A large mouth sterile vial is usually ideal. The technician should wear gloves when handling any body fluids. All vials should have adequate identification.

All plastics are suspect until checked for gametocidal effects. Glassware must be cleaned and rinsed properly. A good approach is to have separate glassware for the cell culture experiments.

The ultimate test for toxic residues is mouse IVF[41] but the mouse two cell embryo assay is often satisfactory,[42] (refer to Chapter 17). Recently a hamster sperm cell assay has been described as a quality control procedure,[43] The assay seems as sensitive as the mouse two cell assay and the results are obtained in a shorter period of time.

Microscope—A microscope with 100, 200, and $400\times$ magnification is required for the examination of sperm samples. Phase contrast optics are helpful.

Columns—Since most of the procedures that are given in this chapter are performed one time per sperm sample, the chromatography columns are disposable. We have designed the columns and the components to be versatile, sterilizable and inexpensive.

D. REAGENTS

Water—Water quality may be one of the most important and possibly most difficult part of any procedure to control. Generally, water quality cannot be too good. There are a number of excellent water purification systems that are marketed which will deliver type 1 water on demand. Even so, the water quality must be constantly monitored. All system users must be informed when the system is to be cleaned or whenever water quality may be compromised. In an emergency, high pressure liquid chromatography (HPLC) water can be substituted.

Chemical—Reagent quality only (and in some cases analytical or tissue culture screened quality) should be used. Chemicals should be stored according to the manufacturer's suggestions. Those that require storage at 4°C or colder should be warmed to room temperature prior to opening the vial to minimize the amount of condensation which may occur and affect shelf-life. All chemicals should be labeled when they are opened and the expiration dates observed.

Antibiotics—Penicillin-G and streptomycin sulfate usually are sufficient for tissue culture techniques. The occasional use of Gentamicin may prevent development of a penicillin resistant bacterial strain. Fungal contamination when it occurs can be debilitating. The routine use of Fungizone is not recommended since it is quite toxic. Mycoplasma contamination of the culture system is not expected due to the short incubation times. However, if the facilities are being shared with long-term culture experiments (such as monoclonal antibody protocols) then screening for mycoplasma infection should be done periodically.

E. GENERAL RECIPES
Baker's phosphate buffered glucose solution

0.2 g sodium chloride
3.0 g D-glucose
0.298 g $Na_2HPO_4 \cdot 2H_2O$ or
0.668 g $Na_2HPO_4 \cdot H_2O$ or
0.354 g Na_2HPO_4 anhydrous
0.03 g KH_2PO_4

Add 100 ml double distilled water and adjust the pH to 7.0. Filter sterilize the buffer through a 0.22 μm filter and store at 4°C. Use portions of the stock on a daily basis. Make fresh buffer every 2 weeks.

Sperm counting solution
5.0 g sodium bicarbonate
1.0 ml 35% formalin

Dilute to 100.0 ml double distilled water and store at room temperature. Do not mouth pipette this reagent.

Locke's Solution—see the X-sperm enrichment method.
Tyrode's Solution—see Y-sperm enrichment method.
Biggers, Whitten, and Whittingham's Medium (BWW)—see ASAP G-200.

REFERENCES

1. **Zavos, P. M.,** Seminal parameters of ejaculates collected from oligospermic and normospermic patients via masturbation and at intercourse with use of Silastic seminal fluid collection device, *Fertil. Steril.,* 44(4), 517, 1985.
2. **Zavos, P. M.,** Characteristic of human ejaculates collected via masturbation and a new Silastic seminal fluid collection device, *Fertil. Steril.,* 43(3), 491, 1985.
3. **Cohen, M. S., Collen, S., and Mardh, P. A.,** Mucosal defenses, in *Sexually Transmitted Diseases,* Holmes, K. K., Mardh, P. A., Sparling, P. F., and Wiesner, P. J., Eds., McGraw-Hill, New York, 1984, 173.
4. **Riedel, H. -H.,** Techniques for the detection of leukocytospermia in human semen, *Arch. Androl.,* 5, 287, 1986.
5. **Wolff, H. and Anderson, D. J.,** Immunohistologic characterization and quantitation of leukocyte sub-populations in human semen, *Fertil. Steril.,* 49,(3), 497, 1988.
6. **Bedford, J. M.,** Significance of the need for sperm capacitation before fertilization in eutherian mammals, *Biol. Reprod.,* 8, 108, 1983.
7. **Rogers, B. J., Perreault, S. D., Bentwood, B. J., McCarville, C., Hale, R., and Sodradahl, D. W.,** Variability in the human-hamster, in vitro assay for fertility evaluation, *Fertil. Steril.,* 39(2), 204, 1983.
8. **Katz, D. F. and Overstreet, J. W.,** Biophysical aspects of human sperm movement, in *The Spermatozoon,* Fawcett, D. W. and Bedford, J. W., Eds., Urban and Schwartzenberg, Baltimore, 1979, 413.
9. **Baker, J. R.,** The spermicidal powers of chemical contraceptives. IV. More substances, *J. Hyg. (Camb.),* 32, 171, 1932.

10. **Jeyendran, R. S., Van der Ven, H. H., Perez-Pelacz, M., Crabo, B. G., and Zaneveld, L. J. D.,** Development of an assay to assess the functional integrity of the human sperm membrane and its relationship to other semen characteristics, *J. Reprod. Fertil.,* 70, 219, 1984.

11. **Alexander, N. J. and Schlaff, W.,** Insemination techniques for overcoming male infertility, *Contemp. Obstet. Gynecol.,* Special issue, 99, 1987.

12. **Kuzan, F. B., Hillier, S. L., and Zarutskie, P. W.,** Comparison of three wash techniques for the removal microorganisms from semen, *Obstet. Gynecol.,* 70(6), 836, 1987.

13. **Clegg, E.,** Mechanisms of mammalian sperm capacitation, in *Mechanism and Control of Animal Fertilization,* Hartmann, J. F., Ed., 1983, 177.

14. **Rogers, B. J. and Brentwood, B. J.,** Capacitation, acrosome reaction and fertilization, in *Biochemistry of Mammalian Reproduction,* Zaneveld, L. J. D. and Chatterton, R. T., Eds., John Wiley & Sons, New York, 1982.

15. **Langlais, J. and Roberts, K. D.,** A molecular membrane model of sperm capacitation and the acrosome reaction of mammalian spermatozoa, *Gamete Res.,* 12, 183, 1985.

16. **Settlage, D. S. F., Motoshima, M., and Tredway, D. R.,** Sperm transport from the external os to the fallopian tubes in women: a time and quantification study, *Fertil. Steril.,* 24, 655, 1973.

17. **Overstreet, J. W. and Tom, R. A.,** Experimental studies of rapid sperm transport in rabbits, *J. Reprod.,* 66, 601, 1982.

18. **Mortimer, S.,** From the semen to oocyte: the long route in vivo and in vitro short cut, in *Human in Vitro Fertilization; INSERM Symposium,* Vol. 24, Testart, J. and Frydman, R., Eds., Elsevier, Amsterdam, 1985, 93.

19. **Florman, H. M. and Storey, B. T.,** Mouse gamete interaction. The zona pellucida is the site of the acrosome reaction leading to fertilization in vitro, *Dev. Biol.,* 91, 121, 1982.

20. **Bleil, J. D. and Wassarman, P. M.,** Sperm-egg interactions in the mouse. Sequence of events and induction of the acrosome reaction by zona pellucida glycoprotein, *Dev. Biol.,* 95, 317, 1983.

21. **Wassarman, P. M.,** Early events in mammalian fertilization, *Annu. Rev. Cell Biol.,* 3, 109, 1987.

22. **Russell, L. D. and Rogers, B. J.,** Improvement in the quality and fertilization potential of a human sperm population using the rise technique, *J. Androl.,* 8, 25, 1987.

23. **Trounson, A. O., Mohr, L. R., Wood, C., and Lecton, J. F.,** Effect of delayed insemination on in-vitro fertilization; culture and transfer of human embryos, *J. Reprod. Fertil.,* 64, 285, 1982.

24. **Fuchs, E. F. and Alexander, N. J.,** Immunologic considerations before and after vasovasostomy, *Fertil. Steril.,* 40, 497, 1983.

25. **Rumke, P., Renckens, C. N. M., Bezemer, P. D., and Van Amstel, N.,** Prognosis of fertility in women with unexplained infertility and sperm agglutinins in the serum, *Fertil. Steril.,* 42, 561, 1984.

26. **Kiser, G. C., Alexander, N. J., Fuchs, E. F., and Fulgham, D. L.,** In vitro absorption of antisperm antibodies with immunobead-rise, immunomagnetic, and immunocolumn separation techniques, *Fertil. Steril.,* 47(3), 466, 1987.

27. **Kiessling, A. A., Loutradis, D., McShane, P. M., and Jackson, K. V.,** Fertilization in trypsin-treated oocytes, in *In vitro Fertilization and Other Assisted Reproduction,* Jones, H. W. and Schrader, C., Eds., *Ann. N.Y. Acad. Sci.,* 541, 614, 1988.

28. **Gordon, J. W.,** Use of micromanipulation for increasing the efficiency of mammalian fertilization, in *In vitro Fertilization and Other Assisted Reproduction,* Jones, H. W. and Schrader, C., Eds., *Ann. N.Y. Acad. Sci.,* 541, 601, 1988.

29. **Mettler, L., Yamada, K., Kuranty, A., Michelmann, H. W., and Semm, K.,** Microinfection of spermatozoa in oocytes, in *In vitro Fertilization and Other Assisted Reproduction,* Jones, H. W. and Schrader, C., Eds., *Ann. N.Y. Acad. Sci.* 541, 591, 1988.

30. **Alexander, N. J., Fulgham, D. L., and Wicklund, R.,** Adrenergic blocking agents inadequate for nonsurgical male contraception, *Fertil. Steril.,* 36, 119, 1981.

31. **Makler, A., David, R., Blumenfeld, Z., and Better, O. S.,** Factors affecting sperm motility. VII. Sperm viability as affected by change of pH and osmolarity of semen and urine specimens, *Fertil. Steril.,* 32, 1981.

32. **Braude, P. B., Ross, L. D., Bolton, V. N., and Ockenden, K.,** Retrograde ejaculation: a systemic approach to noninvasive recovery of spermatozoa from post-ejaculatory urine for artificial insemination, *Br. J. Obstet. Gynecol.,* 94, 76, 1987.

33. **Corson, S. L. and Betzer, F. R.,** Human gender selection, *Semin. Reprod. Endocrinol.* 5, 81, 1987.

34. **Summer, A. T. and Robinson, T. A.,** A difference in dry mass between heads of X- and Y-bearing human spermatozoa, *J. Reprod. Fertil.,* 48, 9, 1976.

35. **Koo, G. C., Stackpole, C. W., Boyse, E. A., Hmarling, V., and Dardis, M. P.,** Topographical location of H-Y antigen on a mouse spermatozoa by immunoelectron-microscopy, *Proc. Natl. Acad. Sci. U.S.A.,* 70, 1502, 1973.

36. **Quinlivan, W. L. G., Preciado, K., Long, T. L., and Sullivan, H.,** Separation of human X and spermatozoa by albumin gradients and Sephadex chromatography, *Fertil. Steril.,* 37, 104, 1982.

37. **Ericsson, R. J., Langevin, C. N., and Nishino, M.,** Isolation of fractions rich in human Y sperm, *Nature London,* 246, 421, 1973.
38. **Zech, L.,** Investigation of metaphase chromosomes with DNA-binding fluorchromes, *Exp. Cell Res.,* 58, 463, 1969.
39. **Sumver, A. T., Robinson, J. A., and Evans, H. J.,** Distinguishing between X,Y and YY-bearing human spermatozoa by fluorescence and DNA content, *Nature New Biol.,* 229, 231, 1971.
40. **Gledhill, B. L.,** Selection and separation of X- and Y-chromosome-bearing mammalian sperm, *Gamete Res.,* 20, 377, 1988.
41. **Fleming, T. P., Pratt, H. P. M., and Braude, P. R.,** The use of mouse preimplantation embryos for quality control of culture reagent in human in vitro fertilization programs: a cautionary note, *Fertil. Steril.,* 47, 858, 1987.
42. **Davidson, A., Vermesh, M., Lobo, R. A., and Paulson, R. J.,** Mouse embryo culture as quality control for human in vitro fertilization: the one-cell versus the two-cell model, *Fertil. Steril.,* 49, 516, 1988.
43. **Tomkins, P. T., Carroll, C. V., and Houghton, J. A.,** Assessment of heterospecific zona-free ovum penetration under fully defined conditions, *Hum. Reprod.,* 3, 367, 1988.

Chapter 12

THE HEMIZONA ASSAY (HZA): ASSESSMENT OF FERTILIZING POTENTIAL BY MEANS OF HUMAN SPERM BINDING TO THE HUMAN ZONA PELLUCIDA

L. J. Burkman, C. C. Coddington, D. R. Franken, S. C. Oehninger, and G. D. Hodgen

TABLE OF CONTENTS

I. BACKGROUND

A spermatozoon's ability to fertilize an egg is dependent on sperm structure, the quality of sperm motility and capacitation. The completion of capacitation is marked by either release of the acrosomal contents[1,2] or, alternatively, binding to and full penetration of the zona pellucida.[3] Sperm function at the site of the zona pellucida is perhaps the ultimate test of fertilizing capacity, since the zona represents the requisite first interaction of egg and sperm. The hemizona assay (HZA) has focused exclusively on the obligatory step of tight sperm binding to the outer surface of the zona pellucida; without tight binding, all subsequent fertilization events cannot proceed.

The optimum human assay would ideally utilize living, fertilizable human oocytes. That approach has been limited by ethical considerations and, pragmatically, by the restricted availability of human oocytes. Until recently, the assays based on human sperm-egg interaction have utilized two substitutes: (1) the zona-free hamster ovum penetration assay,[4-6] and (2) the penetration of nonliving, intact human oocytes.[7-10] There is currently a proliferation of novel sperm function assays: strict morphological assessment,[11] creatine phosphokinase levels,[12] hypoosmotic swelling,[13] sperm ATP content,[14] etc. However, the sperm-egg interaction bioassays may be the most powerful because they assess a spectrum of sperm functions essential to the process of fertilization.

The HZA offers two particular advantages with respect to the use of whole eggs: (1) statistically reliable data are derived when using the matched zona halves from a single egg (the penetration assay typically uses two to four eggs per test),[8] and (2) inadvertent fertilization of a human egg cannot occur, since viability is destroyed during bisection.

A. PURPOSE AND CLINICAL APPLICATION OF THE HZA

The HZA was developed to estimate sperm fertilizing potential, based on the relative binding of spermatozoa from a test patient versus a known fertile control using the matching halves of a nonliving, bisected (hemi) human zona pellucida.[15] The availability of control versus experimental zona hemispheres from the same zona pellucida has very nearly solved the problem of zona-to-zona variations in binding capacity.[16-18] Although the HZA has been utilized most for testing suspected male-factor patients during screening at entry into the Norfolk IVF program, we have broadened the agenda for HZA to include vasectomy reversal patients[19] and the work-up of husbands from infertile couples seeking therapy. The HZA is equally suited for detecting sperm function changes after infertility treatment, or during male contraceptive therapy, or following chemotherapy.

B. DEVELOPMENT AND VALIDATION OF THE HZA

The feasibility of the HZA was examined in four experiments reported previously.[15] We have demonstrated that: (1) the zonae pellucida can be easily bisected into nearly equal halves, using a micromanipulation apparatus; (2) the tissue source for intact zonae (from ovaries at autopsy vs. immature IVF oocytes) did not affect sperm binding; (3) tight binding of sperm to the outer surface of a hemizona was equivalent to binding to the intact zona surface; and (4) tight sperm binding to the surfaces of *matching* hemizonae was equivalent.

Studies on the kinetics of sperm binding to hemizonae (proven fertile donors)[15] showed that tight binding was initiated within one hour of coincubation. Importantly, sperm binding usually peaked at about four hours for proven fertile men. Therefore, a 4 h incubation period was adopted for the HZA. Furthermore, the kinetic curve of sperm binding for subfertile men exhibited the same temporal shape when compared to the data from fertile men (see Reference 23). We have also demonstrated that the sperm binding curves for any two matching hemizonae were nearly identical for both shape and peak value throughout 8.5 h of coincubation (Figure 1).[15]

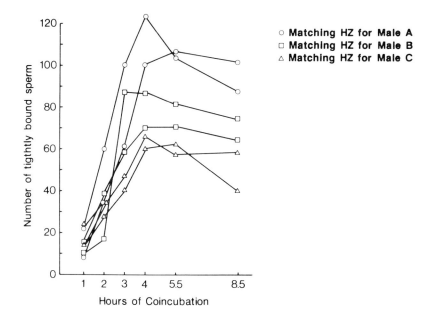

FIGURE 1. The two hemizonae in a matched pair showed similar sperm binding kinetics. In each of three experiments, the same two hemizonae were repeatedly assessed for tight binding throughout 8.5 h of coincubation.[15]

In three different studies, the clinical significance of HZA results was examined using the semen of men who had undertaken IVF treatment at Norfolk. In ten experiments, each using one matched-pair of hemizonae, sperm from fertile men bound more efficiently than sperm from "IVF husbands" who had not achieved fertilization *in vitro* (34.0 ± 8 vs. 5.9 ± 2, respectively).[15] Thus, the concept of the HZA Index was introduced:

$$\text{HZA Index} = \frac{\text{number of test sperm bound to hemizona}}{\text{number control sperm bound to hemizona}} \times 100 \qquad (1)$$

In our hands, the Index values have nearly always ranged between 0 and 150.

The subsequent clinical trials were performed in a blinded fashion. The technician performing the HZA was unaware of patient histories, work-up results, or IVF outcome. In one study, the majority of 36 patients had semen with teratozoospermia as the sole recognized abnormality.[20] Fertilization was achieved in ≥1 of the wife's egg(s) for 27 of these men. As a group, the mean number of sperm tightly bound to the hemizonae was 36.1 ± 7. In contrast, the average number of sperm bound for the nine other cases, where no fertilization occurred during IVF treatment, was 10.4 ± 4 (p <0.05).[20]

Next, a more rigorous study examined a broader spectrum of male factor cases undergoing IVF therapy.[21] Here, proven fertile men (having fathered a child naturally within the past 2 years) provided the control semen. Of 28 cases chosen randomly for HZA testing, the semen of 22 men achieved fertilization *in vitro* with ≥65% of the preovulatory oocytes. The corresponding mean values for number of bound sperm and HZA Index are given in Table 1. For the remaining six cases, fewer than 65% of the preovulatory oocytes were fertilized; the average number of sperm bound and the HZA Index were statistically lower (p <0.02; Table 1). A subjective assessment of the 28 HZA Index values, relative to the IVF outcome, suggested a bimodal distribution, with a cut-off at 36. Based on these two threshold values (65% fertilization and an Index of 36), the HZA accurately predicted the IVF outcome in 26 of the 28 cases. Among the two remaining cases, one case appeared as a false-negative and the other as a false-positive test.

TABLE 1
Hemizona Assay Results After Testing Spermatozoa from Patient-Couples
Undergoing *In Vitro* Fertilization Therapy at Norfolk

	>65% of provulatory oocytes fertilized in IVF	<65% fertilized in IVF
Number of cases (n)	22	6
Number of sperm tightly bound to the hemizona	62.1 ± 10.9	7.3 ± 1.4[a]
HZA Index	120.4 ± 18.3	29.5 ± 7.5[a]
Cases correctly predicted by the HZA[b]	96% (21/22)	83% (5/6)

Note: Semen was received for the HZA at 48 h after the IVF attempt. The 28 cases were grouped according to the percentage of preovulatory oocytes which fertilized *in vitro*.

[a] Significant difference between group means ($p < 0.02$).

[b] Index value of 36 was used as the cut-off.[21]

Initial work with the HZA had been carried-out with frozen-thawed, immature (prophase) oocytes, which were recovered almost exclusively from ovaries obtained at autopsy. All oocytes were stored at $-70°C$ in 2 *M* DMSO. Subsequent experiments have shown that zonae stored in a salt solution reflect an equivalent sperm binding capacity.[22] Whether held at low temperature in DMSO, or stored at room temperature in a concentrated salt solution, these oocytes yielded hemizonae with the same binding kinetics, and equal capacities for assessment of semen samples. Due to simplicity of handling and ease in transportation, storage of zonae in the buffered salt solution is now our preferred method.

II. GENERAL LABORATORY PROCEDURES AND ASSAY PROTOCOL

A. RECOVERY AND STORAGE OF ZONA-INTACT HUMAN OOCYTES (BRIEF EXPLANATION)

Immature human oocytes can be obtained from three possible sources. Ovaries removed at autopsy are held in a chilled medium and dissected within 48 h of receipt. The methods of Overstreet et al.[8] are followed for mincing of tissue and searching for intact zonae. The same recovery procedures are followed when surgically excised ovarian tissue is received. Third, immature, unfertilized oocytes are frequently contributed by a consenting IVF couple if ovarian stimulation results in the collection of four or more "good" metaphase oocytes. The immature oocytes are placed in the concentrated salt solution before removing them from the IVF embryology lab.

B. RINSING AND BISECTING OF THE NONLIVING INTACT OOCYTE (BRIEF EXPLANATION)

In preparation for the HZA, the frozen (DMSO) oocyte is quick-thawed and rinsed; salt-treated oocytes are retrieved from the storage vial and rinsed briefly in culture medium. The cutting blade is attached to the micromanipulator and the cutting dish is mounted on the inverted microscope (see Figure 2). With one intact oocyte held under medium in the cutting dish, the blade is positioned so that it is centered over the egg, then lowered slowly to produce two oocyte halves that are equal in size (Figure 3). After discarding the degenerated ooplasm, the two matching hemizonae are placed in the same holding drop.

C. THE HZA PROTOCOL (BRIEF EXPLANATION, FIGURE 4)

In clinical use, semen is received from a proven, fertile male (control) and one or more

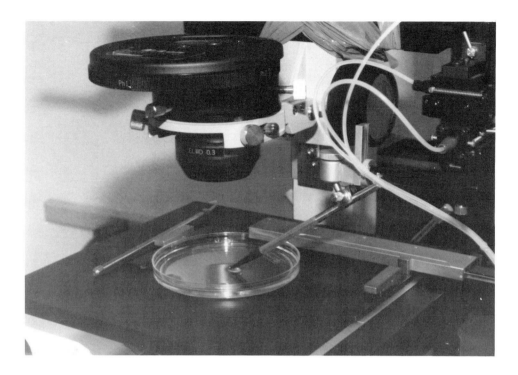

FIGURE 2. Positioning the cutting dish and cutting blade in the microscopic stage, in preparation for bisecting of the zona pellucida.

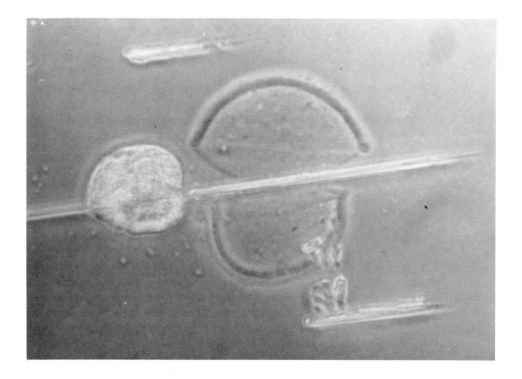

FIGURE 3. Two completely separated zona hemispheres (matching hemizonae). Also shown are the degenerated ooplasmic mass and the groove which was etched into the plastic dish as the blade completed the zona sectioning.

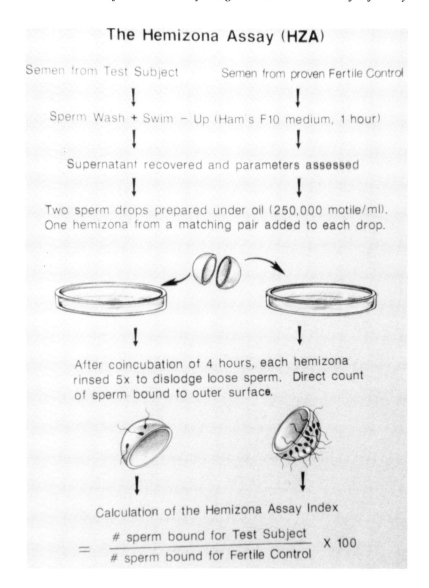

FIGURE 4.   Abbreviated protocol illustrating the major steps in the HZA. See text for more detail.

test patients. After washing with culture medium, motile sperm are allowed to ''swim-up'' during 1 h of incubation at 37°C. (This sperm handling was designed to parallel procedures used in Norfolk's IVF lab). The supernatant sperm are first diluted with medium; a diluted sperm drop is then placed under oil and one hemizona is placed in that drop. In one droplet, the control spermatozoa and a single hemizona are coincubated; a second droplet contains the patient's spermatozoa and the *matching* hemizona. After 4 h of coincubation, each hemizona is removed and rinsed vigorously to detach loosely associated sperm; then the number of sperm tightly bound to the outer hemizona surface is counted (some sperm can bind to the inner surface[15]). The two resulting numbers are then used to calculate the HZA Index for that patient (see Equation 1 above).

III. DETAILED PROCEDURES

A. SUPPLIES, REAGENTS, AND EQUIPMENT

Media—Phosphate buffered saline (PBS; purchased or prepared in the laboratory); Ham's F10 culture medium (Gibco Co.; Grand Island, NY); 0.9% physiological saline with antibiotic (prepared in the laboratory).

Reagents and other factors—Human fetal cord serum (heat-inactivated at 56°C for 1 h, then filter-sterilized), which may be substituted with 3.5% (w/v) human serum albumin (Fraction V, Sigma, St. Louis, MO); dimethylsulfoxide (DMSO, 36 M); magnesium chloride-6 H_2O; (Mallinckrodt Chemical Works, St. Louis, MO); polyvinylpyrrolidone (PVP; MW 40,000, Sigma); Na-HEPES buffer (Sigma); 1.0 N stock solutions of HCl and NaOH (for pH adjustments).

Supplies

Latex tubing with mouthpiece ($\frac{1}{8}''$ and $\frac{1}{4}''$ inner diameters)
Beaver microblades (disposable, K 20-1730, #7530, black, 30°, 3.5 mm; Katena Products, Inc., 4 Stewart Court, Denville, NJ 07834, telephone: 201/989-1600.
Beaver chuck handle (K 20-1920, #1312, round, 7.5 cm) (see note at end of chapter)
Nylon mesh (75 μm openings; sample from Tetko Co., 420 Sawmill River Road, Elmsford, NY 10523)
100 μl glass microcapillary tubes (Corning Co., Corning, NY)
18 and 25 gauge needles, attached to 1-ml syringes
Copper sieves (use the 2 mm and the 300 μm grids from Fisher #14-306A)
15-ml disposable centrifuge tubes with caps (Falcon #2095)
Plastic petri dishes (35 × 10 and 100 × 20 mm, Falcon #3002)
Diamond tip etching pencil (Thomas #5680-D12)
1-ml micro centrifuge tubes and racks
Pasteur pipettes (5 $\frac{3}{4}''$)
Glass microscope slides
Coverslips (22 × 22 mm)
Glass petri dishes (100 × 20 mm)
Pipettors (50—1000 μl range)
Heavy white mineral oil (Sigma)
Large tub for ice, or freezer trays
Alcohol lamp or gas burner
Pen-Strep solution (Sigma #PO 906)
Hemacytometer *
Cell counter *
Laboratory timer
Marker pens
Specimen containers
Scalpels
Large, toothed forceps
Critoseal

* (required for confirming final sperm dilution = 500,000/ml)

Large equipment

Dissecting microscope (illumination within the base is preferable)
Inverted phase contrast microscope
Centrifuge (swing-out buckets)

CO_2 incubator (5% in air; 37°C)

One micromanipulator (Narishige, Leitz, etc.)

B. PROCEDURES FOR OOCYTE RECOVERY, STORAGE, AND CUTTING

1. Concentrated Salt Storage Solution[9,10,22]

Prepare a 30-ml batch using distilled or purified water. Add 0.03 g of polyvinylpyrrolidone (PVP) to 30 ml of water. Stir briefly until the PVP is in solution. Add 40 mM Na-HEPES (0.3 g) and stir briefly. Adjust the pH to 7.4 before using. Store at +4°C or room temperature in a container of your choice (cold storage is preferable).

2. Immature IVF Oocytes

Consenting patient couples may desire to have residual, unfertilized oocytes contributed to the research lab. To assure no accidental abuse, such eggs should not leave the embryology laboratory in a viable state. Therefore, the IVF lab personnel first transfer the oocytes, using a drawn pipette, into a 1-ml microfuge tube (one to five eggs/tube) containing 0.5 ml of the hypertonic salt solution. The oocytes are rendered nonviable by the salt exposure. The eggs should be placed in storage solution within 48 h after retrieval for IVF, since precipitates or follicular matter may coat the zona surface. The capped tubes are kept *upright* in a rack, at either +4° or +25°C, until picked up by the HZA technician. Salt-treated eggs can be stored for about 90 days at ambient temperatures up to 25°C.[10] As a precaution, however, it is best to refrigerate oocytes which may not be used for many months. The storage tubes should not be inverted or unduly disturbed. Each tube should bear a label, stating the date, tissue source and number of oocytes contained.

3. Ooccytes Recovered from Ovarian Tissue

a. Surgically Derived Ovarian Tissue

Following a written informed consent approved by our IRB, surgical cases are selected, where the patient is still ovulating, but is not more than 45 years of age. Ovarian tissue obtained at any stage of the menstrual cycle is acceptable, although the follicular phase may yield a higher number of oocytes.

The tissue is placed in physiological saline (sd with 100 IU/ml Pen-Strep) immediately after excision. The tissue *cannot* be placed in formalin! The specimen is refrigerated at +4°C (never frozen), and should be picked-up within 24 h of surgery. Within 48 h of this ovariectomy, the laboratory personnel should have completed the recovery of oocytes from the tissue.

Using procedures already described,[15] the half or whole ovary is immersed in chilled PBS within a 100 × 20 mm glass petri dish. Any obvious follicles are punctured with a 25-gauge needle attached to a 1-ml syringe, half-filled with PBS. After attempting to aspirate all follicular contents, the tissue is sliced using a scalpel blade into strips that are about $1/_4$" wide. Use large, toothed forceps to anchor the tissue. A 10-min "test" search for oocytes can be made after first cutting the ovarian tissue into strips; if ≤2 eggs are located during this search, the tissue is not promising and could be discarded. (Alternatively, the tissue can be sliced with a set of 6 single-edged razor blades, bolted together in parallel; personal communication from Nick Cross). While one strip is transferred to a new work dish, for further mincing with the blade, and then shredding with 18-gauge needles, all remaining tissue is held aside on ice. After 10 to 15 min of dissection on the first strip, that glass petri dish is carried to a dissecting microscope. Using a total magnification ranging between 10 to 30×, the petri dish is methodically searched. (Alternatively, the suspension is carefully passed through two sieves [2mm and 300 μm openings] so that the oocytes are finally retained on a nylon mesh having 75 μm pores). All zona-intact oocytes, whether denuded or enclosed in granulosa cells, are picked up by mouth suction, using a hand-pulled, small-bore (about 300 μm in diameter) pasteur pipette attached to rubber tubing (pull the glass tips over an alcohol flame; score with the diamond tipped pencil). The oocytes are transferred to a 200 μl holding droplet of PBS held under mineral oil. The holding dish is also kept on ice throughout.

After mincing all strips and searching each dish twice, the accumulated oocytes are stored in concentrated salt solution. On average, one good, whole ovary may yield 20 to 40 potentially useable oocytes (maximum, about 70). From empiric experience, we know that approximately 20% of these will have a very immature zona pellucida, with a markedly limited capacity for binding sperm during the HZA.

b. Storage of Oocytes in DMSO

If frozen storage of oocytes is preferred, the eggs are transferred to 2 ml of PBS in a small petri dish, and placed on ice.[8,15] Every 15 min, two drops (approximately 0.16 ml) of concentrated DMSO (36 M) are added to the petri dish. By the end of 30 min, a total of 0.33 ml has been added (final DMSO concentration should thus equal 2 M). After an additional 15 min, oocyte pairs are transferred with 30 μl of the 2 M DMSO solution into the end of a 100 μl microcapillary tube, using a hand-drawn pipette. Both ends are plugged with Critoseal (or other sealant); a narrow strip of tape is folded over one end (like a flag) and labeled with the number of oocytes, date and tissue source. The tubes are then frozen directly at −70°C.

c. Postmortem Ovarian Tissue

If one provides the tissue-source laboratory with specimen containers filled with the PBS/Pen-Strep solution, the collection of tissue will be facilitated. Ovaries should be recovered within 48 h of the estimated time of death; sooner if possible. All subsequent steps are those given in section (a) above.

4. Retrieving the Oocytes from Storage

If the oocytes have been frozen at −70°C in the DMSO solution, the microcapillary tube is simply retrieved from the freezer and allowed to thaw at room temperature in one step. If one observes that the Critoseal plugs are extruded during the rapid warming, an intermediate step can be added; here, transfer the tube from −70°C to the freezer compartment of a standard refrigerator before bringing the tube up to room temperature. While keeping the tube flat on the stage of a dissecting microscope, score both ends of the glass tube with a diamond-tipped pencil. Snap off each end carefully, tilt the tube vertically over a clean petri dish, and allow the contents to flow out by gravity. Locate the stored eggs and transfer them to rinsing drops of medium, in preparation for zona cutting.

For salt-stored eggs, the storage tube is opened and enough rinse medium is added to nearly fill the tube. Cap it tightly and invert the tube six to eight times in order to suspend the stored eggs in the fluid. Carefully pour the contents into a small 35 × 10 mm petri dish and search for the eggs. Using a drawn pipette, transfer the eggs to a holding drop of medium in preparation for zona cutting.

5. Bisecting of the Intact Zona Pellucida

We utilize an inverted, phase contrast microscope equipped with a micromanipulator on each side (Figure 5). If a *pair* of micromanipulators is used, one has the option of employing an egg-holding pipette for anchoring or moving the oocyte during the cutting procedure (Figure 6). The details for pulling, fire-polishing and shaping such a pipette have been previously published.[15] We have determined that use of the egg-holding pipette is not absolutely necessary; therefore, a simplified procedure is described here, requiring only one manipulator.

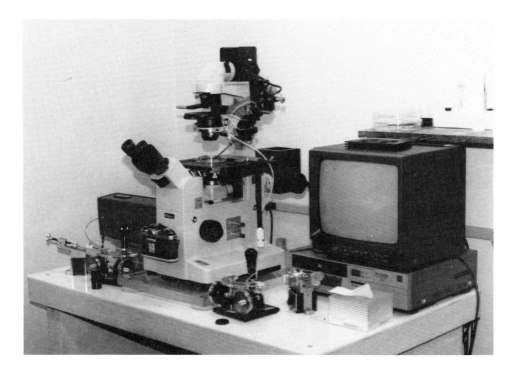

FIGURE 5.   Inverted microscope with attached micromanipulators and support equipment utilized in performing the HZA in the authors' laboratory.

A Beaver chuck handle is fitted with a Beaver micro-sharpe blade. The handle is then clamped to the micromanipulator, over the microscope stage and adjusted to a 45° angle with respect to the stage surface (Figure 2). The blade is further aligned so that its plane is perpendicular to the stage. The top or bottom of a 100 × 20 mm plastic petri dish serves as the cutting chamber. The dish is flooded 3 to 4 mm deep with any balanced salt solution containing 0.3% (or 3.5%) bovine serum albumin, which helps to prevent sticking of the zona. The blade tip is lowered to the petri surface, and a short groove (50 to 100 μm) is etched onto the bottom of the dish (Figure 3). At this time, the technician identifies the precise point along the blade edge where contact is made with the bottom. Later, that same portion of the blade edge will be positioned over the egg. The groove also serves to "grip" the intact egg and keep it from moving during cutting.

The blade is raised slightly (about 200 μm) and the oocyte to be cut is transferred by fine pipette to the working zone immediately next to the groove. The magnification is now increased to ×200. Using the drawn pipette or the flat edge of the blade (or an egg-holding pipette), the oocyte is nudged onto the groove. The correct portion of the blade's cutting edge is positioned slightly above the egg. Lower the blade onto the egg until the zona dimples inward slightly. Using the micromanipulator controls, move the blade slightly along the north/south axis, causing the egg to roll slightly, forward and then back. Choose the position which appears to have the blade edge centered exactly over the egg and could produce two equal halves. Then slowly lower the blade until it cuts through the egg and bites into the plastic of the dish. At this point, manipulate the blade to produce excursions to the left and right, thus yielding two completely separated hemispheres, the two hemizonae. Effective practice in cutting the zona can be achieved by using discarded mouse or hamster ova. Also, we first use a "test" hamster ovum each day to ensure that the blade is properly positioned.

The magnification is then reduced to 100 or 40 ×, and the blade is slowly raised. If one hemizona is stuck to the blade, dislodge it by moving the joystick vigorously left and

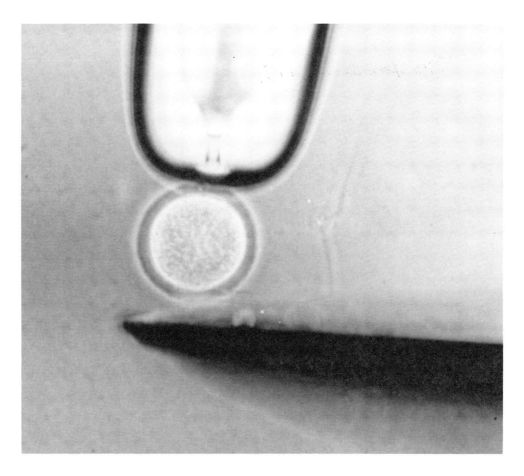

FIGURE 6. Use of two micromanipulators to bisect the zona pellucida. This optional approach (see text for details) utilizes one manipulator to guide the egg-holding pipette and a second manipulator for positioning the cutting blade.

right. Alternatively, gently pull the hemizona free using the tip of a *clean* 25-gauge needle, attached to a 1-ml syringe. Place one or more droplets (100 μl) of rinse medium (any medium containing BSA is acceptable) in a clean petri dish; place the dish on the stage of the dissecting microscope. Using the drawn pipette tip and mouth suction, slowly pick up both hemizonae from the cutting dish, and transfer them to the rinse drop on the dissecting microscope.

If a portion of the degenerated ooplasm is adhering to the inner zona, use a pipette with a very small opening (slightly smaller than the hemizona diameter) and vigorously pipette the hemizona in and out to dislodge the debris. (*Caution*: During any maneuver with the drawn pipettes, make sure that substantial fluid is held in the pipette tip. If all of the medium is inadvertently expelled, bubbles will enter the droplet and the hemizonae can be easily lost). Transfer the two *matching* hemizonae to the same holding drop (100 μl volume of medium or 0.9% saline) under mineral oil. The dish is held at +4°C overnight (or up to 48 h) until the assay is initiated.

C. PERFORMING THE HEMIZONA ASSAY (HZA)
1. Control Semen from Proven Fertile Men
These men have fathered a child naturally within the 2 years previous, and have semen parameters falling within the normal ranges: (1) sperm motility is ≥60% in fresh semen;

(2) the seminal sperm concentration is $\geq 50 \times 10^6/ml$; and (3) the percentage of sperm with normal morphology is $\geq 50\%$ by WHO standards, or $>14\%$ by the new strict method (see Chapter 4). Semen is collected by masturbation after an abstinence period of 1 to 6 days, and delivered to the HZA technician at 15 to 60 min after ejaculation.

Even proven fertile men do not score equally in any assay. Therefore, it is best to screen six to eight potential control donors by testing the binding of their spermatozoa to two pairs of hemizonae. For each man, examine the range for the number of bound sperm per hemizona. It is advisable to avoid any potential donor whose sperm consistently show low zona binding (20 to 30 sperm/hemizona) or very high binding (>120 sperm/ hemizona) under the standard HZA protocol. Either of these conditions will tend to skew the patients' HZA Index values. Also, avoid dependence on just one to two men for providing the control semen. Rely instead on a readily available pool of four to six control men.[24]

2. Sperm Preparation for the HZA

Prepare 4 to 10 ml of Ham's F10 medium, supplemented with 7.5% human fetal cord serum (or 3.5% serum albumin). This medium is, hereafter, referred to as "Ham's medium". Equilibrate the medium for several hours with 5% CO_2 in air ($37°C$). Also, gas-equilibrate 25 ml of *heavy* mineral oil at $37°C$.

Once the patient semen has been received and both ejaculates have liquefied, prepare for the sperm washes and swim-up. Label the appropriate number of 15-ml centrifuge tubes for the control donor and the patient(s). A maximum of three patients can be assayed in a single day. If the patient semen has an adequate concentration and motility, place a 500 μl aliquot of semen in each of two tubes. If the motility is very low ($<30\%$) or the sperm concentration is quite low ($<15 \times 10^6/ml$), use nearly the entire ejaculate, by dispensing 250 μl aliquots into multiple tubes. For the control semen, prepare duplicate tubes, each containing 300 μl of semen.

Mix all semen aliquots with 0.5 ml of Ham's medium, centrifuge at 400 g for 5 to 10 min, and discard the supernatants. Resuspend the pellets in 0.5 ml of Ham's medium, centrifuge again for 5 min and then discard the wash supernatants. For the controls, and for patients having adequate sperm motility and concentration, slowly layer the second pellets with 0.5 ml of Ham's medium. For semen samples requiring multiple tubes, layer each pellet with 0.25 ml of medium.

All tubes are loosely capped and incubated at the same time at $37°C$, with 5% CO_2 in air. After allowing the sperm "swim-up" to proceed for one hour, the tubes are gently removed from the incubator. For each semen sample, the supernatants are carefully removed using a pasteur pipette and pooled. Disturbing the pellets during this particular step will cause some immotile sperm to be included in the swim-up supernatant. For each of the two pooled suspensions (control and patient), the percentage of motile sperm and the concentration are calculated. One can employ standard hemacytometer (for sperm concentration) and slide (sperm motility) methods here, or rely on data obtained from any of several computer-assisted sperm analysis instruments which are now commercially available (see Chapter 6). Calculate the *motile* concentration per milliliter ($= M$).

One milliliter of diluted sperm suspension is then prepared (0.5×10^6 motile/ml) for the HZA coincubation dishes. The following simple equation is useful:

$$\frac{0.5}{M} = \frac{X}{1000 \ \mu l} \quad ; \quad X \ \mu l = \frac{(0.5)(1000)}{M} = \frac{500}{M} \tag{2}$$

Mix the swim-up supernatant, remove the calculated volume (X) and dilute this to 1.0 ml using Ham's medium.

It is critical that the motile sperm concentrations are very close to 500,000 motile/ml for *both* the control suspension and the patient sperm suspension. Therefore, check the motile count again, by placing one drop of the diluted suspension directly onto a hemacytometer chamber. At this point, use of the computer-assisted instruments may result in inaccurate numbers, due to the very low concentration. If the patient vs. control values differ by more than 15% correct the lower suspension by adding a calculated number of sperm from the original (undiluted) swim-up suspension. If the patient's swim-up supernatant does not contain at least 500,000 motile/ml, then either concentrate the supernatant sperm by gentle centrifugation (5 min, 300 *g*), or reduce the sperm number slightly in *both* the control and patient hemizona dishes. However, do not attempt to perform the HZA at motile concentrations below 250,000/ml.

If there is grave doubt concerning the fertilizing potential of sperm from a certain IVF patient, or when the HZA is being repeated due to a failed HZA initially, then a modified HZA could be performed. That is, use the standard hemizona insemination for the control sperm (500,000/ml), but a higher sperm concentration in the patient hemizona dish. If IVF for that patient will be attempted using a tenfold increase in sperm numbers, then the HZA can be performed also using a tenfold increase (i.e., 5×10^6/ml). Is the resulting HZA Index now above 65 (approximately)? If yes, then a simple increase in the insemination concentration has enhanced the patient's fertilizing potential, making it similar to the fertilizing capacity of the control sperm suspension. In those instances, however, where fertilizing potential is to be evaluated for possible *in vivo* conception, then the control and patient hemizona dishes should use the same concentration of motile spermatozoa.

For each patient being tested that day, one pair of *matching* hemizonae must be available. Label the bottom of one 35×10 mm petri dish with the patient name and the hemizona number (egg #1, egg #2, etc.). Place a 100 µl droplet of the diluted control sperm (500,000/ml) in the center of the dish and immediately cover it with warmed mineral oil. Into a second, labeled dish, transfer a 100 µl drop of the patient's sperm and cover it with oil. Using the dissecting microscope, scan both droplets to ensure that they reflect a nearly equal concentration of motile sperm. Now transfer hemizona #1a to the center of the control sperm droplet; add the *matching* hemizona (#1b) to the patient sperm drop. The same procedure is repeated, if two more dishes and two other matching hemizonae are to be used for testing a different patient that day.

All hemizona dishes are then incubated (37°C, 5% CO_2 in air) for 4 h. After completing the coincubation, the two dishes with matching hemizonae are carried to the dissecting microscope. Transfer several drops of chilled rinse medium to a clean petri dish (the cold shock will slow sperm motility and permit easier counting, particularly when the hemizona has a large number of bound spermatozoa). Prepare a drawn pipette such that the opening of the tip is approximately 1.5 times the diameter of the hemizona. Using this narrow-bore pipette and mouth suction, remove the control hemizona from the coincubation droplet and expel it into a rinse drop. Then, vigorously pipette the same hemizona in and out of the pipette tip *five times*, in order to dislodge those sperm which are only loosely attached to the zona surface. After the fivefold rinse, place the hemizona in a labeled drop of clean medium, under oil, and hold it aside for counting.

The rinsing procedure is repeated for the matching hemizona, which had been coincubated with patient spermatozoa. It is likewise transferred to a separate, labeled "counting" drop. Transfer the 35×10 mm petri dishes containing the counting drops to the stage of an inverted microscope. The hemizona is gently nudged and tilted with a clean 25-gauge needle, so that the convex surface of the hemizona is visualized. With practice, one is able to start at the uppermost plane of the convex zona surface and slowly count the bound sperm while focusing down through deeper and deeper planes. One must discriminate between sperm which are tightly bound to the *outer* surface and those few sperm which may bind tightly to the inner surface.[15] It is helpful to evaluate one quarter of the hemizona volume first, then return to the uppermost plane and count through a second quarter of the outer surface, etc. Alternatively, one can flip the hemizona over (concave surface is now up), count *all* of the bound sperm, and then subtract the number of sperm that are bound to the inner surface. The same steps are followed for counting the number of sperm tightly bound to the outer surface of the *matching* hemizona. The value of the HZA Index is then calculated (Equation 1 above) and recorded for that patient.

IV. QUALITY CONTROL

1. The HZA always uses matching hemizonae during a particular assay. This approach provides an internal control and eliminates most of the problems created by zona differences between any two intact eggs.
2. The zona binding of patient spermatozoa is always compared to the binding capacity of sperm from proven fertile men, having reliable semen quality.
3. The motile concentration in both sperm drops (patient and control) is kept very close to 500,000/ml. Multiple counts are performed to ensure that the deviation does not exceed 15%.
4. Periodic assessment of technician error should be carried out. Here two or more HZA technicians should compare their individual counts for motile sperm concentration and, especially, the number of spermatozoa bound tightly to a test hemizona. Due to intertechnician differences in rinsing the hemizonae and counting the bound sperm, the laboratory should minimize the turnover in personnel performing the HZA, and have the same technician perform the final count of bound sperm for any two matching hemizonae, if the Index value is to be valid.
5. One must identify and reject an assay which has used hemizonae of inferior binding quality or used a bad control semen sample. In the authors' laboratory, any assay is rejected if the hemizona that was coincubated with control sperm bound only.[24]
6. The duration of coincubation should not deviate much from the standard 4 h. A very short coincubation period (1 to 2 h) would fall in the early part of the zona binding kinetics curve and may not be reliable for diagnostic purposes.[15]

V. INTERPRETATION OF RESULTS

For a given patient, the HZA Index will indicate sperm fertilizing potential. High Index values represent normal reproductive function, in the context of either *in vivo* or *in vitro* fertilization. One must interpret Index values that fall in the low range as indicative of low to nil fertilizing potential. As a consequence of differences in technician handling and in the quality of control semen utilized, individual laboratories must select and validate their specific HZA Index "cut-off" or "critical region." In our laboratory, HZA Index values falling between 36 and 65 represent our current "critical region." Hence, the physician may choose to have the hemizona assay repeated if a patient response falls into that region.

During the period of assay development, the accuracy of HZA predictions was tested against the actual IVF fertilization outcome for each patient. In over 40 such HZA/IVF comparisons, we have encountered only one instance of a false positive HZA result (i.e., HZA Index was high but the patient's sperm failed to fertilize the ova *in vitro*). Alternatively, that failure might be attributed to a discrepancy in quality between the two semen samples handled, or poor oocyte quality, or a technical error.

Because the HZA, currently, is always performed using an insemination of 500,000 motile sperm/ml, a discrepancy can also arise when patient IVF inseminations are carried out with variable sperm concentrations. For example, many IVF laboratories routinely inseminate oocytes with 50,000 sperm/ml. When handling suspected male factor cases, however, fertilization is maximized by using a three- to tenfold increase in sperm numbers (i.e., 150,000 to 500,000 motile sperm/ml). In contrast, if a standard HZA is performed for such a patient (500,000/ml for both the patient and control hemizona dishes), a false negative HZA prediction may be encountered; that is, the HZA Index was low, thus predicting IVF failure, yet good fertilization was actually achieved *in vitro*.

In our laboratory, if an HZA Index is at the upper end of the critical region (55 to 65) or better, we predict that the patient's sperm will achieve good fertilization *in vitro* when using the *standard* 50,000/ml insemination. However, if the patient's HZA Index is lower than 55, approximately, we recommend that the IVF insemination be carried out using 500,000 motile sperm/ml (refer also to the discussion on HZA insemination concentration found in Section III.C.2).

Based on the technique used in our HZA and IVF laboratories, we are presently examining two approaches that will refine the HZA Index "critical region." (1) What is the range of HZA Index values obtained for patients whose sperm failed IVF even though the IVF insemination was ≥500,000 motile sperm/ml? These data will further document the lower limit of the critical region. (2) What is the range of Index values for hemizona assays which compared the sperm from two proven fertile men? The upper limit of the critical region will be refined with this information.

VI. CONCLUSIONS

To date, we have found the HZA Index to be accurate in predicting IVF outcome to the point of embryo transfer. In time, we will know whether HZA aids in prediction of pregnancy rates and outcome. Equally important will be defining the limits of HZA; that is, situations where reliability is highest vs. conditions where HZA is not useful. We are confident that the HZA offers a genuine technical advance that does assist us in both diagnosis and prognosis. Importantly, given the increased attention to treatment intervention on behalf of male factor cases, the HZA may be a useful tool by which to monitor the progress of therapeutic courses or to select a "better" sperm for microsurgical injection, than would a random choice.

Furthermore, contraceptive effectiveness may be estimated by employing the HZA, again as a functional bioassay. Examples include residual or intermittent oligospermia in men receiving a GnRH antagonist plus testosterone or vaccines employing specific antigens of the sperm or zona pellucida.

AUTHORS' NOTE ADDED IN PRESS

A fine microblade from Feather Industries may offer a better alternative to the Beaver microblade products listed under Supplies in Section III.A. The blades are available in Japan from Feather Industries, Ltd. (Feza-Kogyo Kabushiki Kaisha, Matsumori, Mino-shi Gifu-ken 600-1, Japan). Order the Bio-Cut blades #715 with a 15° angle.

REFERENCES

1. **Bedford, J. M.,** Significance of the need for sperm capacitation before fertilization in Eutherian mammals, *Biol. Reprod.,* 28, 108, 1983.
2. **Yanagimachi, R.,** Mechanisms of fertilization in mammals, in *Fertilization and Embryonic Development In Vitro,* Mastroianni, L. and Biggers, J. B., Eds., Plenum Press, New York, 1981, 81.
3. **Chang, M. C.,** The meaning of sperm capacitation; a historical perspective, *J. Androl.,* 5, 45, 1984.

4. **Yanagimachi, R., Yanagimachi, H., and Rogers, B. J.,** The use of zona-free animal ova as a test system for the assessment of their fertilizing capacity of human spermatozoa, *Biol. Reprod.,* 15, 471, 1976.

5. **Rogers, B. J., Van Campen, H., Ueno, M., Lambert, H., Bronson, R., and Hale, R.,** Analysis of human spermatozoal fertilizing ability using zona-free ova, *Fertil. Steril.,* 32, 664, 1979.

6. **Yanagimachi, R.,** Review article. Zona-free hamster eggs: their use in assessing fertilizing capacity and examining chromosomes of human spermatozoa, *Gamete Res.,* 10, 187, 1984.

7. **Overstreet, J. W. and Hembree, W. C.,** Penetration of the zona pellucida of nonliving human oocytes by human spermatozoa *in vitro, Fertil. Steril.,* 27, 815, 1976.

8. **Overstreet, J. W., Yanagimachi, R., Katz, D. F., Hayashi, K., and Hanson, F. W.,** Penetration of human spermatozoa into the human zona pellucida and the zona-free hamster egg: a study of fertile donors and infertile patients, *Fertil. Steril.,* 33, 534, 1980.

9. **Yanagimachi, R., Lopata, A., Odom, C. B., Bronson, R. A., Mahi, C. A., and Nicholson, G. L.,** Retention of biologic characteristics of zona pellucida in highly concentrated salt solution: the use of salt-stored eggs for assessing the fertilizing capacity of spermatozoa, *Fertil. Steril.,* 31, 562, 1979.

10. **Yoshimatsu, N., Yanagimachi, R., and Lopata, A.,** Zonae pellucidae of salt-stored hamster and human eggs: their penetrability by homologous and heterologous spermatozoa, *Gamete Res.,* 21, 115, 1988.

11. **Kruger, T. F., Acosta, A. A., Simmons, K. F., Swanson, R. J., Matta, J. F., and Oehninger, S.,** Predictive value of abnormal sperm morphology in *in vitro* fertilization, *Fertil. Steril.,* 49, 112, 1988.

12. **Huszar, G., Corrales, M., and Vigue, L.,** Correlation between sperm creatine phosphokinase activity and sperm concentrations in normospermic and oligospermic men, *Gamete Res.,* 19, 67, 1988.

13. **Jeyendran, R. S., Van der Ven, H. H., Perez-Pelaez, M., Crabo, B. G., and Zaneveld, L. J. D.,** Development of an assay to assess the functional integrity of the human sperm membrane and its relationship to other semen characteristics, *J. Reprod. Fertil.,* 70, 219, 1984.

14. **Morshedi, M., Acosta, A., Ackerman, S., and Swanson, R. J.,** Swim-up ATP as a predictor of the outcome of an IVF Program, *J. Androl.,* 9(1), 24P, 1988.

15. **Burkman, L. J., Coddington, C. C., Franken, D. R., Kruger, T. F., Rosenwaks, Z., and Hodgen, G. D.,** The hemizona assay (HZA): development of a diagnostic test for the binding of human spermatozoa to the human hemizona pellucida to predict fertilization potential, *Fertil. Steril.,* 49, 688, 1988.

16. **Chen, C. and Sathananthan, A. H.,** Early penetration of human sperm through the vestments of human eggs *in vitro, Arch. Androl.,* 16, 183, 1986.

17. **Mahadevan, M. M., Trounson, A. O., Wood, C., and Leeton, J. F.,** Effect of oocyte quality and sperm characteristics on the number of spermatozoa bound to the zona pellucida of human oocytes inseminated *in vitro, J. In Vitro Fertil. Embryo Trans.,* 4, 223, 1987.

18. **Oehninger S.,** unpublished data, 1988.

19. **Coddington, C. C., Burkman, L. J., and Hodgen, G. D.,** HZA assessment of spermatozoa from vasovasostomy patients, manuscript in preparation.

20. **Franken, D. R., Oehninger, S., Burkman, L. J., Coddington, C. D., Kruger, T. F., Rosenwaks, Z., Acosta, A. A., and Hodgen G. D.,** The hemizona assay (HZA): a predictor of human sperm fertilizing potential in IVF Treatment, *J. In Vitro Fertil. Embryo Trans.,* 6, 44, 1989.

21. **Oehninger, S., Coddington, C. C., Scott, R., Franken, D. A., Acosta, A. A., and Hodgen, G. D.,** Hemizona assay (HZA): assessment of sperm (dys) function and prediction of *in vitro* fertilization (IVF) outcome, *Fertil. Steril.,* 51, 665, 1989.

22. **Franken, D. R., Burkman, L. J., Oehninger, S. C., Coddington, C. C., Veeck, L. L., Kruger, T. F., Rosenwaks, Z., and Hodgen, G. D.,** The hemizona assay using salt stored human oocytes: evaluation of zona pellucida capacity for binding human spermatozoa, *Gamete Res.,* 22, 15, 1989.

23. **Coddington, C. C., Franken, D. R., Burkman, L. J., Oosthuizen, W. T., Kruger, T., and Hodgen, G. D.,** Functional aspects of human sperm binding to the zona pellucida using the hemizona assay, *J. Andrology,* submitted.

24. **Franken, D. R., Coddington, C. C., Burkman, L. J., Oosthuizen, W. T., Kruger, T. F., and Hodgen, G. D.,** Defining the valid hemizona assay: accounting for binding variability within zonae pellucida and within semen samples from fertile males, *Fertil. Steril.,* submitted.

Chapter 13

CRYOPRESERVATION OF HUMAN SEMEN

J. K. Sherman

TABLE OF CONTENTS

I. INTRODUCTION

A. PURPOSE OF CHAPTER

This chapter is presented in response to the request of the editors for an abbreviated "handbook" manual which can be used "at the bench" by a technician or clinician with a basic knowledge in laboratory procedures. In response to the author's hesitation to place in print, in such a format, only the steps or procedures and techniques of a single method which would be construed as both optimal and requisite to cryobanking of human semen, the existence of a wide spectrum of successful alternate methods is stressed. Examples of several methods with appropriate references are presented to illustrate and reinforce an appreciation of variations acceptable in laboratory practice which satisfy cryobiological principles and authority, as well as standards of professional practice in the clinical application of cryobanking.

There are three salient sources of information on the factors and methods in the cryopreservation of human semen. These are (1) the scientific and clinical literature published by recognized authorities, especially as periodic reviews in symposia and textbooks, as well as papers in such journals as *Fertility and Sterility, Cryobiology, Andrologia, Archives of Andrology, International Journal of Andrology,* etc. (2) on-site observations at a cryobank which has been successful in processing and supplying cryopreserved semen for clinical use, and (3) published guidelines, standards and technical manuals on cryobanking published by the American Association of Tissue Banks.

It is the aim of the author to facilitate the readers efforts to devise their own procedure manual, for the cryopreservation of human semen, one which is tailored to suit the requisite applications, demand, and resources of their laboratory, and which satisfies existing professional practices and standards. Previous publications on appropriate historical background, cryobiological principles and spectrum of methods are excerpted, updated and cited for this purpose. It is not the intention of the author, however, to provide detailed information on aspects other than cryopreservation in the establishment and operation of a cryobank. Those other aspects of cryobanking must be developed by the reader, based on the three sources listed above, especially the second and third. The cryobank's Procedure Manual, once devised, will serve as the guide to its daily and continued operation. This manual will require periodic modification according to new methods and standards of operations, in order to conform with the current state of the art, to better equip the cryobank for successful clinical applications.

B. DEFINITIONS

Cryopreservation is that aspect or branch of cryobiology or low temperature biology, which is concerned with the maintenance of life during prolonged storage in the frozen state at extremely low temperatures.

The underlying principle of preservation of living cells by freezing depends upon control of molecular movement. Life processes require biochemical change realized through movement of molecules in an aqueous medium. If water in and around the protoplasm of a living cell is converted into ice at temperatures low enough to essentially arrest molecular movement, and if the biological system can subsequently be rewarmed without injury, then the life of the cell, held in this state of "suspended animation", can be preserved.

Cryobanks are the vehicles used to realize the clinical and research applications of cryopreserved cells and tissues. A most important component of the cryobank is its Procedure Manual.

The Procedure Manual is a handbook presentation of detailed descriptions of procedures used in cryobanking, prepared as an operation manual for directing technical personnel in the various methods and the activities of a cryobank. It may be based, generally, upon the published "American Association of Tissue Banks (AATB) Standards for Tissue Banking",[1] and the "AATB Technical Manual",[2] but it is tailored specifically to particular semen cryobank laboratory as to its procedures. It does not reflect the spectrum of alternate current and successful protocols in the state of the art but rather only those employed in its cryobank. The Procedure Manual is used to train laboratory personnel and to insure consistency in all phases of operations and step by step procedures in the laboratory.

C. CLINICAL APPLICATIONS

Successful cryobanking of human semen extends and enriches the attributes of artificial insemination of fresh semen in infertility therapy and population effects to include:

1. Timed multiple inseminations of husband semen (AIH) and of donor semen (AID) to coincide better with irregular female cycles or special conditions of the female tract, with the same or naturally optimal number of normal appearing, progressively motile spermatozoa.
2. Storage, pooling, and concentration of many oligozoospermic samples from the husband to increase numbers of progressively motile cells inseminated in AIH.
3. Storage of spermatozoa, whose quality is first improved by *in vitro* treatments, for more potentially fertile use later in appropriately timed AIH; also after treatment for sex preselection, to increase the coincident reduced numbers of cells, by pooling and concentration of stored populations.
4. Retention of fertilizing capacity of husband or donor even in his temporary or permanent absence.
5. Preservation of semen before surgical, chemical, or radiological cancer therapy which endangers reproductive integrity, for subsequent AIH.
7. Therapeutic substitution of carefully screened donor semen for that of the infertile husband in various timed protocols, on demand, from donors selected on the basis of integrity of bodily and genetic characteristics.
7. Production of a family of progeny from the same donor throughout a period of years, on demand, without the presence of the donor.
8. Wide selection of donor semen and ready availability, favoring the voluntary practice of the concept of germinal choice by a couple, to improve upon the genetic attributes of their family directly and of the population indirectly.
9. Restriction of the number of unwanted births through vasectomy which is preceded by cryobanking of semen for possible future potentially successful AIH, if circumstances change regarding desire for progeny.
10. Fertilization of ova *in vitro*, on demand, with cryopreserved spermatozoa of donor or husband, with subsequent embryo transfer in combined programs of such new innovative methods in modern reproductive biology.
11. Microbiological testing of semen or blood for sexually transmitted diseases, e.g., gonorrhea, hepatitis B, and AIDS, prior to insemination, while holding semen in frozen-storage, in quarantine, for release only after the time necessary for favorable screening.

II. HISTORY OF SEMEN CRYOBANKING

A. EARLY PERIOD (1776—1976)

The history of research on frozen human semen is intimately related to the initiation and development of the field of cryobiology.[3] Human spermatozoa were among the first cells to be observed with respect to effects of freezing. The events in the establishment of cryobanks for human semen closely parallel the sequence, if not the degree, of those with

TABLE 1
Highlights of Human Semen Cryobanking (1776—1976)

Contribution	Contributor and date
First low-temperature observations	Spallanzani (1776)
First suggestion of frozen semen bank	Mantegazza (1866)
−269°C survival; storage at −79°C	Jahnel (1938)
Individual variation, aging and thawing	Shettles (1940)
Vitrification principle; foam freezing	Hoagland and Pincus (1942)
Survival better in greater volumes	Parkes (1945)
Glycerol as cryoprotective agent	Polge et al. (1949)
Freezing rates; glycerol; preservation	Sherman (1953—1955)
First progeny from stored spermatozoa; dry ice method	Bunge and Sherman (1953); Bunge et al. (1954)
Sixteen births with stored spermatozoa	Keettel et al. (1956); Keettel (1959 personal communication)
Eleven frozen-semen conceptions in Japan	Iizuka and Sawada (1958); Sawada (1959)
Survival factors; banking applications; nitrogen vapor technique	Sherman (1962—1963)
Four births with nitrogen vapor technique	Perloff et al. (1964)
DMSO unsuitable (toxic) as cryoprotectant	Sherman (1964a)
More births from semen with egg yolk extender	Iizuka et al. (1968)
Metabolic effects; temperature shock, freeze-thawing	Ackerman (1968)
Births from semen stored in plastic straws	Matheson et al. (1969)
Fertility after 3 year storage; mucus test	Fjallbrant and Ackerman (1969)
Stability of DNA, hyaluronidase level, and citric acid in frozen storage	Ackerman and Sod-Moriah (1968—1970)
Normal progeny from semen stored over 10 years	Sherman (1927—1973)
Motility and Y chromosome fluorescence unaltered	Sherman and Char (1974)
Pellet freezing of diluted semen; births	Barkay et al. (1974)
Summary, with clinical results	Richardson (1975)
About 1500 births worldwide; fewer abnormalities and abortions than in normal population	Sherman (1976)

From Sherman, J. K., in *Techniques of Human Andrology,* Hafez, E. S. E., Ed., Elsevier-North Holland, New York, 1977. With permission.

bull semen, which have provided such a stimulus to low-temperature biology as well as to animal breeding.

Highlights in the historical development of low-temperature research and cryobanking of human semen in its most significant period are listed in Table 1. These are detailed and referenced elsewhere.[3-5] The concept of cryobanks for human semen was first proposed in 1866. It was the accidental discovery in 1949 and subsequent use of the polyhydric alcohol, glycerol, as a cryoprotective agent, however, which initiated the establishment of banks for frozen mammalian spermatozoa. Emphasis was placed, at first, on the economically important semen of farm animals, especially the bull. It was not until 1953—1954 that a successful, practical technique for cryopreservation of human spermatozoa was introduced by the author along with the demonstration that the spermatozoa, after being frozen and stored in dry ice (−78°C), were capable of fertilization and the subsequent induced development of normal progeny. From 1953 to 1963, various factors of cryosurvival were evaluated and normal births realized with frozen-stored human semen. During this period, only about 25 births were reported in the U.S. and Japan, all but one from the use of cryopreserved donor semen. This relative inactivity in cryobanking was due perhaps in part to methods and certainly to physicians who were not ready for evaluative application in an atmosphere of relative uncertainty which included the practice of insemination itself. The introduction by the author in 1963—1964 of a method for freezing human semen in the vapor of liquid nitrogen and its storage at −196°C was accompanied by reports of normal births with its use. Later, positive research findings were presented which supported the safety and efficiency of frozen storage of human spermatozoa. Since 1964, more advanced and automated methods have been devised to facilitate large scale cryobanking, but with no significant improvement in cryosurvival. The basic principles in techniques since 1953 have proved suitable for the establishment of clinical cryobanks for frozen human semen which have resulted in normal, healthy offspring in various parts of the world.

Greater appreciation of the applications of cryobanking developed with the wider use of artificial insemination of donor semen (AID) and artificial insemination of husband semen (AIH) in reproductive medicine in the early 1970s. However, warnings about possible dangers in genetic and functional instability of frozen-stored spermatozoa from panels of the American Public Health Association and Planned Parenthood-World Population (which were based on incompletely researched and misleading evaluation) did much to inhibit development. The establishment of much publicized commercial cryobanks in about 1972 was based primarily on the reasonable expectation that millions of men would elect to store their semen as "fertility insurance" before undergoing vasectomy in population control. This has since proved to be an unrealized expectation, the economically important absence of which has slowed considerably the growth of commercial banking.

B. RECENT PERIOD

There is little doubt that since 1976 cryobanking of human semen has received wider and more general acceptance as safe and efficient clinical procedure. This has been noted especially during the last decade for applications which are pertinent to the relatively small but important segment of the reproductive population. Emphasis today is still on cryobanking for AID, but the recent awakening of interest in certain applications of AIH, with unique related benefits of cryobanking, has stimulated more activity in AIH with cryobanked human semen both in research evaluation and in the clinical management of infertility. It has also emphasized the limitations of semen quality in realizing the potential afforded by these applications in infertility therapy, along with the coincident need for improving on both the quality of semen used for AIH and the attendant methods for its frozen-storage.

Cryobanking of human semen is now an established medical procedure which has been growing worldwide in terms of number of births and clinical applications. There are cryobanks in the U.S. and at least 18 other countries. It is generally accepted by cryobiologists and the Reproductive Council of the AATB that cryopreservation of semen is a safe process which maintains the potential reproductive function of human spermatozoa during indefinite storage in liquid nitrogen ($-196°C$).

Updated figures from a worldwide survey of clinical results of cryobanking reported in 1986,[6] now conservatively places the number of births from cryobanked semen used in AID as over 40,000. The longest period of cryopreservation of donor semen which resulted in a birth after artificial insemination (AID) remains at 12 years. There have been over 600 births from artificial insemination of husband semen (AIH) including about 150 from pretherapy and prevasectomy storage. The longest period of cryopreservation which has resulted in a birth after AIH is now 15 years, 9 months.[7]

Continued development of cryobanking is expected in all of its clinical applications, especially in those which involve AIH. The obvious protective benefits of pretherapy storage of semen from cancer patients will be exploited, but it will be a significant success only if oncologists and other involved physicians suggest or prescribe cryobanking at the time of early diagnosis, prior to time-related infertility effects of the disease itself (see Chapter 3).

Cryobanks for human semen are becoming an integral component of many of the rapidly developing centers for reproductive biology in which there are programs for *in vitro* fertilization (IVF) and embryo transplantation (ET). Cryobanks for embryos are being included in such combined IVF-ET centers. In addition, multipurpose banks in tissue and organ transplantation centers and, recently, blood banking facilities are initiating incorporation of semen cryobanking into their expanding programs.

It now appears that the emergence of the dreaded transmitted disease AIDS will have the greatest impact on the accelerated development and use of cryobanked semen in all applications with artificial insemination, as well as with other artificial means of human reproduction involving *in vitro* manipulations with both unfrozen and cryopreserved eggs. The U.S. Food and Drug Administration and the Center for Disease Control have formally recommended that only frozen semen be used in donor inseminations because it permits a quarantine period for retesting donors. Cryobankers of the Reproductive Council of AATB had previously recognized the importance of frozen semen relative to AIDS and have been practicing a quarantine period since 1985. Its AATB standards were the first to formally require a quarantine period for AIDS, as well as hepatitis B testing of semen donors.[8-10]

III. FACTORS IN CRYOPRESERVATION OR CRYOSURVIVAL

A. EARLY LITERATURE

Early cryobiological investigations which were directed toward the development of techniques for cryopreservation of human spermatozoa[6] have included appreciation and investigation of the following factors in cryosurvival:

1. Temperature shock, or the deleterious effects of rapid cooling above the freezing temperature. (Human semen shows little or no susceptibility to temperature shock, but there is individual variation. Egg yolk may reduce its manifestation in semen from some susceptible individuals.)
2. Rates of cooling below the freezing temperature — relative to coincident and induced degree and size of ice formations and dehydration. (Ultrarapid rates (degrees/sec) are lethal to most spermatozoa. Slow rates (1—25°C/min), on the other hand, allow an average of about 70% cryosurvival, in the presence of fewer but larger ice crystallizations and more time for dehydration.)
3. Size, shape, extent and location of ice crystallization — involving aspects of intracellular vs. extracellular ice, as to compatibility with survival, ultrastructural injury and effects of dehydration. (Intracellular ice is not a factor in the death of spermatozoa during successful cryopreservation — slow freezing with glycerol; death is probably caused by solution effects during the dehydration accompanying the extracellular ice formation of slow freezing.)
4. Presence or absence of a cryoprotective agent, such as glycerol — in determining more optimal cryosurvival with a balance, in its concentration, of possible toxicity and degree of cryoprotection. (The use of buffer systems and/or egg yolk extenders may favor its action.)
5. Final temperature reached — which proves to be innocuous in itself, as a favorable storage temperature. (There is no deleterious lower limit for exposure of human spermatozoa and rapid change in temperature from $-75°$ to $-196°C$ and vice versa apparently is innocuous relative to final temperature.)
6. Storage time at the final temperature reached — for the definition of conditions which prevent loss of cells during indefinite periods of cryobanking. (The temperature of liquid nitrogen ($-196°C$) appears optimal in practical long — term cryobanking.)
7. Rates of rewarming or thawing — to determine rates most favorable in recovering viability of cells in their return from the frozen inactive state to the active thawed or rewarmed or unfrozen state. (There is still some controversy, but usually both rapid and slow rates can be used with comparable results in cryosurvival.)
8. Latent cryoinjury, or accelerated loss in functional activities with time after thawing,

compared with unfrozen control cell populations. (Its demonstration stresses the critical importance of proper timing in artificial insemination of cryobanked semen in order to minimize "waiting period" of spermatozoa *in situ*, which could reduce their effectiveness in achieving fertilization.)

B. RECENT LITERATURE

A highlighted history of refrigerants, cryoprotectants, rates of freezing and thawing, and conditions of storage, as factors in the development of methods of cryopreservation of human semen, is presented in detail elsewhere.[6] Examples of more recent contributions from the literature are noted below.

1. The use of 7% glycerol alone was found superior to a mixture of glycerol in egg yolk citrate extender for the cryopreservation of human spermatozoa. An electronic semiautomatic system for pellet freezing was used.[11]

2. Human sperm preservation medium (HSPM), a chemically defined modified Tyrode's solution with glycerol, exhibited an equal or superior capacity to cryopreserve spermatozoa compared to egg yolk citrate medium (ECM) with the same final glycerol concentration. Insemination of patients with semen cryopreserved in HSPM resulted in a higher pregnancy rate than with ECM.[12]

3. Irrespective of the freezing rates, slow thawing of human semen generally resulted in higher cryosurvival than fast thawing methods with HSPM. Storage at $-80°$ to $-85°C$ in a mechanical freezer maintained viability (motility) of frozen spermatozoa as well as liquid nitrogen ($-196°C$) for up to 90 days. Transport of cryobanked semen in solid carbon dioxide therefore, is indicated.[13]

4. A TES-TRIS zwitter-ion buffer system with egg yolk citrate (TESTCY) was evaluated in cryoprotection of human spermatozoa based on post-thaw motility and the zona-free hamster egg penetration test. Results indicated the TESTCY alone is a better cryopreservative than TESTCY with glycerol. It was suggested that glycerol is not an ideal cryoprotectant and that it should be omitted from cryoprotective media.[14]

5. TES-TRIS zwitter-ion buffers (TESTCY) with glycerol were found superior to glycerol alone and to glycerol egg yolk citrate in cryoprotection of human spermatozoa. Inclusion of glycerol as a cryoprotectant in recommended TESTCY media was found crucial for adequate cryosurvival.[15]

6. The within-subject variability of sperm count, total numbers of spermatozoa and pre-freeze and post-thaw motility was studied in 584 ejaculates from 98 normal subjects. The within-subject variances for each variable was found to be similar for all subjects. Sperm count, volume and total number of spermatozoa appeared to increase linearly with the length of abstinence ranging from 1 to 5 days, while pre-freeze and post-thaw motility were not influenced by the abstinence period.[16]

7. The extent of ultrastructural alterations to spermatozoal heads supports the apparent superiority of TESTCY buffer without glycerol over glycerolated semen, as a cryopreservative.[17]

8. Glycerol concentrations of 6,8,12,16, and 24% (by volume) in phosphate buffered egg yolk citrate medium were compared; 12 and 16% gave best cryoprotection in terms of percent and velocity of spermatozoa motility measured by dark-field illumination photography and laser doppler velocimetry.[18]

9. Cryosurvival of spermatozoa in a complex protective medium was the same using a programmable electronically controlled rate freezer (Linde CRC-1) as cryosurvival in a specimen holder in liquid nitrogen vapor (Linde BF-5 biological freezer). The efficiency and simplicity of Sherman's vapor freezing method were confirmed and its use recommended.[19]

10.   No difference in post-thaw spermatozoal viability was demonstrated between semen frozen with a complex egg yolk glycerol cryoprotectant or with glycerol alone, on the basis of the ability of spermatozoa to penetrate zona-free hamster eggs. Thawing at 22°C in air and at 37°C in a water bath was found superior to thawing in a 4°C water bath. Marked individual (donor semen) differences in their cryosurvival rather than differences in cryoprotectant medium were noted in tests of *in vitro* fertilization.[20]

11.   Semen in a modified HSPM was packaged in plastic straws and frozen in an electronically programmable automatic biologic freezer (Planer Product Ltd., Model K204, Essex, England) and thawed in air at room temperature. Data on motility, hamster egg penetration, and acrosome integrity suggested that incorporation of a holding temperature of −5°C for 10 min and seeding may result in a superior method of cryopreservation.[21]

12.   High quality polypropylene plastic is the best biocompatible and stress resistant material to achieve long-term cryopreservation of human semen. Polyethylene and polyethane-base plastic containers show a significant motility depressing effect, while glass is more susceptible to breakage and can be accidentally contaminated by detergents.[22]

C. EXAMPLES OF SIMPLIFIED FREEZING METHODS

1.   A simple manually operated liquid nitrogen freezing apparatus is used to freeze extended semen in plastic straws sealed by polyvinyl chloride sealing powder. Cryoextender consisted of glycerol in modified Tyrode's medium with added fructose, glucose, glycine and human serum albumin.[23]

2.   A simple method of cryopreservation is illustrated which uses glycerol egg yolk citrate medium. Freezing in glass tubes is accomplished in an alcohol bath which is slowly lowered into liquid nitrogen. Method is used successfully for AID and in IVF at the Groote Shuur Hospital in Capetown, South Africa.[24]

D. COMMENTS ON THE LITERATURE

There are statements as conclusions and assumptions in the research literature on cryosurvival of human spermatozoa which illustrate sources for confusion and controversy in selecting a method for cryopreservation. This situation is effected by incomplete appreciation for interrelations of the possible interactions between factors in cryosurvival and related conditions in cryopreservation, especially when results of investigators are contradictory.

Examples of such statements include:

1.   Rates of freezing and thawing — (There is a relationship between rates of freezing and rates of thawing in cryosurvival; there is no such relationship. Rate of thawing is a factor in cryosurvival; it is not a factor in cryosurvival.)

2.   Egg yolk additive — (Egg yolk improves cryosurvival; it does not have any influence on cryosurvival; it is harmful and reduces cryosurvival.)

3.   Glycerol as a cryoprotectant — (Glycerol is essential in a cryoextender or alone as the cryoprotectant; it is not an optimal cryoprotectant; it should be eliminated from all extenders.)

4.   Pre-freeze motility — (There is a relationship between pre-freeze percent motility and cryosurvival; there is no such relationship.)

IV. METHODS OF CRYOPRESERVATION

A. COMPLEXITY IN EVALUATION; CONFLICT IN METHOD SELECTION

The considerable number of variables in the different methods of cryopreservation make valid and meaningful scientific comparisons between the methods quite difficult, if not impossible. The conditions of pretreatment with a cryoprotectant (temperature, time concentration and method of addition), the nature of the cryoprotectant (used alone or within an extender), the nature and components of an extender [buffered zwitter-ion TES-TRIS citrate yolk (TESTCY), phosphate egg yolk citrate (EYC), chemically defined (modified Tyrode's human semen protective medium (HSPM), chemically undefined (egg yolk additives), are examples]. Further, the conditions of freezing and thawing (rates which are constant, varied, programmed or unprogrammed), as well as the type of packaging (straws, ampules or vials) and its position during freezing (horizontal, vertical or angle), may be a basis for differences in results of cryopreservation, as a function of the various conditions of pretreatment with a cryoprotectant. Results of a particular method of cryopreservation, therefore, must be viewed, as to reported comparative performance, by examination and appreciation of all possible interrelationships of the various factors in cryopreservation in each step in the process.

There appears to be no optimal method which clearly stands alone as preferred in successful cryobanking on the basis of a scientific comparison which has experimentally observed and documented such possible factoral interplay whether in laboratory testing or in clinical performance. Instead, there exists an array of modifications which have been devised on the basis of mostly empirically derived data or from procedures and conditions which have been adopted entirely or in part from published methods of cryopreservation of both human and bovine semen.

There is a wide spectrum of conditions and, therefore, techniques, under which cryopreservation of human semen is successful and applicable for cryobanking. However, only those techniques which have been established clinically in the production of populations of normal progeny should be so employed in establishing a cryobank. Excellent cryosurvival of motile spermatozoa, in itself, although most desirable, is insufficient as the sole basis for the selection of a method for clinical use of semen from cryobanks.[2]

B. SUCCESSFUL METHODS OF FREEZING WITH LIQUID NITROGEN VAPOR

The basic, relatively simple, liquid nitrogen vapor freezing technique, which was introduced by the author over 25 years ago,[25] has proved successful over the years in human semen cryobanking. It compares favorably with the newer, more sophisticated, complicated and expensive stepwise programmable and electronically controlled systems. Basic liquid nitrogen vapor freezing is used by most of the large and notable cryobanks. Various rates of freezing (1—25°C/min) and thawing (1—60°C/min) when used with numerous and different simple or sophisticated pretreatment and cryoprotective techniques in cryopreservation, result in satisfactory spermatozoal survival with successful clinical applications.

Various modifications can be used in successful vapor freezing of semen in straws, ampules or cryotubes. A metal container (canister) with cigar tubes, or other holders with straws, or holders or racks with ampules or cryotubes, can be placed directly into liquid nitrogen vapor by using a liquid nitrogen (LN) refrigerator which is large enough to store containers with frozen semen under LN, as well as to allow freezing semen in its vapor above the surface of LN. A biological LN dry shipper also can be used to freeze semen in its vapor, followed by transfer to LN, for storage, in another refrigerator (Figures 1 to 6).

C. GENERAL STEPS IN CRYOPRESERVATION
1. Collection of Semen

Semen is collected by masturbation in a 2 or 4 oz. sterile polypropylene specimen (collection) container (cup or jar), following an abstinence period usually of 3 to 5 days. The abstinence period is designed to favor the use of samples for cryopreservation, generally with more constant and optimal characteristics of the semen profile than under shorter and less regulated periods prior to collection.

STRAWS

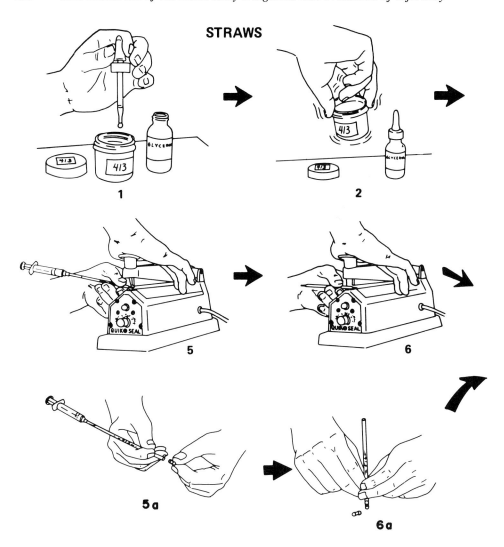

FIGURE 1.   Schematic representation of the major steps in the cryopreservation of human semen in polypropylene plastic straws. Addition of cryoprotectant (glycerol) to semen (1,2); filling of straws (3,4); packaging by heat sealing (5,6) and nylon plugging (5a,6a); air freezing at −80°C to −85°C (8,9) or liquid nitrogen vapor freezing in sealed canister (10); and storage in open canister in liquid nitrogen (10). Refer also to Figures 2, 3, and 4 for illustration of glass ampules, packaging units and a vapor freezing canister.

Liquid semen is ejaculated but, normally, it immediately coagulates into a gel. When the coagulated semen liquefies, usually within 30 min, its volume is measured. Processing for cryopreservation of liquefied semen is initiated within 1 h after collection, to favor greatest cryosurvival from the ejaculate.

2. Measurement of the Volume

This measurement is made by using a calibrated pipette or a 5 ml calibrated syringe with an 18 gauge needle. It is sometimes calculated with values of weight of collection jar with and without semen. An aliquot of about 0.1 to 0.2 ml is removed for semen analysis (percent and quality of motility, cell concentration, etc.; see Chapter 3). Other aliquots, usually are also removed at this time for tests in screening for certain sexually transmitted disease organisms, such as *Neisseria gonorrhoeae* as appropriate (see Chapter 14).

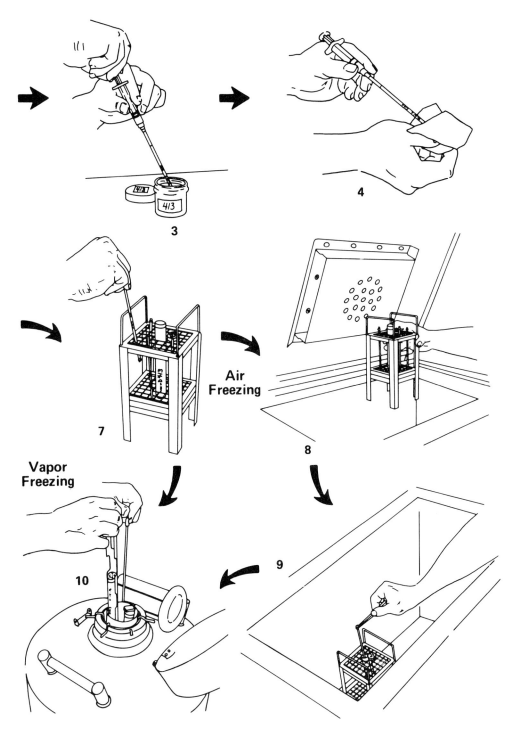

FIGURE 1 (continued)

3. Glycerolation

Glycerol, the cryoprotective agent, is added directly to neat (untreated) semen in a stepwise fashion, with subsequent mixing, after each addition and 1-min intervals between additions, or indirectly as a component of an extender or medium which is mixed in aliquots of dilution with extended semen, usually in a stepwise fashion. Over 40% of notable banks,

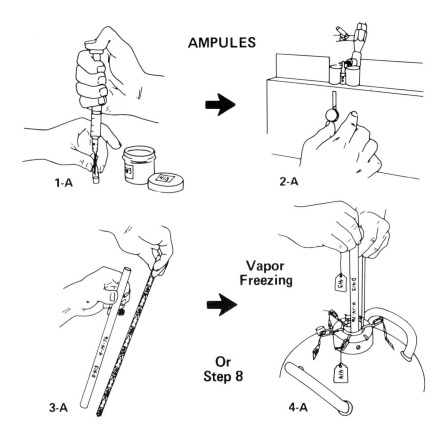

FIGURE 2.   Schematic representation of major steps in filling, sealing (packaging) and freezing in the cryopreservation of semen in glass ampules. See Figure 1 for glycerolation and the alternate freezing method (step 8).

notable banks, member-associated with AATB (Table 2) still use glycerol alone, with an increasing number of new cryobanks using an extender, especially a zwitter-ion buffer system, with glycerol.

Conditions for glycerolation may or may not involve special conditions of temperature (other than room temperature) and time of exposure (other than time necessary for addition and mixing). One extender which is used by one notable cryobank, contains no glycerol, because of a report in which *in vitro* observations suggested that removal of glycerol may be harmful to survival of frozen-thawed semen *in situ*.[14]

4. Packaging; Viability Observations

Glycerolated semen is drawn into plastic straws (sealed by a powder sealant, by heat, or with nylon plugs), or placed into glass ampules (sealed by flame), or into plastic cryotubes (cryovials) which are screw-capped. The volume of cryoprotected semen in each package is usually from 0.4 to 0.8 ml, which is designated as a unit for artificial insemination. More than one unit can be used in AI, of course, as appropriate. It is important to process semen for cryopreservation in a container or package which is easily labeled, handled, stored and recovered for use, as well as being biocompatible and stress resistant. High quality polypropylene straws or vials seem best suited in meeting these criteria without the drawback of glass in breakability and accidental contamination by detergents.[22]

In addition to units of semen packaged for freezing and storage, a quality control test unit is prepared for measurement of cryosurvival prior to storage in liquid nitrogen. Observations, usually on percent and quality of motility of spermatozoa, are made on untreated

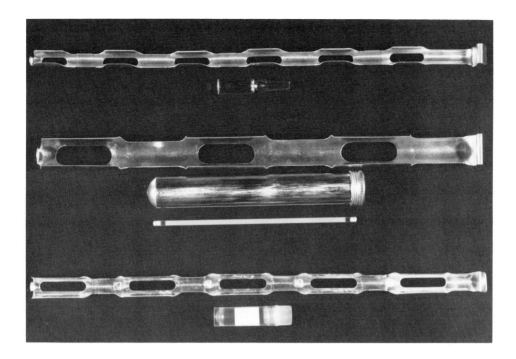

FIGURE 3.   Three sets of packaging units in the cryopreservation of semen are shown in this photograph. From top to bottom: a 1 ml capacity glass ampule with its aluminum cane; a 0.6 ml capacity plastic nylon plugged straw with its aluminum tube and cane; and a 1 ml plastic cryotube with its aluminum cane.

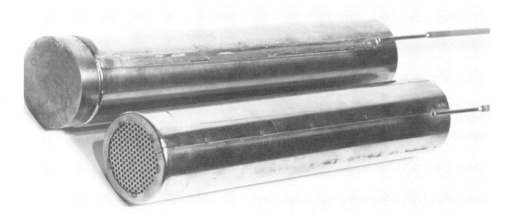

FIGURE 4.   Pictured is the usual open liquid nitrogen storage canister (below) and the specially sealed and weighted canister, modified for vapor freezing. A machined brass plate was soldered on the bottom as a weight to prevent floating of the canister in the liquid nitrogen. (From Sherman, J. K., in *Techniques of Human Andrology*, Hafez, E. S. E., Ed., Elsevier-North Holland, New York, 1977. With permission.)

semen after collection, on semen after treatment with the cryoprotectant, and after freeze-thawing prior to storage. These observations trace survival during stages in cryopreservation and ensure the storage of semen with known survival potential which will be realized after proper storage in liquid nitrogen.

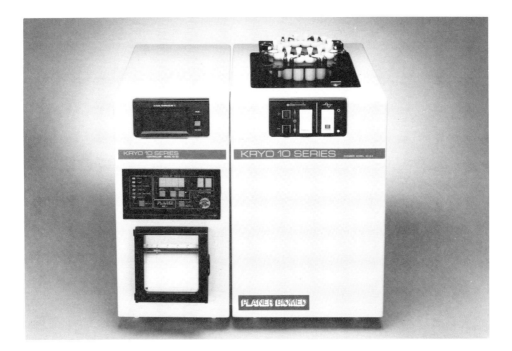

FIGURE 5.   This controlled rate embryo and semen freezer is an example of a sophisticated automated state of the art instrument which is used in the majority of *in vitro* fertilization and embryo transfer centers.

5. Freezing

Semen in straws, ampules of cryotubes (cryovials) as separate units or packaged in groups, is placed in a vertical (usual), horizontal or a slanted (angular) position, usually in liquid nitrogen vapor, or sometimes in refrigerated air of a mechanical (electrical) freezer. Cooling and freezing is accomplished with a manual static or stepwise regime, or in an electronically automated and programmed liquid nitrogen-fed system. Most often, the vapor phase of a liquid nitrogen storage container is used for manual freezing at one (static level) or at various levels in a stepwise regime. A biological dry shipper with an asbestos lining which is absorbed with liquid nitrogen can also be used for freezing in its vapor, followed by transfer into a storage container, in the liquid phase.

6. Storage

Specimens, as packaged units, are submerged and maintained under the surface of liquid nitrogen in metal canisters, boxes, canes or compartments within appropriate liquid nitrogen refrigerators (tanks). Provisions (mechanical and/or electronic) for monitoring the liquid nitrogen level are made to prevent loss of functional activity of spermotozoa if stored above the temperature of liquid nitrogen ($-196°C$) during long-term storage. The common mechanical (manual) method used in monitoring is a calibrated dip-stick upon which a frost-line forms after removal from liquid nitrogen to indicate its level. Various sophisticated electronic local and remote warning systems are commercially available. A few cryobanks, on the other extreme, used only regular visual checks with a flashlight. ''AATB Standards for Tissue Banking'' requires only a workable program for monitoring which will ensure continuous storage below the surface of liquid nitrogen. The cryobiologists' position and the author's experience, along with others, is that there is some loss in percent motility of spermatozoa during the initial freezing process which is detected by thawing of a test sample before storage. However, there is no further loss in motility in the population of frozen

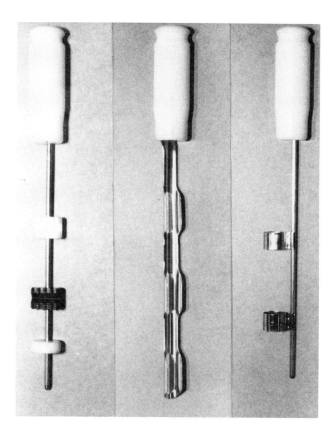

FIGURE 6. Holders for packaged specimens during freezing in the unit pictured in Figure 5. Left to right — for plastic straws, for glass ampules, and for plastic cryotubes.

spermatozoa which is then stored at $-196°C$ under the surface of liquid nitrogen. It has been established that cryosurvival of the spermatozoal population in semen of pre-therapy cancer patients is often poor (reduced percent post-thaw motility) when tested after freezing prior to storage. However, this reduced motility is maintained, not lost, during long-term storage.

Of the 42 AATB member-associated banks (Table 2) surveyed recently, only 2 reported instances of loss, during long-term storage of semen (donor and/or pre-therapy clients) and the literature reveals only one report of loss after 3 years. The accepted view is that such reported losses are due to either errors in motility measurements or, more probably, to less than optimal storage conditions.

7. Thawing

Rewarming from the frozen to liquid state is realized by exposure of the package with frozen semen, either to air or water, usually at room temperature, but also at other temperatures, according to alternate methods devised by cryobanks.

8. Disposition

Aliquots (units) of cryopreserved semen generally are sent from a commercial or university-based bank to physicians which request semen for clinical use. Units are packaged in special shipping containers containing liquid nitrogen or solid carbon dioxide (dry ice). However, cryobanked semen is not always shipped. Units are sometimes thawed and provided

TABLE 2
AATB-Associated Human Semen Cryobanks in the U.S. and Canada[a]

Andrology Laboratory
Dept. Obstetrics & Gynecology
Mt. Sinai Medical Center
1 Mt. Sinai Drive
Cleveland, OH 44106
216-421-5884
Director: Leon Sheean, Ph.D.

Andrology Laboratory
Box 668
Dept. Obstetrics & Gynecology
University of Rochester
601 Elmwood Avenue
Rochester, NY 14642
313-434-4766
Director: Grace Centola, Ph.D.

Ann Arbor Reproductive Medicine Assoc.
4990 Clark Road, Suite 100
Ypsilanti, MI 48197
313-434-4766
Director: E. P. Peterson, M.D.

Arizona Fertility Institute
2850 N. 24th Street, Suite 500
Phoenix, AZ 85008
602-468-3840
Director: Robert H. Tamis, M.D.

Astarte Lab, Inc.
Jacksonville Hospital
P.O. Box 0070
Jacksonville, AL 36265
205-453-3953
Director: Carol S. Armone, M.D.

Biogenetics Corp.
950 Sanford Avenue
Irvington, N.J. 07111
1-800-942-4646
Director: Albert Anouna

California Cryobank, Inc.
1019 Galey Avenue
Los Angeles, CA 90024
213-553-9828/800-223-3588
Co-Directors: Charles Simes, M.D.
                      C. M. Rothman, M.D.

Cleveland Clinic Sperm Bank
Cleveland Clinic Foundation
A-1-191
9500 Euclid Avenue
Cleve'and, OH 44195-5020
216-444-2488
Director: Susan Rothmann, Ph.D.

Cryo Laboratory Facility
100 E. Ohio-Suite 268
Chicago, IL 60601
Director: Alfred Morris

Cryogenic Laboratories, Inc.
2233 Hamline Avenue, North
Roseville, MN 55113
612-636-3792
Director: John H. Olson, M.S.

Cryo-V, New York, Inc.
88 University Place, 9th Floor
New York, NY 10003
212-627-7450
Director: Mitchell Essig, M.D.

Evanston/Glenbrook Hospital
Dept. Obstetrics & Gynecology
2050 Pfingsten Road, Suite 350
Glenview, IL 60025
312-729-6450
Director: Marybeth Gerrity, Ph.D.

Fairfax Cryobank
A Division of the Genetics and IVF Institute
3020 Javier Road
Fairfax, VA 22031
703-698-8605
Director: Edward Fugger

Fertility Institute of Southern California
1125 E. 17th Street, W-120
Santa Ana, CA 92701
714-953-5683
Director: Linda Sullivan

Genetic Semen Bank
University of Nebraska Med. Ctr.
42nd and Dewey Avenue
Omaha, NE 68105
402-559-5070
Director: Warren Sanger, Ph.D.

Hoxworth Blood Center
University of Cincinnati Medical Center
3231 Burnet Avenue—M.L. #5
Cincinnati, OH 45267
513-569-1100
Director: Charles Mayhaus

TABLE 2 (continued)
AATB-Associated Human Semen Cryobanks in the U.S. and Canada[a]

Idant Laboratory
645 Madison Avenue
New York, NY 10022
212-935-1430
Director: Joseph Feldschuh, M.D.

International Cryogenics, Inc.
189 Townsend—Suite 203
Birmingham, MI 48011
313-644-5822
Director: Mary Ann Brown

Jefferson Semen Bank
Dept. Of Urology
Jefferson Medical College
1025 Walnut Street
Philadelphia, PA 19107
215-928-6961
Director: Irvin Hirsch, M.D.

The Life Bank
P.O. Box 1094
Manhattan Beach, CA 90266-8094
213-546-7418
Director: Raymond Klemp

Midwest Fertility Foundation and Laboratory
3101 Broadway-Suite 650A
Kansas City, MO 64111
816-756-0040
Director: Elwyn Grimes, M.D.

Newton Andrology and Cryoperservation Center
2014 Washington Street, Pratt Bldg.
Newton, MA 02162
617-332-1228
Director: Robert A. Newton, M.D.

Northern California Cryobank
5821 Jameson Court
Carmichael, CA 95608
916-486-0451
Director: Marvin Kamras, M.D.

Paces Cryobank and Fertility Service
3193 Howell Mill Road—Suite 322
Atlanta, GA 30327
404-350-5561
Director: Diane Snoey

Pennsylvania Sperm Bank, Inc.
c/o Personal Doctor Care
7215 Frankfort Avenue
Philadelphia, PA 19135
215-624-7704
Director: Sharon Miller

Regional Andrology Facility
University of Ottawa
501 Smyth Road
Ottawa, Canada K1H86
613-737-8559
Director: Arthur Leader, M.D.

The Repository for Germinal Choice
P.O. Box 2876
Escondido, CA 92025
619-743-0772
Director: Robert Graham

Reproductive Genetics Group
Swedish Hospital
747 Summit Avenue
Seattle, WA 98104
206-386-2483
Director: Lawrence Karp, M.D.

Reproductive Resources
200 W. Esplanade
Kenner, LA 70065
504-464-8725
Director: Brenda Bordson, Ph.D.

Rocky Mountain Cryobank
P.O. Box 2156
Jackson, WY 83001
307-733-9170
Director: William Racow

Chicago IVF & Fertility Institute
Grant Hospital of Chicago
550 West Webster Avenue
Chicago, IL 60614
312-883-3870
Director: W. Paul Dmowski, M.D.

Southwest Fertility Center
3125 N. 32nd Street
Phoenix, AZ 85108
602-956-7481
Director: Sujatha Gunnala, Ph.D.

Drs. Sparr, Stephens, & Assoc.
8160 Walnut Hill Lane
Dallas, TX 75231
214-691-0924
Director: Stacy Stephens, M.D.

The Sperm Bank of Northern California
3007 Telegraph Avenue, Suite 2
Oakland, CA 94609
415-444-2014
Director: Barbara Raboy

TABLE 2 (continued)
AATB-Associated Human Semen Cryobanks in the U.S. and Canada[a]

Tyler Medical Clinic
921 Westwood Boulevard
Los Angeles, CA 90024
213-208-6765
Director: Stanley Friedman, M.D.

University of Arkansas for Medical Sciences
Semen Cryobank—Slot 708
4301 W. Markham
Little Rock, AR 72205
501-660-2098
Director: J. K. Sherman, Ph.D.[b]

University of Missouri
Columbia School of Medicine
Dept. Urology/Surgery
Health Sciences Center N510
One Hospital Drive
Columbia, MO 65212
314-882-1151
Director: Jawad Ali, Ph.D.

University of Wisconsin
Clinical Sciences Center
Dept. Obstetrics & Gynecology
600 Highland Avenue
Madison, WI 53705
608-263-1217
Director: Sander Shapiro, M.D.

Washington Fertility Study Center
2600 Virginia Avenue, N.W. #500
Washington, D.C. 20037
202-333-3100
Director: Sal Leto, Ph.D.

Western Cryobank
210 E Bijou
Colorado Springs, CO 80909
303-578-9014
Director: Charles Johnson, D.O.

Xytex Corporation
1100 Emmett Street
Augusta, GA 30904
800-214-9700
Director: Armand Karow, Ph.D.

ZyGen Laboratory
6047 Tampa Avenue #101
Tarzana, CA 91356
818-344-7777
Director: Cyrus Milani, M.D.

[a]   List includes only those notable cryobanks with directors as individual members of AATB who practice AATB
     Standards, and which participate in AATB questionnaires on clinical applications and results with cryobanked
     semen.
[b]   Dr. Sherman is also Chairman, AATB Reproductive Council.

for use within a clinic with its own cryobank or by a physician in a nearby office. Thawing
of units of semen at the cryobank permits the added dimension of quality control in assessing
cryosurvival, once again, this time prior to release for clinical use.

D. SPECIFIC STEPS IN CRYOPRESERVATION (SHERMAN METHOD)

Unless specified, all steps or treatments are conducted at room temperature ($\pm 22°C$).
Figure 1 depicts the basic steps in several techniques which have been and are used in
cryopreservation, as well as some of the special equipment and materials employed by the
author, including the techniques in the current method described.

1. Collection of Semen

Masturbation into a 4 oz. sterile polypropylene plastic specimen container after 3—5
days of abstinence provides the semen which is then completely processed for cryopreservation, frozen and stored, with appropriate observations and measurements, within 90 min.

2. Measurements of Volume

When the coagulated semen liquefies, its volume is measured by drawing it up into a calibrated 5 ml syringe with an 18 gauge needle. It is then returned to the specimen container for glycerolation. A small aliquot (± 0.2 ml) can be removed at this time for semen analysis (observations on percent, type, and duration of motility, viability staining, cell density and abnormalities), culturing for sexually transmitted diseases and the like.

Depending on the technician's preference relative to work load and schedule, observations and measurements of cell density and abnormalities as well as culturing for organisms can be made with semen from the quality control test straw after being thawed for cryosurvival (motility) determination. This can be performed at a selected, convenient and unlimited time following the freezing cycle as long as the straw is in liquid nitrogen (see 4. Packaging). Viability staining and its measurement, however, always is made in both pre-freeze and post-thaw samples, along with observations on motility.

3. Glycerolation

Glycerol is added to semen from a plastic dropping bottle, coincident with rotational mixing of the container, with about 1 min holding time between stepwise additions. The measure of two drops of glycerol per milliliter of semen yields the 8 to 10% glycerol concentration by volume which is employed. Exact quantitation is unnecessary as the same cryosurvival is realized in this concentration range. No consistent difference in cryosurvival has been found in this laboratory between concentrations of 5 to 10%.

4. Packaging

A number, determined by semen volume, of 0.6 ml capacity polypropylene plastic straws is appropriately labeled, with a permanent black ink pen, with the code identification and date for semen donor or client depositor. This can be done following measurement of semen volume after collection of semen, or prior to collection, based upon average volume of measurements from previous collections of regular donors or depositors. In addition to straws with semen for storage, a test straw with a smaller volume (± 0.3 ml) is prepared for quality control of percent cryosurvival before storage. Observations on percent and quality of motility of spermatozoa are made after collection of fresh untreated semen, after exposure to the cryoprotectant and after freeze-thawing prior to storage to document the extent and stage during which loss occurs and to measure cryosurvival.

A 2 or 3 ml plastic syringe fitted with a short tygon tube adaptor with a ± 3 mm inside diameter is used to hold the straw during its filling. Glycerolated semen is drawn into the straw to the designated or desired level. The free or exposed end is wiped dry with tissue paper in preparation for the sealing process. Each straw is first sealed at its free or exposed end with a solid nylon plug which is first inserted with the thumb and index finger and then pressed into place and firmly seated by a downward vertical pressure of the straw on the counter top (Figure 1, steps 5a and 5b). The same steps in sealing are then repeated for the other end which is removed from the syringe, now protected from the possibility of loss of semen in handling the straw, because one end has been sealed. Enough space is left in the straw during filling with cryoprotected semen, to allow for sealing by plugs in the described manner. If no space is allowed between plug and semen, it is possible that expansion of ice during freezing could, in isolated cases, lift the plug from its seating with possible loss or contamination of semen during subsequent thawing. "Measured" straws may be marked with a pen in aliquot groups before use, with a line or dot, guided by a ruler across the row of straws, to indicate the filling level which allows for maximum capacity with sufficient room for plugs and expansion during freezing. In our laboratory, experience makes such marking of straws unnecessary. Sealing with nylon plugs easily adapts to partial filling when appropriate, as for preparation of test samples, for quality control and screening. It is rare to experience any problems with this simple and efficient method of packaging, in filling, sealing, freezing, storing or thawing. Use of straws favors maximum efficiency in use of storage space.

5. Freezing

Sealed labeled straws with glycerolated semen are placed in a metal rack with a similarly labeled (coded) aluminum cigar tube which subsequently will hold the straws during storage. The tube is perforated by a hole at the bottom end, to allow entrance of liquid nitrogen for bathing the enclosed straws during storage.

Freezing is accomplished by either of two techniques. One is in refrigerated air about −83°C in a mechanical (electrical) freezer; the other in the vapor above the level of nitrogen in a refrigerator (storage) container; both for a period of 30 to 60 min. Split-sample comparisons have revealed no difference in cryosurvival between the two methods, but the liquid nitrogen vapor method is simpler, less expensive and the equipment required is portable for processing at local or distant locations outside of the laboratory. It can be used with various size liquid nitrogen containers with or without a modified "freezer" canister (Figure 4) as long as samples are suspended or held in the vapor phase during freezing. Modifications of the liquid nitrogen vapor freezing are used in many laboratories but, in principle, they are the same whether straws or other packages are suspended or held in vapor above the liquid in racks, trays, tubes or canisters, whether vertically, horizontally or at an angle, or whether at one level or passed through various programmed levels. Results appear successful in all cases.

6. Storage

Straws which have been frozen in air at about −83°C in a mechanical (electrical) freezer are quickly placed with pre-cooled forceps into the appropriately labeled aluminum cigar tube which is capped and clipped to a pre-cooled appropriately labeled aluminum cane which is quickly transferred to a storage canister in liquid nitrogen, at a designated and recorded inventory position in the refrigerator. Straws in cigar tubes which were frozen on aluminum canes in liquid nitrogen vapor are stored in the same fashion by quickly transferring the cane with tube to a canister with a mesh "open" bottom for storage of canes under the surface of liquid nitrogen (Figure 4). Labeling must clearly and accurately identify the stored units of semen for prompt recovery in the inventory system employed.

7. Thawing

Semen frozen in straws is thawed by immersion of straws in tap or distilled water or merely by exposure to air, both at room temperature (±22°C). Split-sample comparisons in this laboratory have revealed no difference in cryosurvival between the two options.

V. EXAMPLES OF VARIATIONS IN METHODS OF CRYOPRESERVATION

Variations from the author's specific methods or techniques are illustrated in the following examples of comparisons with those of four other cryobanks. Differences reside chiefly in (1) the nature of the cryoprotectant in that glycerol is not used alone but rather within an extender medium containing ingredients of a zwitter-ion buffer with egg yolk, and (2) to a lesser extent in certain details of freezing and packaging which also exist between these four cryobanks as variations which are noted in Table 3 and in the cited text of their Procedure Manuals.

There is an increasing trend toward the use of a zwitter-ion buffer system with egg-yolk as an extender with the cryoprotectant glycerol, as well as toward the use of plastic tubes

TABLE 3
Examples of Variation in Aspects of Cryopreservation Between Cryobanks

CRYOBANKS[a]

ASPECTS	I	II	III	IV	V
Cryoprotective medium	TESNaK-EYG with glucose without citrate 7—10% glycerol 16—19% extender	TESNaK-EYG with glucose without citrate ±7% glycerol ±26% extender	TEST-EYG without glucose with citrate 7% glycerol 26% extender	TEST-EYG without glucose with citrate 7.7% glycerol 2.3% extender	No extender 8—10% glycerol
Special post-glycerolation conditions	7½ min at +4°C before freezing	Cooling to 0°C before freezing technique #1; none before #2	15—30 min room temperature before freezing	15 min at room temperature before freezing	None before freezing
Freezing technique	Vapor of liquid nitrogen (levels of decreasing height above liquid)	1. Controlled rate programmed freezing machine or 2. Vapor of liquid (levels of decreasing height above liquid)	Vapor of liquid nitrogen	Vapor of liquid nitrogen	1. Referigerated −83°C air or 2. Vapor of liquid nitrogen
Packaging	Plastic straws (0.4 ml/straw) heat-sealed	Plastic cryotubes (0.75 ml/tube) screw-capped	Plastic cryotubes (0.8-1 ml/tube) screw-capped	Glass ampules (0.4 ml/ampule) flame-sealed	Plastic straws (0.6 ml/straw) nylon-plugged

[a] I = Genetic Semen Bank, University of Nebraska; II = International Cryogenics, Inc.; III = California Cryobank, Inc.; IV Cryogenic Laboratories, Inc.; V = Semen Cryobank, University of Arkansas for Medical Sciences.

TABLE 4
Materials Used in Cryopreservation

SUPPLIES

Item[a]	Source[b]
Aluminum canes; glass ampules	Minnesota Valley Engineering 407 7th Street New Prague, MN 56071
Aluminum (cigar) tubes (0.78″ × 5 3/8″)	Victor Industries 810 North Main Harrisonburg, VA 22801
Cellulose nitrate membrane	Nalge Co. P.O. Box 20365 Rochester, NY 14602-0365
Cryotubes, NUNC	Interlab 2373 Teller Road, Suite 103 Newburg Park, CA 91320
Egg yolk (pathogen free)	Local Chicken Egg Supplier
Goblets (JE 1993); marking pens; plastic straws (heat sealing); vapor trays (SUC-1)	Edwards Agricultural Supply Box 65 Baraboo, WI 53913
Plastic straws, nylon plugs	Continental Plastic Corp. Box C Delevan, WI 53115
TES, TRIS, other chemicals	Sigma Chemical Co. 3050 Spruce Street St. Louis, MO 63178
TEST yolk buffer (prepared)	Irvine Scientific 2511 Daimler Street Santa Ana, CA 92705-5588

EQUIPMENT

Ampule sealer (Model HS-1)	Cozzoli Machine Co. 401 East 3rd Street Plainfield, NJ 07060
Controlled rate freezers CryoMed (Model 1010)	CryoMed 51529 Birch Street New Baltimore, MI 48047
Planer Biomed (KRYO 10 Series)	T.S. Scientific P.O. Box 198 Perkasie, PA 18944
Centrifuge; mixer; osmometer; rotator	Fisher Scientific Corporate Headquarters 113 Hartwell Lexington, MA 02173-3190
Liquid nitrogen canisters;[c] liquid nitrogen refrigerators;[d] liquid nitrogen dry shippers[d]	Southland Cryogenics, Inc. 2424 Lacy Lane Carrollton, TX 75006
Low temperature (−94°C) (mechanical) freezer	So-Low Environmental Equipment Co., Inc. 10310 Spartan Drive Cincinnatti, OH 45215
Thermal impulse sealer	Lorvic Corp. 8810 Frost Avenue St. Louis, MO 63134

[a]   Only the more specialized items are listed.
[b]   There are other sources for the same or equivalent items.
[c]   Sealed for vapor freezing by local machine or welding shop.
[d]   Manufactured by Minnesota Valley Engineering, 407 7th Street, New Prague, MN 56071

or vials especially in newly established cryobanks as revealed in a recent survey by the author. Tes-Tris (TEST) buffer extenders with egg yolk are used by about 25% of AATB member-associated cryobanks. It was confirmed that glycerol used alone, however, is still the most widely used cryoprotectant in cryobanking.[15] The four notable and successful cryobanks chosen for comparison, employ the buffer system with glycerol with differences in the nature and amount of certain components and/or in the techniques in its preparation.

Sections on cryopreservation in the Procedure Manuals of the four cryobanks compared were generously provided by their directors for unrestricted use in this chapter. Portions have been excerpted with only minor modifications, for a more valid representation. Treatment of techniques in aspects of cryoprotection and freezing in cryopreservation are presented to illustrate differences, not only in the techniques employed but also in the detail and style in the descriptive texts. The Procedure Manual cannot be expected to be the same from laboratory to laboratory even though its use proves satisfactory in the laboratory and successful in clinical applications. Differences primarily are due to individuality as to input according to specific laboratory requisites and limitations in techniques as viewed and determined by the cryobank director whose sources in experience and literature determines such formulation. Each Procedure Manual, however, should reflect adherence to standards established by the Reproductive Council of the AATB.

A. GENETIC SEMEN BANK, UNIVERSITY OF NEBRASKA
1. Preparation of Cryoprotective Medium (TESNaK-EYG)

a. Dissolve 74.4 g TES in distilled water to make 100 ml. Adjust to 325 milliosmoles (mOsm) by adding water or TES, as appropriate.

b. Dissolve 9.1 g KOH in distilled water to make 100 ml. Adjust to 650 mOsm by adding water or KOH, as appropriate.

c. Dissolve 6.5 g NaOH in distilled water to make 100 ml. Adjust to 650 mOsm by adding water or NaOH, as appropriate. Combine with KOH solution to make NaK solution.

d. Titrate NaK solution to the TES solution to a pH of 7.2 (approximately 2.5 ml TES to 1 ml NaK solution) to make TESNaK solution.

e. Dissolve 12 g glucose in 200 ml distilled water to make 6% glucose which is adjusted to 325 mOsm.

f. Mix TESNaK with glucose (9:1) to make 0.6% glucose. Hold for egg yolk (EY) addition.

g. Separate yolks from eggs, placing each yolk on an 11 cm Whatman #1 filter paper. Prick yolk near base, tip filter paper toward mouth of 500 ml graduated cylinder, collecting yolk while leaving membranes behind. Add 400 ml TESNaK glucose to 100 ml yolk (about 8 egg yolks).

h. Cover graduated cylinder with parafilm and shake vigorously.

i. Pour solution into appropriate size beaker. Using a magnetic stir bar and a combination hot plate/stirrer, bring solution to the boiling point, with constant stirring. (Caution must be taken not to vigorously boil the solution; it should slowly be brought to the temperature at which coagulation of the egg yolk protein is observed).

j. Strain this solution with cheesecloth. Make a square several layers thick which is placed over the top of a beaker, then push the center of the square approximately $1/3$ of the way into the beaker, allowing for cheesecloth over the edges. Pour slowly or solution will be absorbed up into the cheesecloth and drip over the edges.

k. Centrifuge the filtrate at approximately 12,000 rpm for about 20 min to remove the remaining coagulated egg yolk protein. Repeat if ultracentrifuge is unavailable, 40 min at 6000 rpm is satisfactory, with repetition.

l.   Filter by utilizing many small funnels and paper toweling for filters. Set up as many small funnels in 100 ml bottles as possible. Change filter paper often. Allow 2 h/500 ml for this step.

m.   After filtering has been accomplished and the filtered buffer has been pooled, the osmolality should be 325 ± 10 mOsm and the pH should be 7.2. If the osmotic pressure is higher than 325, distilled water can be added until the optimum osmolality of 325 has been obtained.

n.   Add approximately 5 ml or 2 ml aliquots of the TESNaK yolk buffer to appropriate glass ampules.

o.   Seal each ampule with a flame ampule sealer.

p.   Place ampules in H_2O and bring to boiling point. Let boil for 2 to 5 min and remove from heat.

q.   Check for and discard leaking ampules.

r.   Store ampules at $-10°C$ until use.

2. Addition of Cryoprotective Medium

a.   To insure the required minimum of 50×10^6 spermatozoa per straw, the amount of glycerol and TESNaK-EY buffer to be added to the semen is determined by utilizing the following equation:

$$\frac{\text{Total Semen Count}}{52} = A$$

$(A) \times 0.5 = B$
$(B) \times 0.08 = C$
$(C) + \text{Semen Volume} = D$
$(B) - (D) = E \text{ (amount of buffer to be added in ml)}$

Note: If E is less than 0.05 then disregard equation and add 0.05 ml of buffer. Do not add less than 0.05 ml of buffer.

$(E) + \text{Semen Volume} = F$
$(F) \times 0.08 = \text{(amount buffer to be added in ml)}$

b.   Example: Total Semen Count $= 353 \times 10^6$

Semen Volume $= 2.7$ ml

$$\frac{353 \times 10^6}{52} = 6.79 \text{ (A)}$$

$6.79 \times 0.5 = 3.39 \text{ (B)}$
$3.39 \times 0.08 = 0.27 \text{ (C)}$
$0.27 + 2.7 = 2.97 \text{ (D)}$
$3.39 - 2.97 = \underline{0.42 \text{ ml of buffer}} \text{ (E)}$
$0.42 + 2.27 = \underline{3.12} \text{ (F)}$
$3.12 \times 0.08 = \underline{0.25 \text{ ml of glycerol}} \text{ (G)}$

c.   Using a 1 ml syringe with 18 gauge needle, mix the buffer with the glycerol.

d.   Slowly add the buffer-glycerol mixture to the semen and swirl gently to completely mix.

e.   Label the straws with the donor number or client depositor name and number, and the date.

f.   The straws used for cryopreservation are filled to about $5/6$ capacity by utilizing a 2 ml syringe with rubber tubing attached to the end.

g.   The final straw for each specimen should be filled with remaining portion of sample for quality control post-thaw analysis.

h.   The ends of the straws are sealed by utilizing a thermal impulse sealer. (Figure 1, steps 5 and 6)

i.   The straws containing semen are then placed on a rack in the refrigerator at $+4°C$ for $7\ 1/2$ min.

3. Freezing Procedure

a.   The straws with cryoprotected semen, which are cooled at $+4°C$, are rapidly suspended on the rack approximately 12 cm above the liquid nitrogen level, in a styrofoam freezing box, so that the rate of cooling is approximately 3 to 5°C per minute, for 7 $^1/_2$ min.

b.   Straws are brought to the second level (5 cm) for 5 min. and to the third level (3 cm) for 3 min. After the 3 min, the post-thaw straw is placed on the slide warmer for 9 min for microscopic observation in quality control.

c.   After the straws have reached $-80°C$ or lower, they are immersed in the liquid nitrogen.

d.   Goblets and canes, which have been pre-labeled with name or donor number and date, must be placed in the liquid nitrogen with the straws and the desired number of straws may be placed in each goblet. This should be done in the liquid phase of the nitrogen to prevent a rise in temperature.

e.   The canes must then be transferred immediately to the permanent liquid nitrogen storage tank, under the surface of liquid nitrogen.

f.   Straws, goblets, and canes can be easily handled in liquid nitrogen with pre-cooled cryopreservation forceps.

g.   The cryopreservation process must be initiated within 1 hour of ejaculation.

B. INTERNATIONAL CRYOGENICS, INC.

1. Preparation of Cryoprotective Medium

a.   Dissolve 72.0 gm TES with 2.0 g glucose (TES-glucose buffer) in deionized water, to a final volume of 1 liter; osmotic pressure is approximately 325 mOsm.

b.   Dissolve 3.64 gm KOH and 2.60 g NaOH in deionized water, to a final volume of 100 ml; osmotic pressure, is approximately 650 mOsm.

c.   Titrate TES-glucose buffer to pH of 7.3—7.4 with KOH-NaOH titrant. Measure and adjust osmotic pressure, as appropriate, with deionized water, to 320—325 mOsm, of the TESNaK.

d.   Sterilize TESNaK buffer by filtration through 0.20 μm cellulose titration membrane.

e.   Obtain albumin-free egg yolk (EY) by carefully rolling yolk, separated with its sac, along a paper towel, to remove surrounding membranes.

f.   Prepare cryoprotectant medium by mixing 50% TES-glucose buffer, 29.4% egg yolk and 20.6% glycerol (G). Centrifuge at $10,000 \times g$ for 30 min at room temperature. Remove supernatant and freeze ($-10°C$) overnight.

g.   Thaw and centrifuge at $10,000 \times g$ for 30 min to remove cold labile proteins. If desired, add 100 μg/ml of streptomycin sulfate as an antibiotic.

h.   Store until use at $-10°C$ as 10 ml aliquots in 15 ml sterile screw cap glass culture tubes.

2. Addition of Cryoprotective Medium

Determine the volume of liquefied semen to the nearest 0.1 ml with a calibrated pipette. Using a 250 μl fixed volume precision pipettor and disposable tips, add room temperature extender in increments of 500 μl/ml of semen as follows: after adding each 500 μl increment of extender, rotate the semen/extender mixture at room temperature for 2 min. Add additional extender at the same rate until a final 2:1 sample: extender ratio is achieved. This gives a final glycerol concentration of approximately 7%.

3. Freezing Technique

Technique #1: Liquid Nitrogen, Electronically Controlled Rate, Freezing Machine (Similar to Figure 5)

a.   Turn on the controlled rate freezer and bring freezer chamber to 0°C. Divide the samples of glycerolated extended semen into 0.75 ml aliquots in 1 ml cryotubes (Figure 3).

b. Place the cryotubes into the chamber of the freezer, insert the ''sample temperature'' thermocouple into one cryotube and bring the temperature of the samples to the chamber temperature.

c. When the sample and chamber temperature have equilibrated, begin the program following the instructions of the manufacturer.

d. Cool the samples at 1°C/min to -30°C and then at 5° C/min to -80°C. Program should compensate for latent heat so that the cooling curve remains linear. Programs will need to be adjusted with changes in volume.

e. When samples have reached -80°C, quickly transfer to liquid nitrogen storage. Do not allow samples to be exposed to room temperature for more than a few seconds.

Technique #2: Liquid Nitrogen Vapor

After dividing the specimen into cryotubes as above, place the cryotubes in alternating slots of a plastic rack and cool in liquid nitrogen vapor 3.5 inches above the liquid surface for 15 min. Lower the rack to 0.5 inches above the liquid surface for an additional 2 h before submersion in the liquid nitrogen. Maintain the samples below the surface of the liquid nitrogen until shipping in liquid nitrogen dry shippers or thawing for use.

C. CALIFORNIA CRYOBANK

1. Preparation of Cryoprotective Medium (TEST-EYG)

a. Dissolve 2.2 g TES, 0.5 g TRIS, 0.2 g fructose and 1.0 g citric acid in 50 to 60 ml distilled water to make TEST.

b. Add 20 ml egg yolk (EY) to TEST mix and bring up to 100 ml with distilled water.

c. Centrifuge mixture at 2500 $\times$ *g* and decant supernatant into a 500 ml beaker.

d. Add glycerol (G) to make 21% (v/v) and mix well.

e. Titrate with 1% TRIS to a pH 7.2 to 7.6

f. Store in about 10 ml aliquots in 15 ml plasic conical centrifuge tubes with screw caps, at about -10°C, until use.

2. Addition of Cryoprotective Medium

a. Using a sterile volumetric pipette, add 0.5 ml of cryoprotective medium (cryoextender) for each 1 ml of semen. Slowly rotate cup containing semen and cryoextender for 5 min. Insure that cryoextender is brought to room temperature prior to addition of semen.

b. Extended semen is now dispensed by pipette into cryotubes (Figure 3), 0.8 to 1.0 ml per cryotube depending on cell concentration. Place 0.2 ml into a cryotube as the labeled test cryotube (for quality control of cryosurvival).

3. Freezing Technique

a. A minimum of 15 min and a maximum of 30 min should elapse between addition of cryoextender and exposure to vapor freezing. Place labeled cryotubes onto aluminum canes and label top of cane with donor or client depositor identification and date.

b. Place cane into the vapor chamber of the upper section of a liquid nitrogen refrigerator (MVE-A-7000), or a liquid nitrogen dry shipper.

c. After 30 min the cane is quickly transferred from the upper chamber to the lower liquid section for immersion in the same refrigerator, or from the shipper to a liquid nitrogen refrigerator.

D. CRYOGENIC LABORATORIES, INC.

1. Preparation of Cryoprotective Medium (TEST-EYG)

a.   Dissolve 51.8 g TES in 700 ml distilled water.

b.   Dissolve 15.6 g TRIS in 400 ml distilled water.

c.   Titrate TES with TRIS to a stable pH of 7.2 which makes the solution (TEST) about the desired 320 mOsm.

d.   Mix the TEST with 20% egg yolk (EY), bring mixture to a boil and filter first through gauze, then through a millipore filter using sterile technique.

e.   Adjust pH of TEST-EY to 7.2 with TRIS.

f.   Mix 77 ml glycerol (G) with 23 ml of buffer using sterile technique.

g.   Store resulting medium (TEST-EYG) as 10 ml aliquots in sterile 15 ml glass culture tubes at about $-10°C$, until use.

2. Addition of Cryoprotective Medium

a.   After analysis is complete, determine the volume of the cryoprotective medium required by calculating 10% of the specimen volume.

b.   Draw the calculated amount of cryoprotective medium into a 3 ml syringe with an 18 gauge needle, wiping the excess off the needle.

c.   Add the medium dropwise to the semen specimen, mixing constantly on slow speed of a Vortex mixer, or by gently shaking the specimen container.

d.   Allow the specimen to equilibrate for at least 15 min.

e.   In the meantime, label the ampules with the specimen number (twice) and the client depositor's initials or the donor's number (twice). Bake the markings onto the ampules for 5 to 10 min. Allow the ampules to cool thoroughly.

f.   Label the storage canes with the specimen number, patient's initials, and visit number or in the case of a donor, just the specimen number and donor number. Bake the canes also and allow them to cool completely.

g.   Once the ampules and canes have cooled, use the syringe to deposit 0.4 ml of prepared semen specimen into each ampule.

h.   Flame seal the tops of the ampules using a flame ampule sealer (Figure 2), taking care that there are no holes in the seal.

3. Freezing Technique

a.   Place the ampules on the canes (6 per cane or distributed as evenly as possible given the final number of ampules). Reserve one ampule as a test ampule (for post-freeze analysis) and place it on a test cane.

b.   Place the loaded canes into the vapor tray in the vapor phase of the liquid nitrogen storage tanks, at a 30° angle. After at least 2 h of vapor cooling, submerge the canes into the liquid nitrogen within a canister and record the location. Immerse the test cane into the liquid nitrogen, allowing it to reach liquid nitrogen temperature, and remove it for thawing and examination of semen for the quality control test of cryo-survival. Cover the ampule immediately upon the removal from the tank with a cloth to prevent injury from rare but potential explosion of the ampule.

VI. STANDARDS IN CRYOBANKING

A. BACKGROUND

Our present level of technology in cryopreservation has been proven adequate to establish cryobanks of human semen on a scale of considerable clinical importance. There has been and still is concern, however, about necessary standards in genetic selection of donors, screening of semen, testing for venereal (sexually transmitted) diseases and pathogenic microorganisms, as well as the methods for freezing and storage in cryopreservation. Regulations in terms of acceptable scientific and ethical practices seem warranted in cryobanking of human semen initially through peer groups themselves and later, in appropriate areas, through peer-group input to appropriate governmental agencies.

The American Association of Tissue Banks (AATB) was chartered in 1976 with cell and tumor, musculoskeletal, ocular, renal, skin, tissue banks, and reproductive councils. AATB has published the first "Standards for Tissue Banking".[1] This publication has fostered a self-disciplined adherence to a uniform set of standards devised by peers in cryobanking for more beneficial clinical and research applications, as well as a close association of AATB with concerned professional societies and governmental agencies in the continuing process of reevaluation and modification of these standards.

The standards of the Reproductive Council for cryobanking of human semen stress donor procurement, screening, and selection as well as analysis and evaluation of semen as to suitability for cryopreservation and inseminations. The most recent revision of "AATB Standards for Tissue Banking" will be published in 1989.

B. EXAMPLES OF STANDARDS

Excerpts from the Reproductive Council Addendum of the "AATB Standards for Cryobanking" (1987)[1] which relate specifically to cryopreservation of donor semen and pertain to the techniques discussed here include.

1. Semen Analysis

This is the most important laboratory tool in evaluation of male infertility and proposed therapy and one which requires expertise and thoroughness.

Semen shall be collected by the donors ejaculation into a chemically clean container such as a 2 oz glass or plastic ointment jar. Collection shall occur at the semen bank.

In screening a potential donor for cryobanking three separate ejaculates shall be examined initially for evaluation and initial storage. Each ejaculate collected shall be preceded by a period of 3 to 5 days of abstinence. Observations and tests of semen analysis shall include: color, odor, obvious inclusions, coagulation, liquefaction, viscosity, volume, cell count (density), percentage of motility, movement (kind, activity, speed, duration), percentage of viability, abnormal-appearing cells, foreign cells, glycerol (osmotic) sensitivity, and cryosensitivity (percentage of survival during freezing and thawing).

The minimum acceptable values shall be: liquefaction, 50 M/cc, 50% progressive motility, average or better quality of movement, below 30% abnormalities of sperm head and neck, percentage of viability within 10% of motility, relative insensitivity (no more than 5% motility loss) to glycerol (osmotic) shock, and at least 50% cryosurvival on the basis of progressive motility before and after freezing and thawing.

2. Semen Culturing

Semen shall be screened for scientifically established important sexually transmitted diseases using validated tests and procedures which can be performed routinely in a clinical laboratory. Each semen sample shall be cultured for the detection of *Neisseria gonorrhoeae*.

3. Blood Testing

Blood samples shall be tested initially for syphilis and hepatitis B surface antigen. (Periodic testing of blood samples, as appropriate, is necessary for long-term active donors). Blood from the prospective donor shall be screened for HIV (HTLV-III/LAV) antibody and hepatitis B surface antigen, using FDA-required tests. Cryobanked semen shall be released for use only if results of these tests are negative for the prospective donor after a quarantine period for his stored semen of at least 6 months.

4. Examination and Donor Acceptance

Only the density, motility, and cryosurvival need be measured in samples after initial screening and acceptance of donor semen, but all requisite microbiological tests shall be performed on aliquots of every sample which is to be frozen and stored.

5. Processing

Collection of semen shall occur at the semen bank or within the institution in which it is housed and processing of liquefied semen shall be initiated within 1 h of collection after small aliquots are removed for semen analysis and microbial examination.

Tests and measurements used in steps in semen cryobanking shall be performed with appropriate checks such as duplicate readings. To control accuracy, it is desirable that microscopic observations of semen specimens be made just prior to their use in insemination.

6. Preservation and Storage Methods

Several methods are available which have been demonstrably successful in cryopreservation. There is no basis, therefore, for rigidity in selecting one as preferred.

The level of liquid nitrogen in storage and shipping containers shall be adequate to satisfy the low temperature requirements of long-term maintenance to prevent loss of functional activity during storage. The samples shall be immersed in liquid nitrogen in approved storage containers with a system for monitoring levels during storage.

Semen processed for frozen storage shall be placed in containers such as plastic straws and glass ampules which are sealed to prevent possible contamination.

C. FROZEN SEMEN AND TESTING FOR AIDS

In December 1985, the American Association of Tissue Banks Task Force (AATB) on "The Role of Semen in Transmitting Human T-Lymphotrophic Virus III Infection", recommended the use of frozen semen as the optimal and safest means of testing for AIDS in semen donors. Most semen cryobankers of the AATB Reproductive Council already were practicing a 3-month quarantine period for retesting donors before semen release, a practice which was formally adopted as a AATB standard in 1986 and published in the 1987 revision of "AATB Standards for Tissue Banking". Recently,[10] FDA and CDC recommended the use of frozen semen instead of fresh with a quarantine period of at least 6 months prior to donor AIDS retesting and use of cryobanked semen. The Reproductive Council recommended in 1988 that AATB Standards for the Reproductive Council be modified, accordingly, as of September 1989. A formal revision of standards is awaiting publication along with other actions approved by the AATB Board of Governors in 1989. Most AATB-associated cryobanks (Table 2) already were, or now are, practicing the 6 months quarantine program, prior to approval of the standard.

VII. REGULATION OF SEMEN CRYOBANKING

Since 1976 there has been a close and watchful association between the FDA and the AATB, specifically its Reproductive Council, regarding semen cryobanks. The FDA has taken the position that cryobanking has been adequately self-regulated on a voluntary basis through the development of standards, education and cryobank certification programs of the Reproductive Council of AATB through AATB.

The danger now exists, however, that a few uninformed and misinformed state and municipal legislatures may pass bills to regulate and perhaps severely restrict or even eliminate cryobanking of human semen. These bills have been introduced by well-intentioned legislators primarily in response to lay and quasi-medical reporting and letters to the editor in journals on sexually transmitted disease, donor payment, and donor screening rather than after input by the experts in medical societies especially the Reproductive Council of AATB. Lacking background information of the state of the art knowledge of the mature posture assumed by the FDA, the legislators fail to properly evaluate the consequences of regulation, especially with poorly researched and devised, scientifically inaccurate, and untenable sections of proposed legislation. Adherence to the text of the bills the author has seen could reduce the beneficial aspects of cryobanks on our society.

Even if regulation of semen cryobanking was warranted and accurately formulated into legislation, it would be relatively ineffective as the regulation would address and control the wrong segment of the medical community. The focus should be on the recognized clinical practice of artificial insemination rather than cryobanking. Cryobanking is merely a vehicle through which cryopreserved semen is obtained for a growing fraction of the inseminations performed in the U.S. Many inseminations still do not involve cryobanked or cryopreserved semen, but rather freshly ejaculated semen. Actually, cryobanked semen already allows for the microbiological screening of semen or blood during a quarantine storage period which is not feasible with fresh semen.

The author suggests that appropriate scientific evaluation, in concert with input from the FDA be undertaken by legislators regarding an approach, if appropriate, to state or federal regulation of the clinical practice of artificial insemination of human semen. Premature and ill-conceived regulatory laws directed at semen cryobanks not only would do little to protect public safety in artificial insemination but could establish the danger of stifling the innovation and availability of the health products contributed by cryobanks.

VIII. SUMMARY

Highlights of the background, including history and cryobiological principles, in the cryopreservation of human spermatozoa, were presented. The value and requisites for a Procedure Manual were noted and the basis for the formulation of sections on cryopreservation was outlined with examples of sources in its unique tailoring for each cryobank. Emphasis was placed upon the complexity of scientific evaluation of methods, the resulting conflicts in the literature, and the wide spectrum of variations in procedures in cryopreservation which, nevertheless, result in successful clinical applications of cryobanked semen.

The author hopes that his brief contribution will be of value in both the establishment and the continuation of high standard cryobanks for human semen which will beneficially serve the infertile couple.

ACKNOWLEDGMENT

The author wishes to acknowledge, with appreciation, members of the Reproductive Council of the American Association of Tissue Banks (AATB) who responded to surveys and inquiries concerning their experiences in cryobanking. Special recognition is made to the directors of the following cryobanks who provided portions of their Procedure Manuals for this purpose:

- Warren Sanger, Ph.D.—Genetic Semen Bank, University of Nebraska, 42nd and Dewey Ave., Omaha, NE 68105
- Mary Ann Brown—International Cryogenics, Inc., 189 Townsend Suite 203, Birmingham, MI 48011
- Steve Broder—California Cryobank, Inc., 1019 Galey Avenue, Los Angeles, CA 90024
- John Olson, M.S.—Cryogenic Laboratories, Inc., 2233 Hamline Ave., North Roseville, MN 55113

The assistance of Joy Thompson, especially in proofing the manuscript, is gratefully acknowledged.

REFERENCES

1. American Association of Tissue Banks, *Standards of Tissue Banking,* Arlington, VA, 1989.
2. American Association of Tissue Banks, *Technical Manual for Tissue Banking,* Arlington, VA, 1987.
3. **Sherman, J. K.,** Low temperature research on spermatozoa and eggs, *Cryobiology,* 1, 103, 1964.
4. **Sherman, J. K.,** Synopsis of the use of frozen human semen since 1964: state of the art of human semen banking, *Fertil. Steril.,* 24, 397, 1973.
5. **Sherman, J. K.,** Cryopreservation of human semen, in *Techniques of Human Andrology,* Hafez, E. S. E., Ed., North Holland, New York, 1977, chap. 24.
6. **Sherman, J. K.,** Current status of clinical cryobanking of human semen, in *Andrology; Male Fertility and Sterility,* Paulson, J. D., Negro-Vilar, A., Lucena, E., and Martini, L., Eds., Academic Press, New York, 1986, chap. 30.
7. **Olson, J. H.,** personal communication, 1988.
8. **Sherman, J. K.,** Frozen semen: efficiency in artificial insemination and advantage in testing for aquired immune deficiency syndrome, *Fertil. Steril.,* 47, 19, 1987.
9. American Association of Tissue Banks, *Standards of Tissue Banking,* Arlington, VA, 1985.
10. Centers for Disease Control, Semen banking, organ and tissue transplantation and HIV antibody testing, *MMWR,* 37, 57, 1988.
11. **Phillip, M., Hermoni, D., and Potashnik, G.,** Comparison of post-thaw sperm motility after freezing in liquid nitrogen with protective media of either glycerol or glycerol-egg-yolk-citrate, *Int. J. Fertil.,* 28, 156, 1983.
12. **Mahadevan, M. and Trounson, A. O.,** Effect of cryoprotective media and dilution methods on the preservation of human spermatozoa, *Andrologia,* 15, 355, 1983.
13. **Mahadevan, M. and Trounson, A. O.,** Effect of cooling, freezing and thawing rates and storage conditions of preservation of human spermatozoa, *Andrologia,* 16, 52, 1984.
14. **Jeyendran, R. S., Van der Ven, H. H., Kennedy, W., Perez-Pelaez, M., and Zaneveld, L. J. D.,** Comparison of glycerol and a zwitter-ion buffer system as cryoprotective media for human spermatozoa, *J. Androl.,* 5, 1, 1984.
15. **Prins, G. S. and Weidel, L.,** A Comparative study of buffer systems as cryoprotectants for humans spermatozoa, *Fertil. Steril.,* 46, 147, 1986.
16. **Heuchel, V., Schwartz, D., and Price, W.,** Within subject variability and the importance of abstinence period for sperm count, semen volume and pre-freeze and post-thaw motility, *Andrologia,* 13, 479, 1981.
17. **Heath, E., Jeyendran, R. S., Perez-Palaez, M., and Sobrero, A. J.,** Ultrastructural categorization of human sperm cryopreserved in glycerol and in TESTCY, *Int. J. Androl.,* 8, 101, 1985.
18. **Pilikian, S., Czyba, J. D., and Guerin, J. F.,** Effect of various concentrations of glycerol on post-thaw motility and velocity of human spermatozoa, *Cryobiology,* 19, 147, 1982.
19. **Thachil, J. V. and Jewett, M. A. S.,** Preservation techniques for human semen, *Fertil. Steril.,* 35, 546, 1981.
20. **Cohen, J., Felten, P., and Zeilmaker, G.H.,** *In vitro* fertilizing capacity of fresh and cryopreserved human spermatozoa: a comparative study of freezing and thawing procedures, *Fertil. Steril.* 36, 356, 1981.
21. **Critser, J. K., Huse-Benda, A. R., Aaker, D. V., Arneson, B. W., and Ball, G. D.,** Cryopreservation of human spermatozoa. I. Effects of holding procedure and seeding on motility, fertility ability, and acrosome reaction, *Fertil. Steril.,* 47, 656, 1987.
22. **Balerna, M., Nutini, L., Eppenberger, U., and Campana, A.,** Technology and instrumentation for semen analyses and AIH/AID. Effect of plastic and glass on sperm motility, pH, and oxidation, *Arch. Androl.,* 15, 225, 1985.
23. **Ing, R. M. Y.,** A simplified liquid nitrogen vapour method for the cryopreservation of human sperm. *Clin. Reprod. Fertil.* 1, 137, 1982.
24. **Roner, J., Boschieter, J., Leving, M., and Wiswedel, K.,** A simple method for cryopreservation of human sperm, *SAMT DEEL,* 69, 755, 1986.
25. **Sherman, J. K.,** Improved methods of preservation of human spermatozoa by freezing and freeze-drying, *Fertil. Steril.,* 14, 49, 1963.

Chapter 14

MICROBIOLOGICAL EXAMINATION OF THE INFERTILE COUPLE

Michael P. O'Leary and Ruth M. Greenblatt

TABLE OF CONTENTS

I. INTRODUCTION

There is little controversy regarding whether or not to treat the infertile male or female with an active genital infection. However, in the case of asymptomatic individuals presenting for infertility, the decision to use diagnostic tests should be based upon the association between the test outcome and a disease state, and the reversibility of the disease state based upon treatment indicated by the test outcome. In this chapter, we will consider the value of detecting infections in the assessment of infertile couples. Evaluation of the male and female will be considered separately. The association between various infections and infertility, the reversibility of infertility, and the value of diagnostic tests in detecting infection will be discussed. Finally, we will make recommendations regarding the evaluation of infertile couples and research questions which remain unanswered.

II. MALE FACTOR INFERTILITY

Considerable controversy exists as to what role infection plays as a cause of infertility in males, although consensus does acknowledge the association of pelvic inflammatory disease with female factor infertility.[1] This will be discussed in greater detail later in the chapter. Several large series have failed to indicate infectious causes in males who present with infertility.[2,3] In reporting on their experience with 1294 patients who presented with infertility, Dubin and Amelar identified no cases in which infection played a role. Although no mention is made of a specific attempt to isolate an infectious etiology, 5.4% of these were identified as "unknown."[3] Greenberg et al. indicate the possibility that infection may contribute to "idiopathic subfertility" but offer no suggestions regarding diagnosis or treatment.[2] Nevertheless, up to one quarter of all males evaluated for infertility are classified as having idiopathic infertility;[4] it is in this group that an infectious etiology may most likely be present.

There are potentially four ways genital infection can lead to infertility in the male: (1) by having a direct deleterious effect on sperm production, (2) by causing alteration in sperm storage and transport in the secretory glandular system, (3) by causing inflammation with subsequent sclerosis of the tubular transport system, and finally (4) by causing immunologically mediated infertility. We will discuss each of these, and outline a method for diagnosis and treatment. In addition, the male may be the source of infection in the female.

Bacterial attachment to spermatozoa has been demonstrated with several organisms including *Escherichia coli, Neisseria gonorrhoeae,* and *Ureaplasma urealyticum.*[5,6] The proposed mechanism of bacterial interference with sperm metabolism or sperm tail motility is not clear, but a significant decrease in sperm motility has been demonstrated when normal sperm concentrations were exposed to greater than 100,000 colonies/cc of *E. coli.*[7] Gnarpe and Friberg studied 36 men with unexplained infertility and 23 fertile controls.[8] T-mycoplasmas were isolated from semen specimens of 30 infertile men (85%) but only 6 of the controls (23%), a difference that was statistically significant ($p < 0.001$).[8] However, De-Louvois and colleagues studied 109 infertile couples and isolated T-mycoplasmas from one or both partners in 57.% while this organism was also isolated from 53% of 38 fertile controls.[9] Prostatic and seminal vesicle infection may alter the secretory function of these glands and at least transiently, alter fertility. Additionally, sexually transmitted diseases, such as syphilis, can result in seminiferous tubular damage, while epididymal infection may result in ductal obstruction with impaired sperm transport particularly in the case of infection with mycobacteria. Perhaps the best example of specific infectious agents resulting in infertility is that of mumps orchitis in the post-pubertal male which may result in permanent infertility if it is bilateral. However, it is not thought to be of epidemiologic importance.[10]

The spermatozoa itself is highly antigenic, but it is isolated from the host immune surveillance system by the blood testis barrier. Alterations in this barrier which occur during active infection such as epididymitis may result in the formation of anti-sperm antibodies.[11] These autoantibodies could result in sperm agglutination followed by infertility.

There is controversy regarding the importance of male genital tract infection in the etiology of infertility, but since the possibility that infection may impair fertility cannot be ruled out, males presenting for evaluation should undergo thorough evaluation.

A. EXAMINATION OF THE MALE

A detailed history is the first and perhaps most important step in evaluating the sub-fertile male. Symptoms of acute infection are usually obvious: dysuria, urgency, frequency, urethral discharge suggesting urethral infection, irritative voiding symptoms accompanying perineal or low back pain suggesting prostatic inflammation, scrotal pain with or without swelling suggesting epididymal or testicular infection. However, symptoms of chronic or sub-acute infection may be much more subtle or absent entirely. Thus a high index of suspicion is required. A previous history of any sexually transmitted disease, tuberculosis, or mumps orchitis should be identified. Male patients should be questioned about infections in any previous sexual partner, and the possibility of sub-clinical chronic infection should be considered. The standard evaluation of the sub-fertile male is covered in detail elsewhere in this text. Semen analysis is performed at least twice and particular attention is paid to motility and forward progression. Asthenozoospermia or asthenoteratozoospermia may be caused by infection and should lead the clinician to consider this possibility particularly if a varicocele has been ruled out.

A standardized routine should be used in evaluating men with suspected infection. If there is a history of urethral discharge, a urethral swab should be obtained. Gram stain and routine culture for *N. gonorrhoeae* and *C. trachomatis* should be performed. *C. trachomatis* is probably the most common of all the etiologies of urethritis and may coexist with *N. gonorrhoeae*. The asymptomatic patient may also harbor *N. gonorrhoeae* or *C. trachomatis*. Unfortunately, recovery of chlamydia can be difficult because the organism does not grow in standard culture media. Two direct methods have recently been developed however that simplify the detection of *C. trachomatis*. Chlamydiazyme (Abbott Labs, North Chicago, IL) is a solid phase enzyme immunoassay which is capable of detecting chlamydial antigen in swabs collected from the urethra. Sensitivity has been reported between 73 and 80% in males, while specificity exceeds 95%.[12] A direct immunofluorescence test has also been developed (MicroTrak, Syva Co., Palo Alto, CA) which employs a fluorescein labeled monoclonal antibody specific for chlamydia. Sensitivity has been reported as 90% with specificity of 95%.[12] However, one might expect the prevalence of chlamydial infection in a population of males presenting with infertility to be low thus decreasing the predictive value of these tests.

Rather than having a urethral discharge or other symptoms, the typical infertility patient often has few if any symptoms referable to the genitourinary tract. In the asymptomatic patient, the possibility of lower tract infection should be considered. Localization studies, as first proposed by Meares and Stamey in 1968[13] (Figure 1), are simple and invaluable in the diagnosis of lower tract infection in the male. If uncircumcised, the prepuce is retracted. The glans is carefully cleansed and dried. The first 10 cc of voided urine is collected in a sterile container and labeled VB 1 (voided bladder 1). The patient continues to void, and a midstream aliquot is obtained in a sterile container labeled VB 2. The patient is then carefully examined in the standing position. The size and consistency of the testes is noted with careful palpation for the presence of varicocele. The patient should be asked to Valsava at this point. Any epididymal tenderness may indicate infection. A rectal exam is then performed noting the presence of any tenderness with prostatic massage to obtain secretions which are labeled EPS (expressed prostatic secretions). The patient then voids a final 5 cc for the VB

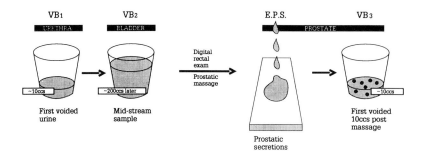

FIGURE 1. Lower tract localization studies. (Adapted from Meares, E. M., Jr. and Stamey, T. A., *Invest. Urol.,* 5, 492, 1968. With permission.)

3. Portions of the VB 1 and 2 samples are centrifuged and examined microscopically. The presence of >5 WBCs/hpf on the VB 1 is evidence of significant inflammation and likely urethral infection. The patient may have chlamydial infection with negative culture by routine methods and should be treated with a tetracycline. Evidence of pyuria in the VB 2 and positive bacterial culture suggests chronic infection as persistent bacteriuria is the hallmark of chronic bacterial prostatitis. This patient's urine should be sterilized with a urinary antimicrobial such as nitofurantoin for several days prior to further localization studies.

A drop of fluid from the EPS on a glass slide with a coverslip should be examined microscopically. Fewer than 12 WBCs/hpf are present in normal prostatic fluid after a period of sexual abstinence of at least two days. After ejaculation, an increase in the number of white blood cells in prostatic secretions occurs and 20 WBC/hpf is considered the upper limit of normal.[14] A larger number suggests infection. Negative routine bacteriologic cultures in the presence of >12 WBCs/hpf on the EPS suggests the likelihood of infection with chlamydial organisms and tetracycline therapy should be initiated. In those patients in whom prostatic massage does not yield fluid, a urethral washout specimen (VB 3) should be obtained.

Finally, the semen itself is analyzed. The existence of pyospermia has been recognized for some time, but the significance of this finding has been unclear. For example, Fowler and Kessler have reported the leukocyte concentration in seminal fluid of 50 fertile men compared with that of 50 men with idiopathic infertility[15]. The infertile men had a mean white cell count of 2.1 × 10⁶/ml while the control group had even higher counts with a mean of 2.3 × 10⁶/ml raising doubt concerning the role of pyospermia in infertility. On the other hand, Berger and associates reported improvement in sperm penetration assay in 50% of infertile men with pyospermia. An increased conception rate occurred in the partners of those treated for 20 days with doxycycline compared with similar untreated controls.[16] Thus, the significance of pyospermia is unclear. However, because of the generally benign nature of tetracycline therapy, an empiric course of 500 mg, q.i.d. for 2 weeks is reasonable when no other source for infertility can be identified.

B. SUMMARY

An association between infection and "idiopathic" male factor infertility has not been proven. Nonetheless, evidence of infection may be uncovered in the careful evaluation of the infertile male and, under these circumstances, warrants treatment.

III. EVALUATION OF THE FEMALE

A. INTRODUCTION

The decision to use diagnostic tests should be based upon the association between the test outcome and a disease state, the reversibility of the disease state based upon treatment indicated by the test outcome, or the value of prognostic information provided by the diagnostic test. In this part of the chapter, we will consider the value of detecting infections in the assessment of infertile women. The association between various infections and infertility, the reversibility of infertility, and the value of diagnostic tests in detecting infection will be discussed. Finally we will make recommendations regarding the evaluation of infertile women and research questions which remain unanswered.

B. THE ASSOCIATION BETWEEN INFECTION AND INFERTILITY

Several kinds of infection have been associated with infertility in the female. Most of these infections can be transmitted via sexual activity and are therefore considered sexually transmitted diseases (STDs). STD etiologies which may be associated with female infertility include *C. trachomatis, N. gonorrhoeae, Mycoplasma hominis,* and *U. urealyticum.* Of the STD syndromes, pelvic inflammatory disease (PID) appears to have the closest association with infertility in women. The current 20 year epidemic of cervicitis and urethritis has been followed by increases in the incidence of PID and the prevalence of infertility.[17,18] Approximately 15% of all infertility is due to dysfunciton of the Fallopian tubes.[19] STDs clearly play a large role in the etiology of tubal damage and the infertility that often follows.[17,18] Thus, it is appropriate to consider the value of testing infertile women for STD pathogens.

C. PELVIC INFLAMMATORY DISEASE

Cohort studies of PID patients have identified a 2.8- to 5-fold higher incidence of infertility and a 6- to 10-fold higher incidence of ectopic pregnancy than among women without PID.[1,18] One fifth of all PID patients go on to experience involuntary infertility.[20] It has been estimated that between 30 to 50% of all cases of female infertility and ectopic pregnancy are caused by PID related tubal damage.[18] The fact that the occurrence of tubal damage and related infertility is proportional to the total number of PID episodes gives further weight to evidence that a causal relationship exists between PID and some cases of tubal factor infertility.[21]

C. trachomatis may be more likely to result in tubal damage and subsequent infertility than other etiologies of PID, such as *N. gonorrhoeae,*[20,22,23] Serologic evidence of previous chlamydial infection was closely associated with tubal factor infertility (TFI) in a series of case control studies.[24-27] In one study this association was found to be independent of number of sexual partners and age at first intercourse.[28]

While a strong epidemiologic link between previous PID and TFI exists, the role of acute infection in infertility has not been defined. Several studies of tubal pathology among women with TFI have failed to identify active infection with chlamydial or other pathogens or evidence of acute inflammation.[29] For example, Sellors and colleagues found that only 4 of 52 women with tubal factor infertility had evidence of acute PID (vs. chronic damage) at laparotomy and chlamydial organisms were not recovered from tubal biopsy specimens.[27] In contrast, Henry-Suchet and co-workers isolated *C. trachomatis* from 13 of 69 women with TFI undergoing tuboplasty[30] and in a later study from 48 of 162 such patients undergoing laparoscopy.[23] Cleary and Jones reported an association between the recovery of *C. trachomatic* from endometrial biopsies and female infertility.[31] So the proportion of women in whom infertility can be attributed to active chlamydial infection is not clear. Thus, the potential benefit of detecting chlamydial infection among infertile women is currently not known.

D. INFECTIONS WITH GENITAL MYCOPLASMAS

Some investigators have suggested that chronic cervical or endometrial infection with genital mycoplasmas (*M. hominis* or *U. urealyticum*) may be related to reversible infertility in women.[32,33] *M. hominis* but not *U. urealyticum* has been identified as a cause of PID.[34] Any association of *U. urealyticum* with infertility is not absolute since the organism has been isolated from cervical mucus in fertile as well as infertile women.[9] Henry-Suchet reported the isolation of *U. urealyticum* from laparoscopic specimens among women with TFI but not significantly more often than among women in a control group.[30] Cassell and associates[35] identified a group of women whose infertility was associated with a particular male partner. These women were more likely to have *U. urealyticum* isolated from the lower genital tract than other infertile women.

E. THE EFFICACY OF ANTIBIOTIC THERAPY IN THE TREATMENT OF INFERTILITY

1. Pelvic Inflammatory Disease

Despite the close association of PID with subsequent female factor infertility, there is no evidence that anti-infective treatment can reverse established TFI. Successful efforts for the prevention of the sequelae of PID, such as the Swedish program, focus on intensive treatment and follow-up of persons with chlamydial infections and PID to prevent tubal damage rather than reverse existing damage.[36] The effect of detection of acute PID or chlamydial infections and subsequent treatment on reproductive function is not known. Since most patients with TFI show evidence of chronic disease, it is unlikely that antibiotic treatment would often lead to the reversal of infertility. On the other hand, the treatment of proven chlamydial infection is always indicated. Such treatment may prevent the added damage to Fallopian tubes produced by recurrent episodes of PID.

2. Infections With Genital Mycoplasmas

Antibiotic treatment can be followed by conception in couples who have been previously infertile.[29,32,37] Gnarpe and Friberg[37] reported a high (29%) conception rate in an uncontrolled trial of doxycycline in the treatment of infertile couples. Harrison and colleagues[38] conducted a controlled trial of doxycycline among 88 couples with infertility of unknown etiology. Despite the fact that this treatment was found to have eliminated genital mycoplasma infections, only 16% of the doxycline group subsequently conceived, a rate not significantly different from that of the control group which did not receive antibiotic treatment. Overall the role of genital mycoplasmas in female infertility remains controversial. Taylor-Robinson called for continued caution in assessing the value of antibiotics in the treatment of infertility.[39]

F. DIAGNOSTIC TESTS

One approach to estimating the potential value of diagnostic tests for STDs among infertile women is to extrapolate from data on the utility of the tests in the general population of sexually active women. Since 1979, the U.S. has pursued a national policy of identifying all women with gonorrhea. This policy was partially a response to the recognition of the serious morbidity related to PID and the association between PID and gonorrhea. Curran noted that screening for gonorrhea should be performed because it is inexpensive and that treatment is highly effective.[40] The recent increase in the incidence of antibiotic resistant *N. gonorrhoeae* has highlighted the need for identification of cases.[41] Cervical culture for *N. gonorrhoeae* has become routine in the U.S. since adoption of the national control policy. Culture remains the standard for detection of gonococcal infections, the test has a sensitivity of 80 to 95%.[42] Recently, enzyme immunoassay techniques have been applied to a test for the detection of gonococcal infection.

Many infertile women are involved in stable monogamous relationships and may therefore face a very low risk of acute gonorrhea. On the other hand, some infertile women are more likely to have had STDs in the past. In addition the risk of morbidity due to gonorrhea during a pregnancy, if conception were to occur, is high. Thus, considering recent national policy and the high morbidity of gonococcal infection, it would seem appropriate to screen infertile women for gonococcal infections despite the fact that this process is very unlikely to result in reversal of established infertility.

Even though chlamydial infections are several times more common than gonorrhea, routine screening for this infection has not been widely adopted probably reflecting the relatively high cost and cumbersome nature of chlamydia detection via culture. Recently new tests for the detection of chlamydial infections have been developed. These include fluorescent antibody tests (FA) and enzyme immunoassays (EIA). They are highly sensitive and specific (sensitivity ranges from 61 to 93% and specificity from 94 to 99% in females).[43-47] These tests are much less expensive and cumbersome than culture techniques. Indeed several recent studies have found that chlamydia screening would be cost effective if the new tests were used in populations with a prevalence of chlamydial infection of 7/100 or greater.[48,49] In many populations, chlamydial infections are highly prevalent. Among women presenting to a variety of outpatient medical settings (not including STD facilities), recent studies have identified chlamydial infection in 5 to 22%.[47,50-52] Many of these infected women were asymptomatic.

Genital chlamydial infections are much more common than gonorrhea, and the potential morbidity in infertility secondary to chlamydial infections is at least as great as that associated with gonorrhea. So it seems reasonable to provide routine chlamydia screening to sexually active women. A more aggressive approach to case finding has been called for.[53] Because women who present with infertility are usually sexually active and may have a greater chance of having had chlamydial infection at some point in time, it may be reasonable to advocate the screening of these women. On the other hand, it is not clear that the treatment of infertile women who have chlamydia infection would be effective in reversing established infertility.

The points in favor and against screening for genital mycoplasmas are even less clear than for chlamydia and gonorrhea because the association of mycoplasmas with infertility is less certain. Cultures for *M. hominis* and *U. urealyticum* can be obtained from the vaginal pool, cervix, endometrium, or tubal structures.[54] However, a 30-day therapeutic trial of antibiotics (such as doxycycline or erythromycin) may be of equal value and less costly.

The potential benefits of STD screening with antibiotic treatment as a public health measure and the small chance of reversing infertility must be weighed against the potential costs and side effects of antibiotic treatment as well as the psychologic distress associated with being diagnosed with an STD. More research, such as randomized, placebo controlled, longitudinal studies, is needed to establish the efficacy of antibiotic therapy in infertile couples. Studies of the cost-benefits of STD diagnostic screening and treatment are also needed since infertility is a common problem and decisions regarding the implementation of screening and treatment are likely to become far reaching and have significant economic impact. Currently we would recommend culture for *N. gonorrhoeae* and a chlamydia detection test in women with TFI, evidence of acute cervicitis or PID, in sexually active women who have not undergone these tests during the previous year, or in the partners of men with urethritis, epididymitis, or a positive screening test. The use of culture in screening for genital mycoplasmas or therapeutic trial should be considered in women with evidence of PID, endometritis, or a sexual partner with pyospermia.

REFERENCES

1. **Cates, W.,** Sexually transmitted organisms and infertility: the proof is in the pudding, *Sexually Trans Dis.,* 11, 113, 1983.
2. **Greenberg, S. H., Lipshultz, L. I., and Wein, A. J.,** Experience with 425 subfertile male patients, *J. Urol.,* 119, 507, 1978.
3. **Dubin, L. and Amelar, R. D.,** Etiologic factors in 1294 consecutive cases of male infertility, *Fertil. Steril.,* 22, 469, 1971.
4. **Lipshultz, L. I. and Howards, S. S.,** Evaluation of the subfertile man, in *Infertility in the Male,* Lipshultz, L. I. and Howards, S. S., Eds., Churchill Livingstone, New York, 1983, 187.
5. **Teague, N. S., Boyarsky, S., and Glenn, J. F.,** Interference of human spermatozoa motility by *Escherichia coli, Fertil. Steril.,* 22, 281, 1971.
6. **Toth, A., Swenson, C. E., and O'Leary, W. M.,** Light microscopy as an aid in predicting ureaplasma infection in human semen, *Fertil. Steril.,* 30, 586, 1978.
7. **Del Porto, G. B., Derrick, F. C., Jr., and Bannister, E. R.,** Bacterial effect on sperm motility, *Urology,* 5, 638, 1975.
8. **Gnarpe, H. and Friberg, J.,** Mycoplasma and human reproductive failure, *Am. J. Obstet. Gynecol.,* 114, 727, 1972.
9. **DeLouvois, J., Harrison, R. F., Blades, M., et al.,** Frequency of mycoplasma in fertile and infertile couples, *Lancet,* 1, 1073, 1974.
10. World Health Organization, The epidemiology of infertility, Tech. Rep. No. 582, Geneva, 1975.
11. **Bronson, R. A., Cooper, G. W., and Rosenfeld, D. L.,** Correlation between regional specificity of antisperm antibodies to the spermatozoon surface and complement mediated sperm immobilization, *Reprod. Immunol.,* 2, 222, 1982.
12. **Needham, C. A.,** Rapid detection methods in microbiology, *Med. Clin. North Am.,* 71, 591, 1987.
13. **Meares, E. M., Jr. and Stamey, T. A.,** Bacteriologic localization patterns in bacterial prostatitis and urethritis, *Invest. Urol.,* 5, 492, 1968.
14. **Jameson, R. M.,** Sexual activity and the variations of the white cell content of prostatic secretions, *Invest. Urol.,* 5, 297, 1967.
15. **Fowler, J. E. and Kessler, R.,** Genital tract infections, in *Infertility in the Male,* Lipshultz, L. I. and Howards, S. S., Eds., Churchill Livingstone, New York, 1983, 283.
16. **Berger, R. E., Smith, W. D., Critchlow, C. W., Stenchever, M. A., Moore, D. E., Spadoni, L. R., and Holmes, K. K.,** Improvement in the sperm penetration assay results after doxycycline treatment of infertile men, *J. Androl.,* 4, 126, 1983.
17. **Mosher, W. D. and Aral, S. O.,** Factors related to infertility in the United States, 1965—1976, *Sex. Transm. Dis.,* 12, 117, 1985.
18. **Westrom, L.,** Incidence, prevalence, and trends of acute pelvic inflammatory disease and its consequences in industrialized countries, *Am. J. Obstet. Gynecol.,* 138, 880, 1980.
19. **Moore, D. E. and Spadoni, L. R.** Infertility in women, in *Sexually Transmitted Diseases,* Holmes, K. K., Mårdh, P.-A., Sparling, P. F., and Wiesner, P. J., Eds., McGraw-Hill, New York, 1984, chap. 65.
20. **Westrom, L.,** Effect of acute pelvic inflammatory disease on fertility, *Am. J. Obstet. Gynecol.,* 122, 707, 1975.
21. **Westrom, L.,** Influence of sexually transmitted diseases on sterility and ectopic pregnancy, *Acta Eur. Fertil.,* 16, 21, 1985.
22. **Svensson, L., Mårdh, P.-A., and Westrom, L.** Infertility after acute salpingitis with special reference to *Chlamydia trachomatis, Fertil. Steril.,* 40, 322, 1983.
23. **Henry-Suchet, J., Ultzmann, C., De Brux, J., Ardoin, P., and Catalan, F.** Microbiologic study of chronic inflammatoin associated with tubal factor infertility: role of *Chlamydia trachomatis, Fertil. Steril.,* 47, 274, 1987.
24. **Punnonen, R., Terho, P., Nikkanen, V., and Meurman, O.,** Chlamydial serology in infertile women by immunofluorescence, *Fertil. Steril.,* 31, 656, 1979.
25. **Jones, R. B., Ardery, B. R., Hui, S. L., and Cleary, R. E.,** Correlation between serum antichlamydial antibodies and tubal factor as a cause of infertility, *Fertil. Steril.,* 38, 553, 1982.
26. **Moore, D. E., Spadoni, L. R., Foy, H. M., et al.,** Increased frequency of serum antibodies to *Chlamydia trachomatis* in infertility due to distal tube disease, *Lancet,* ii, 574, 1982.
27. **Sellors, J. W., Mahoney, J. B., Chernesky, M. A., and Rath, D. J.,** Tubal factor infertility: an association with prior chlamydial infection and asymptomatic salpingitis, *Fertil. Steril.,* 49, 451, 1988.
28. **Brunham, R. C., Maclean, I. W., Binns, B., and Peeling, R. W.,** *Chlamydia trachomatis:* its role in tubal infertility, *J. Infect. Dis.,* 152, 1275, 1985.

29. **Cevanini, R., Possati, G., and LaPlaca, M.,** *Chlamydia trachomatis* infection in infertile women, in *Chlamydial Infections,* Mårdh, P.-A., Holmes, K. K., Oriel, J. D., et al., Eds., Elsevier Biomedical Press, Amsterdam, 1982.

30. **Henry-Suchet, J., Catalan, F., Loffredo, V., Sanson, M. J., Debache, C., Pigeau, F., and Coppin, R.,** *Chlamydia trachomatis* associated with chronic inflammation in abdominal specimens from women selected for tuboplasty, *Fertil. Steril.,* 36, 599, 1981.

31. **Cleary, R. E. and Jones, R. B.** Recovery of *Chlamydia trachomatis* from the endometrium of infertile women with serum antichlamydial antibodies, *Fertil. Steril.,* 44, 233, 1985.

32. **Knudsin, R. B., Falk, L., Hertig, A. T., and Horne, H. W.,** Mycoplasma, chlamydia, Epstein-Barr, herpes I and II, and AIDS infections among 100 consecutive infertile female patients and husbands: diagnosis, treatment, and results, *Int. J. Fertil.,* 31, 356, 1986.

33. **Stray-Pederson, B., Eng, J., and Reikvan, T. M.,** Uterine T-mycoplasma colonization in reproductive failure, *Am. J. Obstet. Gynecol.,* 130, 307, 1978.

34. **Mårdh, P.-A.,** Mycoplasmal PID: a review of natural and experimental infections, *Yale J. Biol. Med.,* 56, 529, 1983.

35. **Cassell, G. H., Younger, J. B., Brown, M. B., et al.,** Microbiologic study of infertile women at the time of diagnostic laparoscopy: association of *Ureaplasma urealyticum* with a defined subpopulation, *N. Engl. J. Med.,* 310, 937, 1983.

36. **Westrom, L.,** Treatment of pelvic inflammatory disease in view of etiology and risk factors, *Sex. Transm. Dis.,* 11, 437, 1984.

37. **Gnarpe, H. and Friberg, J.,** T-mycoplasmas as a possible cause for reproductive failure, *Nature,* 242, 120, 1973.

38. **Harrison, R. F., Blades, M., DeLouvois, J., and Hurley, R.,** Doxycycline treatment and human infertility, *Lancet,* i, 605, 1975.

39. **Taylor-Robinson, D.,** Evaluation of the role of *Ureaplasma urealyticum* in infertility, *Pediatr. Infect. Dis.,* 5, S262, 1986.

40. **Curran, J.,** Prevention of sexually transmitted diseases, in *Sexually Transmitted Diseases,* Holmes, K. K., Mårdh, P.-A., Sparling, P. F., and Wiesner, P. J., Eds., McGraw-Hill, New York, 1984, chap. 79.

41. **Whittington, W. L. and Knapp, J. S.,** Trends in resistance of *Neisseria gonorrhoeae* to antimicrobial agents in the United States, *Sex. Transm. Dis.,* 15, 202, 1988.

42. **Handsfield, H.H.,** Gonorrhea and uncomplicated gonococcal infection, in *Sexually Transmitted Diseases,* Holmes, K. K., Mårdh, P.-A., Sparling, P. F., and Wiesner, P. J., Eds., McGraw-Hill, New York, 1984, chap. 19.

43. **Tam, M. R., Stamm, W. E., Handsfield, H. H., et al.,** Culture-independent diagnosis of *Chlamydia trachomatis* using monoclonal antibodies, *N. Engl. J. Med.,* 310, 1146, 1984.

44. **Lipkin, E. S., Moncada, J. V., Shafer, M.-A., et al.,** Comparison of monoclonal antibody staining and culture in diagnosing cervical chlamydial infection, *J. Clin. Microbiol.,* 23, 114, 1986.

45. **Stamm, W. E., Harrison, H. R., Alexander, E. R., et al.,** Diagnosis of *Chlamydia trachomatis* infection by direct immunofluorescence staining of genital secretions: a multicenter trial, *Ann. Intern. Med.,* 101, 638, 1984.

46. **Kiviat, N. B., Wølner-Hanssen, P., Peterson, M., et al.,** Localization of *Chlamydia trachomatis* infection by direct immunofluorescence and culture in pelvic inflammatory disease, *Am. J. Obstet. Gynecol.,* 154, 865, 1986.

47. **Shafer, M.-A., Vaughan, E., Lipkin, E. S., et al.,** Evaluation of fluorescein-conjugated monoclonal antibody test to detect *Chlamydia trachoamtis* endocervical infections in adolescent girls, *Pediatrics,* 108, 779, 1986.

48. **Phillips, R. S., Aronson, M. D., Taylor, W. C., and Safran, C.,** Should tests for *Chlamydia trachomatis* cervical infection be done during routine gynecologic visits?, An analysis of the costs of alternative strategies, *Ann. Intern. Med.,* 107, 188, 1987.

49. **Nettleman, M. D. and Jones, R. B.,** Cost-effectiveness of screening women at moderate risk for genital infections caused by *Chlamydia trachomatis, J. Am. Med. Assoc.,* 260, 207, 1988.

50. **Schachter, J., Stoner, E., and Moncada, J.,** Screening for chlamydial infections in women attending family planning clinics: evaluations of presumptive indicators for therapy, *West. J. Med.,* 138, 375, 1983.

51. **Saltz, G. R., Linnemann, C. C., Brookman, R. R., and Rauh, J. L.,** *Chlamydia trachomatis* cervical infections in female adolescents, *J. Pediatr.,* 98, 981, 1981.

52. **Thompson, S. E. and Washington, A. E.,** Epidemiology of sexually transmitted *Chlamydia trachomatis* infections, *Epidemiol. Rev.,* 5, 96, 1983.

53. **Washington, A. E., Johnson, R. E., and Sanders, L. L.,** *Chlamydia trachomatis* infections in the United States: what are they costing us?, *J. Am. Med. Assoc.,* 257, 2070, 1987.

54. **Mårdh, P.-A.,** Bacteria chlamydiae, and mycoplasmas, in *Sexually Transmitted Diseases,* Holmes, K. K., Mårdh, P.-A., Sparling, P. F., and Wiesner, P. J., Eds., McGraw-Hill, New York, 1984, chap. 69.

Chapter 15

STATISTICAL METHODS FOR SERUM HORMONE ASSAYS

Ajit K. Thakur

TABLE OF CONTENTS

I. INTRODUCTION

Serum hormone assay techniques have become important tools for diagnostic methods as well as for new drug development. Many workers in the field still use nonoptimal graphical means for investigative work in the field. Furthermore, often there is no attempt made to ensure the precision and accuracy of the assays used. Particularly, since there is easy access to computers and specific programs are available for accurate characterization and validation of such systems, there should be no excuse to avoid them and instead rely on techniques which have been shown to be inappropriate.

We will use the term radioimmunoassay (RIA) to include a very broad class of assay methods. With some variations in specific assays, the present discussion will still hold as general principles for new assay techniques such as competitive immunoassays, noncompetitive (sandwich) immunofluorometric assays (IFMA), etc. which are widely used especially in sex hormone assays for HCG, LH, FSH, prolactin, and others.[1-3]

The physical chemical nature of many RIA-related reactions are very well understood. Specifically, for the thermodynamic equilibrium case it is possible to derive the mathematical expressions for many complex reactions using statistical mechanical or thermodynamic principles. These expressions allow one to understand and investigate the physicochemical nature of the system under study. They may further elucidate the biological nature of the system which may be important in many cases for understanding a disease process as well as for development of drugs. These expressions may be called mechanistic models.

On the other hand, if the purpose of the investigation is not to go into details of the mechanistic principles of such a system but to make use of some local behavior of the system under study, one can resort to some empirical models. Often these empirical models are easier from computational and statistical standpoints. Also, for many of the time-resolved fluorometry based assay and similar nonequilibrium techniques,[1-3] modeling and curve fitting with mechanistic expressions are numerically much more difficult. As a consequence, routine work related to these assays is easier to perform with empirical models.

In our discussion we will briefly describe both techniques and expand on the empirical methods to provide further statistical examination of the data.

II. MECHANISTIC DESCRIPTION OF RIA DATA

The equilibrium description of a binding system assumes that the system is at complete thermodynamic equilibrium and the free and bound receptor concentrations are completely separable. If there is nonspecific binding present, it is not considered as part of the reaction scheme and is accounted for by an additional parameter. A general case of such binding has been presented elsewhere.[4-6] For simplicity, let us take the example of the binding of homogeneous hormones to heterogeneous and cooperative bivalent receptors. For many RIAs these assumptions will be valid. The binding isotherm can be described as follows:[4-6]

$$B/F = \sum_{j=1}^{n} [R_j K_j (1 + CK_j F)/(1 + 2K_j F + CK_j^2 F^2)] \tag{1}$$

where

B = Bound hormone concentration
F = Free hormone concentration
R_j = Concentration of the jth receptor site

K_j = Affinity of the jth receptor site

C = Cooperativity factor

    C = 1: No cooperativity

    C >1: Positive cooperativity

    C <1: Negative cooperativity

$R_o = \sum\limits_{j=1}^{n} R_j$ = total receptor concentration over all sites

n = Number of distinct receptor sites

When n = 1, there is only one homogeneous receptor site with affinity K and total receptor cencentration R_o. In this case, Equation 1 can be rewritten in the Scatchard coordinates (B/F vs. B)[7] as:

$$B/F = K\{(R_0 - 2B) + [(R_0 - 2B)^2 + 4CB(R_0 - B)]^{1/2}\}/2 \qquad (2)$$

Equation 2 is the Scatchard form of a cooperative system. When C = 1, Equation 2 simplifies to the well-known Scatchard equation[7] for a homogeneous noncooperative site:

$$B/F = K(R_0 - B) \qquad (3)$$

When C = 1, and n >1, the system is noncooperative but heterogeneous and Equation 1 simplifies to:

$$B/F = \sum\limits_{j=1}^{n} [R_j K_j/(1 + K_j F)] \qquad (4)$$

The general form of Equation 4 in the Scatchard or any other coordinates requires solution of a polynomial equation.[9] However, for the special case when n = 2 (two independent receptor sites with affinities K_1 and K_2 and receptor concentrations R_1 and R_2), Equation 4 can be rewritten in the Scatchard coordinates as follows:

$$B/F = \{X + [X^2 + 4K_1 K_2 B(B - R_0)^{1/2}\}/2 \qquad (5)$$

where

$$X = K_1(R_1 - B) + K_2(R_2 - B) \text{ and}$$
$$R_o = R_1 + R_2$$

Many people still prefer to present experimental data in Scatchard coordinates[7] where the quantity B/F is plotted on the ordinate and B on the abscissa in arithmetic scales. A detailed examination of several other coordinates as well as variations of Equation 1 appear in previous works.[8-13] In many cases, these people also use graphical techniques in these plots to estimate the binding parameters, etc. There are serious statistical problems associated with such methods:

A.   If the curve-peeling or graphical techniques are used during or after visual examination of Scatchard plots or any other plots, there is bound to be subjectivity and bias in the estimation of the parameters.

B.   One does not get any measure of uncertainty of the parameters from these techniques.

C.   Presence of nonspecific binding distorts the true shape of the curves and as a result, there may be serious inaccuracies in the graphical estimates.

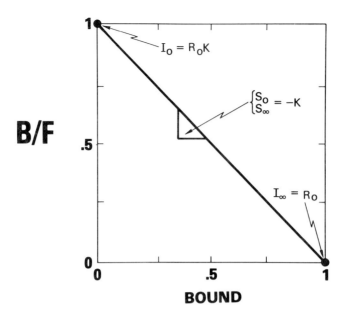

FIGURE 1.   Scatchard plot of homogeneous receptors with no cooperativity ($n = 1$, $C = 1$).

D.   The range and number of data points of the linear segments of these plots are limited.
       This makes the resolution of the segments difficult. As a result, the error in the
       parameter estimates will be further magnified.
E.   There are some serious statistical problems with the Scatchard and related coordinate
       systems which will be discussed in a later section.

Despite all the problems with graphical and curve-peeling techniques, it is a good idea to
use them as preliminary exploration of the binding data. In some cases such plots may
provide us clues as to the approximate nature of the binding curve. They may also offer
good initial estimates for the parameters of interest for further statistically valid evaluation
of data. Here we will discuss an objective way of utilizing such graphs with the idea that
parameters estimated by these means will not be the final estimates. The graphical exploration
we prefer to have should be based on the slopes, intercepts and some other characteristics
of the binding curves. Specifically, in the Scatchard coordinates, the two limiting slopes
and intercepts will provide us with all the necessary estimates for most cases. Figures 1 to
4 indicate the locations of the slopes and intercepts. The necessary mathmatical expressions
relating these limiting slopes and intercepts with the binding constants are presented in
Appendix I. Details of the derivation as well as other graphical presentation techniques can
be found elsewhere.[8-13]
       Once one obtains initial estimates of the binding parameters, one must resort to nonlinear
curve fitting techniques to obtain the final parameter values. The question is how to approach
such procedures? This topic has been addressed in details in the literature of RIA.[14-17] We
will briefly summarize some of the observations here. Even though the problems we address
here are specific for the Scatchard coordinates, i.e., B/F vs. B, many of them apply equally
well to several other coordinates.

A.   Both B/F and B are subject to errors.
B.   The errors in B/F and B are highly correlated. As a consequence, errors in the estimates
       of B/F are associated with errors in B in the same direction.

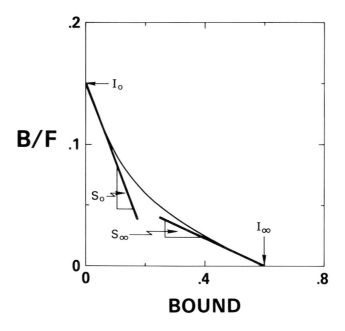

FIGURE 2. Scatchard plot of homogeneous receptors with negative cooperativity (n = 1, C < 1).

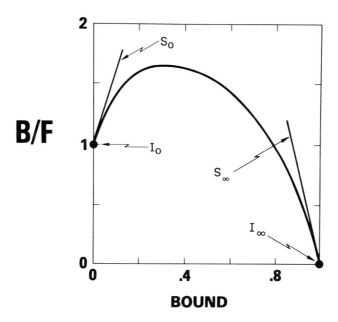

FIGURE 3. Scatchard plot of homogeneous receptors with positive cooperativity (n = 1, C > 1).

C. Neither B nor B/F can be considered a true independent variable as a result.
D. There is serious nonuniformity of variances in this and several other coordinates. This
   problem becomes worse when nonspecific binding is estimate d using the total binding
   as is customary in many assays.

Although it may be possible to use an appropriate weighted nonlinear least squares and

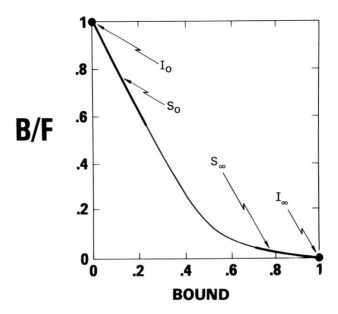

FIGURE 4.   Scatchard plot of heterogeneous receptors with no cooperativity ($n = 2$, $C = 1$).

TABLE 1
Estimates of Binding Parameters by
Graphical Methods in Three Coordinate
Systems

	B/F vs. F	Scatchard (B/F vs. B)	Dose-response (B/T vs. T)
K	105.0	133.0	99.9
R_0	96.5	90.0	103.0
C	93.8	66.5	87.2

Note: Parameters used: $K = 10^6$, $R_0 = 10^{-6}$, $C = 10$ (tenfold positive cooperativity) and 5% normal error in B (Bound). Results expressed as % of true value.

methods which allow for errors in both independent and dependent variables to circumvent many of the above problems, it is desirable to seek for a better coordinate system for such curve fitting. As has been shown in the past,[14-17] B or B/T vs. T or log(T) is a better coordinate system for this purpose. The variable T may be properly regarded as an independent variable in most assays. The pipetting and/or counting error in T is very small in most assays[14] in comparison to similar errors in B or B/T. Also the error correlation at different dose levels is small in this coordinate system. Even in this coordinate system, there may be some small systematic trend in the variance of B or B/T.[14] As a result, weighting is still desirable in this coordinate system. Appropriate weighting functions to be used will be described in the next section.

Let us examine the magnitudes of errors in different coordinates for a representative simulated study using graphical methods. As Table 1[8] indicates, even with only 5% normal error in B and with no nonspecific binding, the Scatchard plot provided the worst estimates of the three parameters in question. In this example, B was much smaller than F which was in excess. As a result, the two coordinates, B/F vs. F and B/T vs. T provided similar estimates of the parameters. If F were not in such an excess, the B/F vs. F coordinates would have behaved similar to the Scatchard coordinates. In the presence of nonspecific binding, the estimates would have been much worse in all three coordinate systems by graphical techniques. On the other hand, either one of the techniques will provide us with good intial estimates for an appropriately weighted curve fitting for this example.

Curve fitting for RIA could be accomplished with any standard non-linear curve fitter.[18-23] With the advent of PCs the choices are even wider. However, from a practical standpoint, it is better to have a customized package, one reason being that conversion of the binding model in terms of B or B/T vs. T or log(T) for complex systems will require some implicit solution of polynomial equations numerically. For example, Equations 2 and 3 when converted to B/T vs. T will require rather complex cubic equations to be solved.[8] The program LIGAND[24] is an excellent customized package developed for this purpose. This program will estimate parameters of many complex hormone binding problems using the most appropriate weighting function as well as coordinates. Recently it has been converted for PCs.

Before we digress to the next topic, we will discuss briefly the question of heterogeneity in receptor sites. If there are a few discrete receptor populations, say two to three, and if the range of data permit, one can effectively estimate the parameters using LIGAND or similar methods. One must remember, with two such discrete receptor sites, one has to estimate K_1, K_2, R_1, R_2 and at least one additional parameter representing nonspecific binding in most cases. With standard RIAs there may not be enough data covering a wide enough range to allow one to perform curve fitting for any more complex models. If there are more discernible receptor sites, one may be able to use a continuous approximation of the affinities and reconstruct its distribution as a spectrum by finite difference or similar methods.[25-26] If measurement error exceeds 5% or so, particularly in the presence of appreciable nonspecific binding, such reconstructions may not be effective in many cases.

III. EMPIRICAL DESCRIPTION OF RIA DATA

Nonlinear curve fitting with mechanistic models generally require human-machine interaction and thorough knowledge and regard for the method and the data. Statistical input and interpretation becomes absolutely essential. Several problems arising in such endeavors have been addressed previously.[14-17]

If the purpose of the assay is not specifically to understand the inherent thermodynamic behavior of the system, an elegant alternative is to use some well-behaved empirical function for this purpose. If the dose-response curve (B or B/T vs. T or log(T)), is conceptually monotonic, it may be represented by a sigmoidal function in the case of many RIAs. These approaches will allow one to characterize and compare subjects in terms of estimated median effective dose (ED_{50}) or the slope of the linear segment from such an empirical fitted function. Many of the RIA and other types of dose-response curves can usually be described by logistic curves. The form often used in RIA data processing in the presence of nonspecific binding or activity is called the four-parameter logistic curve:

$$Y = (a-d)/[1+(X/c)^b] + d \qquad (6)$$

where

a = Expected response at $X = 0$
b = Slope factor (= the slope of the logit-log plot)
c = ED_{50} (the dose at which the expected response = $(a + d)/2$)
d = Nonspecific binding (the response at infinite dose)

When the reaction is not at thermodynamic equilibrium, some of these parameters may have different physical implications. After all, Equation 6 is an empirical description of many varieties of sigmoidal response curves.

The logistic curve is continuous, smooth, and possesses a desirable property of being numerically stable for between-point interpolation. Its properties have been investigated in great detail in literature.[16,17,27,28] As implemented in SIGMOID,[29] from a nonlinear curve fitting standpoint, the logistic equation poses less convergence problems than any of the mechanistic models. This feature allows this model to be used on a routine basis for RIA estimation and precision testing. If an RIA dose-response curve indicates true nonmonotonicity, the logistic method may not produce meaningful results. In such cases there may still be lessons to be learned from logistic curve fitting. Even though true nonmonotonicity may arise due to multiple receptor sites with one or more possessing considerable positive cooperativity, often it may be due to inadequacies and errors in experimental techniques. Some recent work with splines in conjunction with a logistic transformation[30,31] may have made curve fitting even simpler for RIA data. This technique should allow one to investigate nonsigmoidal as well as nonmonotonic RIA curves more efficiently. When performing parallel line assays using the four-parameter logistic model, it is necessary to compare the three parameters, a, b, and d for the different curves under study for their homogeneity before combining them to obtain pooled estimates. This would lead to reestimation of the residual variance, c and finally the point estimate and confidence limits of the relative potencies. Although one can perform all these exercises with standard statistical packages such as SAS and BMDP, an RIA worker may be better off using a program like SIGMOID which has been specifically designed for this purpose.

As mentioned in the previous section, depending on the assays, the dependent variable, B/T, may show significant nonuniformity of variance from the low-dose toward the high-dose region. As a result, weighted regression should be the rule, not an exception for all RIAs.[14-17] The weight used for such regressions is inversely proportional to the variance of the observed counts. In reality, we do not know the true variance, we only know the sampling variance. A better estimate of the true variance can be obtained if we do the assays in replicates (five to 10, more the better) at each of the dose levels and calculate the variances at each of these levels. We can then use a smoothing function to fit these variances and get a good approximation for the variance at each dose level. These variances then can be used inversely as weights for the curve fitting. The following power function has been proposed as a smoothing function for variances in RIA:[14,15]

$$\sigma^2(Y) = a_o Y^J \tag{7}$$

where a_o and J are two empirical parameters of the smoothing function to be estimated by regression of variance of Y over Y.

Equation 7 can be linearized easily for estimating a_o and J by simple linear regression as follows:

$$\log[\sigma^2(Y)] = \log a_0 + J \log Y \tag{8}$$

In many assays, a_o and J are close to 1 and can be fixed as such. This is not surprising because of the Poisson nature of Y in many assays. However, one should not automatically accept this assumption for all assays. One should test this for each individual assay system. Once again, these features are built into programs such as SIGMOID although a statistically sophisticated person can perform all these analyses with SAS, BMDP, or MLAB.

Let us now briefly summarize the information one needs from curve fitting of RIA curves for evaluation of assays:

A. Dose interpolation for unknown samples with measures of uncertainty such as standard deviation (SD) or standard error (SE), % coefficient of variation (%CV), confidence limits, etc.

B. Potency estimate and its %CV based on the standards.

C. Mean, SD, or SE and %CV for the samples, if in replicates.

D. Potency estimates with confidence limits.

E. Test for parallelism and parallel line potency estimation when appropriate.

F. In the case of nonparallelism, ED_{50} ratio.

G. Estimates of a_o, J, and the residual variance for assay validity and precision testing, to be discussed later.

H. Some type of residual plot to examine the appropriateness (goodness of fit) of the model used. A formal statistical test for this purpose is not essential; a visual examination for trend, etc. in the residuals will generally suffice. Such plots will also help detect any irregularities in the assay and improve the design for future assays.

I. A plot of the observed and fitted values and their confidence intervals, preferably as a function of log(X). Both plots in (H) and (I) are useful diagnostic tools for model validation as well as for outliers.

J. The possibility of mapping the fitted curve back in the Scatchard coordinates. Also should try to estimate the actual thermodynamic parameters of the system.

K. Calculation of the minimal detectable dose (MDD).[32,33] This can be defined as the dose producing a response which is $t(1-\alpha;df)$ times the standard error of the zero dose response more than the zero dose response itself, where $t(1-\alpha;df)$ is one-tailed Student's t with df degrees of freedom.

IV. ASSAY PRECISION AND QUALITY CONTROL

Quality control (QC) is one of the most important aspects of RIA. Based on analysis of variance (ANOVA) techniques, QC allows one to investigate the precision and reliability of assays. If the assays have good accuracy and precision, one can compare them globally. For example, one can examine the variations between assays, between technicians, between reagents, between laboratories, etc. Details of QC of RIA are in previously published works.[34-40] Here we will briefly summarize the techniques and in Appendix 2 the arithmetic of QC of RIA will be described in full detail for easy implementation. The actual QC computations are very simple and can be performed even on a calculator; although we will suggest the use of some sort of a computing device with some storage and recall capabilities. Once a QC mechanism is set up, it should be mandatory to use it on a routine basis. For new drug development, bioequivalence testing and even in carcinogenicity/toxicity testing, RIAs are playing important roles and different regulatory agencies are requiring at least some minimal QC checks.

QC of RIA is performed on certain characteristics of the dose-response curves. For example, in the case of a mechanistic model of hormone binding, the actual binding parameters such as the receptor concentrations, the affinities or equilibrium binding constants, and the ED_{50}s can be used for QC checks. Similarly, for an empirical model such as the four-parameter logistic function, QC can be performed on the four parameters, a, b, c, d, and some statistical aspects of the assays such as the residual variance, etc. For on-line routine RIAs, this last method, once again, may be more convenient and requires the least human-machine interactions. Henceforth, we will then concentrate on QC of RIA using the four-parameter logistic model, although the same methods will apply to any other model one wishes to implement.

Let us briefly discuss the procedure of QC of RIA now. Ideally one should have a large number of standard curves (20 or more) for each assay. Let us suppose one is using the four-parameter logistic model to fit the data on these standard curves. One then pools the four parameters, a, b, c, and d; a_o and J from the weighting function and the residual variance (s_o^2) and calculates the mean, SD, and %CV of these parameters. These 20 or so standard curves are saved as a QC file. One then compares the results of the current assay with the pooled results from the previous QC file by Student's t-test. One should also examine the %CVs to assure that they are within reasonable limits. These limits will depend on the experience gathered from previous assays and the type and purpose of the assay. The %CVs may be given scores for evaluation on a variable scale depending on the assay type. As a second step, one should now combine the current estimates of the parameters with the pooled values from the QC file and calculate updated estimates of the previously mentioned statistics. One should then calculate the minimum %CV for replicates and its corresponding X and Y values as shown in Appendix 2. A working or acceptable range for the assay is estimated by calculating 1.5 times the minimum %CV and the corresponding X values (Appendix 2). The constant 1.5 in the above expression is arbitrary and can be changed a priori to something else for a particular assay. The X values or concentrations ($= X/volume$), %(B/B), SD, and %CV of X for the entire dose range are calculated. Between-assay and within-assay %CVs of the QC samples are calculated by random effect (variance components or Model II) ANOVA (Appendix 2). Finally one generates a precision profile by plotting the predicted %CV of X as a function of X (preferably vs. log X) and superimposes the between- and within-assay %CVs as points on such a curve. This precision profile is extremely educating as to the working range of a given assay.

The precision profile provides meaningful working range for a particular assay. The low and high-dose regions of the profile corresponds to excessively high %CV of the unknown, and as a result, should be avoided for all assays. The approximately flat region of the profile should be taken as the working or acceptable range of an assay. All samples above the higher acceptance region should be diluted and reanalyzed. On the other hand, if the sample falls below the working range, one may try several alternatives, such as concentrating the sample by extraction, reassaying with a higher volume, using a higher number of replicates or improving the sensitivity of the assay.

One can reduce the within-assay variability (%CV) by increasing the number of replicates. This may not have any appreciable effect on the between-assay variability. The latter can be minimized by optimizing the assay steps, such as extraction, chromatography, counting and whatever other steps may be involved. Change in any one of these techniques or a change in technician will increase between-assay variability. In either one of the above cases, a single factor Model II ANOVA will not be valid any more. One will have to introduce additional factors in the analysis making it rather complex statistically.

Precision (reproducibility) of an assay does not necessarily produce validity and accuracy of the assay. However, a lack of precision may provide some insights into the reasons why there may be lack of the latter. In other words, a better design may emerge by investigating the source of any lack of precision.

The observed and the expected %CVs should not differ much ideally given their respective sampling errors. In reality, the between-assay %CV should be slightly larger than the within-assay %CV. If there is a significant difference between them, there should be reasons to investigate the assay techniques carefully.

In order to avoid systematic bias in the assay, it is desirable that the QC samples and the assay curves all have the same number of replicates. Although there may be occasional accidental breaking of tubes, etc., such a balanced design should always be strived for. This is particularly true for more complex situations where one may have multicenter and multitechnician RIAs.

Some of the reasons for discrepancy between the observed and the predicted %CVs can be investigated easily. For example, if the observed within-assay %CV is less than the predicted %CV, any one or combination of the following may have taken place:

A. Extra care taken for the QC samples — Should not treat the QC samples any differently from the standards.
B. Improved stability and precision of QC samples — This may be due to the presence of serum or plasma in the QC samples as opposed to purified standards in the buffer. If that is the case, the fact should be taken into consideration while comparing the two sources of variability.
C. Use of an inappropriate model — If there is reasonable lack of fit (can be detected from residual plots or formal ANOVA-type tests), the estimate of root mean square (RMS) would be biased, thereby affecting the computation of the predicted %CV from the standard curves. An example is the linear logit-log model when the logit-log plot seems to be inherently nonlinear. Try to find a better model to compute the predicted %CV under such situations.

On the other hand, if the observed within-assay %CV is significantly larger than the predicted %CV, one should investigate the following:

A. Extra care given to the standards — Once again, should be avoided as before.
B. Presence of serum or plasma in QC samples — There may be increased variability due to the presence of serum or plasma. Must keep that in mind while comparing the within-assay %CV with predicted %CV.

V. AN EXAMPLE

We will use a typical cortisol assay system as an example here. The QC file for this example consisted of 20 assays, all in duplicates. All 20 assays were analyzed by SIGMOID to obtain values for the four-parameters of the logistic function and a_o, J and s_o^2. The between- and the within-assay %CVs were obtained using random effect ANOVA from triplicates at three dose levels. Only the first and the 20th assays are shown in Table 2 along with the results of the QC analysis described here. The precision profile with the between- and the within-assay %CVs superimposed on it is shown in Figure 5. For this example, the minimum %CV/duplicates was 4.9%, which can be rated as outstanding. This minimum took place at Y = counts = 3081 and X/Volume = 14.02. The 1.5 × minimum %CV was 7.39. As a result, the ideal working range for this cortisol system may be taken as between 3.8 and 57.4. Even though the RMS is significantly different in the current assay compared to the previous 20 assays, the pooled %CV for this quantity (27.23%) is still considered to be good for the cortisol assay system. On the other hand, even though the nonspecific binding for the current assay is not statistically different from the previous assays ($p = 0.952$), the rather high %CV of both the previous assays (55.28%) and the pooled assays (53.9%) dictate a warning for improvement of the assay system. For this particular system, the estimated nonspecific binding (d) ranged between 198 and 886 which would be indicative of considerable heterogeneity in this parameter. Given such a wide range for this parameter, the current assay should be accepted and the QC file should be updated by including it.

We have earlier mentioned some recent developments in serum assay techniques where the assay sensitivity may be increased by as much as a hundred-fold.[1-3] The scoring system for the %CVs for such assay system may need to be more stringent than the ones used for classical RIAs.

TABLE 2
Partial Results of QC Analysis of the Cortisol Example

Assay No.	a	b	c	d	a	J	s_0^2	$s_0(=RMS)$
1	8488	1.070	458	290	1	1	1.996	1.413
—	—	—	—	—	—	—	—	—
—	—	—	—	—	—	—	—	—
20	6856	1.110	360	399	1	1	4.349	2.096
Mean	7700.1	1.088	421.1	444.2	1	1	5.381	2.245
S.D.	828.5	0.056	44.4	245.5			3.022	0.599
%CV	10.76	5.15	10.54	55.3			56.18	26.690
Current assay	7565	1.060	382	429.0	1	1	2.472	1.572
t	0.163	0.501	0.881	0.062				3.747
Probability	0.872	0.622	0.389	0.952				0.001
Conclusion	NS	NS	NS	NS				**
Pooled result	7693.3	1.09	419.15	443.4	1	1	5.236	2.288

** = significant at 1% level.

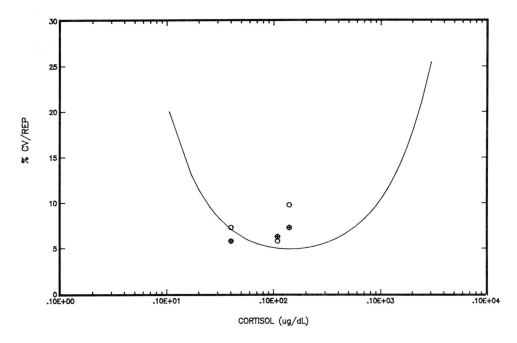

FIGURE 5. Precision profile of the cortisol example. Open circles are within and crossed circles are between-assay %CVs.

VI. APPENDIX 1
DERIVATION OF BINDING PARAMETERS FROM SCATCHARD PLOTS

A. Single Class of Noncooperative Sites:

$$I_0 = R_0K, \; S_0 = -K, \; I_\infty = R_0, s_\infty = -K$$

The best graphical estimates for the two parameters are obtained from:

$$K = (I_0/I_\infty) \text{ and } R_0 = I_\infty$$

B. Single Class of Cooperative sites:

$$I_0 = R_0K, \; S_0 = (C-2)K, \; I_\infty = R_0, \; S_\infty(K_{AMP2-}) = -CK$$

The best graphical estimates of the three parameters are obtained from: $K = (I_0/I_\infty)$, $C = 2 + (S_0/I_0)I_\infty$ and $R_0 = I_\infty$. (From the expresssion for S_0 it is obvious that when $C>2$, the plot will be nonmonotonic with an initial "bump". In practice, C has to be quite a bit larger than 2 before this "bump" is visible because of error in data. How much larger, will depend on the magnitude of error. Because of nonspecific binding in many assays, it may also be possible to have a "bump" at the low region of B on a Scatchard plot without positive cooperativity).

C. Multiple Classes of Noncooperative Sites:

$$I_0 = R_0<K>, \; S_0 = -<K^2>/<K>, \; I_\infty = R_0, \; S_\infty = -1/<K^{-1}>$$

where $< \; >$ = Moment of the distribution around the origin; for example, $<K>$ = mean, $<K^2>$ = second moment, etc.

The graphical estimates of the parameters of interest are

$$<K> = I_0/I_\infty, \text{ Variance of K} = -(I_0/I_\infty)[S_0 + (I_0/I_\infty)] \text{ and } R_0 = I_\infty$$

For the special case of two independent noncooperative sites:

$$I_0 = R_1K_1 + R_2K_2, \quad S_0 = -(R_1k_1{}^2 + R_2K_2{}^2)/(R_1K_1 + R_2K_2), \quad I_\infty = (R_1 + R_2), \text{ and}$$
$$S_\infty = -[K_1K_2(R_1 + R_2)]/(R_1K_2 + R_2K_1).$$

The graphical estimates of the four parameters, K_1, K_2, R_1, and R_2, are

$$K_1 = [A + (A^2 - 4BE)^{1/2}]/(2E), \quad K_2 = A/E\text{-}K_1, \quad R_1 = (I_0\text{-}I_\infty K_2)/(K_1\text{-}K_2), \text{ and } R_2 = (I_\infty K_1\text{-} I_0)/(K_1\text{-}K_2), \text{ where } A = S_\infty\text{-}S_0, B = S_\infty(S_0 + I_0/I_\infty) \text{ and } E = 1 + S_\infty(I_\infty/I_0).$$

Graphical estimates of binding parameters can be obtained in other coordinates in many cases using similar limiting slopes and intercepts. Specifically in the coordinates B/T vs. T or B/F vs. F, I_∞ and S_∞ do not exist and one has to resort to some additional characteristics of the graphs such as ED_{50} or EF_{50}, i.e., total or free hormone concentration producing 50% response in the B/T or B/F variable. Also, similar analysis can be performed using other models such as the Adair model.[12] For more details, see Thakur et al.[a]

One must remember that unless nonspecific binding can be approximated efficiently, the estimates of these parameters by such methods or by other curve peeling techniques may not be meaningful.

VII. APPENDIX 2
COMPUTATIONAL STEPS IN QC OF RIA

A. Input: Assay type, assay name, assay volume, total number of standard curves (20 or more), and the number or numbers of replicates.
B. Input: a, b, c, d, a_0, J and $s_0{}^2$ for each of the above curves.
C. Input: Potency estimates from each of the above curves.
D. Compute: Mean, SD, and %CV for each of the seven parameters and of s_0:

$$\text{Mean} = \Sigma x/n$$
$$\text{SD} = [\Sigma(x \text{-}\bar{x})^2]^{1/2}$$
$$\%\text{CV} = (\text{SD/Mean}) \times 100$$

where x is the specific parameter in each case.
E. Compare: Logistic parameters from the current assay (P_{curr}) using two-tailed Student's t-test (since the direction of the difference is not known a priori) against the pooled parameters from the previous assays (P_{pool}). It is preferable to compare s_0 (Root Mean Squares or RMS) instead of $s_0{}^2$ (Residual Variance) since the latter may not be normally distributed in many cases with possible nonuniformity of variance:

$$t = \text{abs}(\bar{P}_{pool} - \bar{P}_{curr})/\text{SD}(\bar{P}_{pool})$$
$$\text{df} = \text{Number of assays pooled} - 1$$
$$t \sim \text{Student's } t(1\text{-}\alpha;\text{df}).$$

Evaluate the statistical significance of the observed difference to see whether it happened due to chance alone:

If Pr(t) ≤0.01 : Conclusion = **
If Pr(t) >0.01 but ≤0.05 : Conclusion = ★

Depending on the type and the purpose of the assay, a small probability like 0.01 may be taken as not being serious. On the other hand, for some assays one may want to use a rather large probability such as 0.10 as being objectionable. If the computations are performed on any type of computers, it is desirable to compute the exact probability instead of using critical values.

F.   Include: The same parameters from the current assay along with the parameters from the QC file and recompute the mean, the SD, and the %CV in each case. Evaluate the magnitude of the %CV for this step using some preassigned scoring system. The scoring system should be pre-determined and may depend on previous knowledge and/ or experience with the assay and the nature of applications. The following scoring system was used in a cortisol assay previously and may be used for guidelines:

%CV	Magnitude	Score
a,b,c	≤ 5	Excellent
	≤ 10	Good
	≤ 15	OK
	≤ 25	Warning
	≤ 50	Poor
	> 50	Censored
d	≤ 15	Excellent
	≤ 25	Good
	≤ 50	OK
	≤ 75	Warning
	≤ 100	Poor
	> 100	Censored
s_0	≤ 25	Excellent
	≤ 50	Good
	≤ 75	OK
	≤ 100	Check
	> 100	Excessive

G.   Print: Results and interpretations from the previous steps.

H.   Compute: Expected values of counts (Y) for given values of B/B and their corresponding expected X values with the combined estimates of all the parameters (current assay included). Also, calculate the basic statistics for X:

$$X = \bar{c}[(\bar{a}-Y)/(Y-\bar{d})]^{1/\bar{b}}$$
$$abs(slope) = |dY/dX| = abs[\bar{b}(\bar{a}-Y)(Y-\bar{d})/\{X(\bar{a}-\bar{d})\}]$$
$$Var(X) = (s_0^2 a_0 Y^2)/(slope)^2$$
$$Var(X)/Replicate = Var(X)/r$$
$$SD(X)/Replicate = [Var(X)/r]^{1/2}$$
$$\%CV(X)/Replicate = \{[Var(X)/r]^{1/2}/X\} \times 100.$$

for a<Y<d and where r is the number of replicates. If the number of replicates is not the same in each case and if they do not differ much from each other, one can take the geometric mean (GM) of the different replicates to get r:

$$GM(r) = (\prod_{j=1}^{n} r_j)^{1/n}$$

I.   Compute: Y_{min} from the $\%CV(X)$ equation:

$$Y_{min} = \{(2\text{-}\bar{J})(\bar{a} + \bar{d}) + [(2\text{-}\bar{J})^2(\bar{a}+\bar{d})^2 + 4\overline{adJ}(4\text{-}\bar{J})[2(4\text{-}\bar{J})r^{1/2}]$$

for $J \neq 4$

Now substitute Y_{min} in the expression for X in (8) to obtain the corresponding X_{min} value. Similarly, substitute Y_{min} in the expression for $\%CV(X)$ to get the minimum $\%CV$.

J.   Compute: Working or acceptable range as the range of concentration such that $\%CV/$ Replicates $= 1.5 \times \%CV(X)$. The factor 1.5 is somewhat arbitrary and may be modified for particular assays depending on the magnitude of $\%CV$. The $\%CV(X)$ may be scored in a fashion similar to the one in (F). For our cortisol case, the following scoring was used:

Magnitude of $\%CV(X)$	Score
<5	Outstanding
<7.5	Excellent
<10	Good
<15	Marginal
<25	Poor
<50	Bad
>50	Reject

K.   Compute: Within- and between-assay $\%CV$ using Model II ANOVA[41] with the QC samples:

$$Var(within) = [\sum_j\sum_i X_{ij}^2 - \sum_j (T_j^2/r_j)]/(\sum_j r_j -n)$$

$$r^1 = (\sum_j r_j - \sum_j r_j^2/\sum_j r_j)/(n\text{-}1)$$

$$Var(between) = [\sum_j (T_j^2/r_j) - \Sigma\, T_j^2/\sum_j r_j]/(n\text{-}1) -Var(within)/r^1$$

where

n	=	number of assays
i	=	replicate number index
j	=	assay number index
X_{ij}	=	replicate i of assay j
T_j	=	sum of all the Xs in assay j
r_j	=	number of replicates in assay j

Finally, compute within- and between-assay $\%CV(X)$:

$$\%CV(within) = \{[Var(within)]^{1/2}/X\} \times 100$$
$$\%CV(between) = \{[Var(between)]^{1/2}/X\} \times 100$$

L.   Plot: Predicted $\%CV(X)$ vs. log(concentration) as a continuous curve and superimpose within- and between-assay $\%CVs$ as points.

M.   Update: QC file by deleting the first curve and including the current one if all the evaluations are satisfactory.

All of the above steps should be easy to program even for a nonstatistician. If it seems difficult, contact the present author for the availability of such a program.

The computational steps for QC described here are identical for any type of assay system. They are, by no means, specific for RIA or related procedures. However, if one wishes to use, for example, mechanistic models such as Equations 2, 4, 5, or more complex ones, computational steps for obtaining %CV, etc., or dose interpolation may become difficult. For many of those cases one may have to resort to numerical or analytical approximations for some of the required quantities. Since the purpose of QC is validation and precision of an assay, any empirical description of the response function, such as the four-parameter logistic, is optimal as well as desirable.

VIII. APPENDIX 3
COMPUTER PROGRAMS FOR RIA DATA EVALUATION

A. SIGMOID: Analyzes RIA dose-response curves using the four-parameter logistic model. Contact: Dr. David Rodbard, Laboratory of Theoretical and Physical Endocrinology, National Institute of Child Health and Human Development, NIH, Bethesda, Maryland.
B. LIGAND: Analyzes mechanistic models; can accomodate multiple ligands simultaneously. Contact: Dr. Peter J. Munson, the same address as Dr. Rodbard's.
C. LIMIT: A program to estimate binding parameters graphically. Contact: Dr. Ajit K. Thakur.
D. RELAX: A program to construct affinity spectra with the assumption of continuous distribution for heterogeneous receptors. Contact: Dr. Ajit K. Thakur.
E. FLEXIFIT: A curve fitting program for families of curves of similar shape. The program has the capability of fitting and comparing the four-parameter logistic model as well. Contact: Dr. Peter J. Munson.
F. RIAQC: Performs the QC analysis described in this chapter. Contact: Dr. Ajit K. Thakur.

ACKNOWLEDGMENT

The author thanks Drs. David Rodbard and Vojislav Resanovic for critical reviews and Terry Horner for her careful preparation of the manuscript. Thanks are also due all the authors of previous works in the field.

REFERENCES

1. **Leuvering, J. H. W., Thal, P. J. H. M., and Schuurs, A. H. W. M.,** Optimization of a sandwich sol particle immunoassay (SPIA) for human chorionic gonadotrophin (hCG), *J. Immunol. Meth.,* 62, 75, 1983.
2. **Hemmila, J.,** Fluoroimmunoassays and immunofluorometric assays, *Clin. Chem.,* 31, 359, 1985.
3. **Barnard, G. J. R., Williams, J. L., Paton, A. C., and Shah, H. P.,** Time-resolved fluoroimmunoassay, in *Complementary Immunoassay,* Collins, W. P., Ed., John Wiley & Sons, New York, 1987, 149.
4. **Thakur, A. K. and DeLisi, C.,** Theory of ligand binding to heterogeneous receptor populations: Characterization of the free-energy distribution function, *Biopolymers,* 17, 1075, 1978.
5. **DeLisi, C.,** Characterization of receptor affinity heterogeneity by Scatchard plots, *Biopolymers,* 17, 1385, 1978.
6. **Thakur, A. K. and Rodbard, D.,** Graphical aids to interpretation of Scatchard plots and dose-response curves, *J. Theoret. Biol.,* 80, 383, 1979.
7. **Scatchard, G.,** The attractions of proteins for small molecules and ions, *Ann. N.Y. Acad. Sci.,* 51, 660, 1949.
8. **Thakur, A. K., Jaffe, M. L., and Rodbard, D.,** Graphical analysis of ligand-binding systems: evaluation by Monte Carlo studies, *Analyt. Biochem.,* 107, 279, 1980.

9. **Klotz, I. M. and Hunston, D. L.,** Properties of graphical representations of multiple classes of binding sites, *Biochemistry,* 10, 3065, 1971.
10. **Klotz, I. M. and Hunston, D. L.,** Protein affinities for small molecules: conceptions and misconceptions, *Arch. Biochem. Biophys.,* 193, 314, 1974.
11. **Lineweaver, H. and Burk, D.,** The determination of enzyme dissociation constants, *J.Am. Chem. Soc.,* 56, 658, 1934.
12. **Adair, G. S.,** The haemoglobin system: VI. The oxygen dissociation curve of haemoglobin, *J. Biol. Chem.,* 63, 529, 1925.
13. **Hill, A. V.,** The possible effects of the aggregation of the molecules of haemoglobin on its dissociation curves, *J. Physiol. (London),* 40, IV, 1910.
14. **Rodbard, D., Munson, P. J., and Thakur, A.K.,** Quantitative characterization of hormone receptors, *Cancer,* 46, 2907, 1980.
15. **Finney, D. J.,** Response curves for radioimmunoassay, *Clin. Chem.,* 29, 1762, 1983.
16. **Rodbard, D.,** Lessons from the computerization of radioimmunoassay: an introduction to the basic principles of modeling, in *Computers in Endocrinology,* Vol. 14, Rodbard, D. and Forti, G., Eds., Raven Press, New York, 1984, 75.
17. **Rodbard, D., Munson, P. J., and De Lean, A.,** Improved Curve-fitting, Parallelism Testing, Characterization of Sensitivity and Specificity, Validation and Optimization for Radioligand Assays, Paper IAEA-SM-220/58, Proc. Symp. Radioimmunoassay and Related Procedures in Medicine, Vienna, 1977.
18. BMDP Statistical Software, University of California Press, Berkeley, CA, 1985.
19. SAS, SAS Institute Inc., Cary, NC, 1985.
20. **Knott, G. D.,** MLAB-An On-line Modeling Laboratory-Applications Manual, National Institutes of Health, Bethesda, MD, 3rd ed., 1981.
21. **Knott, G. D.,** MLAB-An On-line Modeling Laboratory-Reference Manual, National Institutes of Health, Bethesda, MD, 9th ed., 1980.
22. **Berman, M. and Weiss, M. F.,** SAAM-27: User's Manual, NIH-78-180, National Institutes of Health, Bethesda, MD, 1978.
23. **Metzler, C. M. and Weiner, D. L.,** PCNONLIN User's Guide, Version V02, Statistical Consultants, Inc., Edgewood, KY, 1986.
24. **Munson, P. J. and Rodbard, D.,** LIGAND: A versatile computerized approach for characterizatoin of ligand binding systems, *Anal. Biochem.,* 107, 220, 1980.
25. **Thakur, A. K., Munson, P. J., Hunston, D. L., and Rodbard, D.,** Characterization of ligand-binding systems by continuous affinity distributions of arbitrary shape, *Anal. Biochem.,* 103, 204, 1980.
26. **Tobler, H. J. and Engel, G.,** Affinity spectra: A novel way for the evaluation of equilibrium binding experiments, *Naunyn-Schmiedebergs Arch. Pharmacol.,* 322, 183, 1983.
27. **Rodbard, D. and Hutt, D. M.,** Statistical Analysis of Radioimmunoassays and Immunoradiometric (Labelled Antibody) Assays: A Generalized, Weighted, Iterative, Least-squares Method for Logistic Curve Fitting, Proc. Symp. Radioimmunoassay and Related Procedures in Medicine, IAEA, Vol. 1, Vienna, 1974, 165.
28. **Rodbard, D., Lenox, R. H., Wray, H. L., and Ramseth, D.,** Statistical characterization of the random errors in the radioimmunoassay dose-response variable, *Clin. Chem.,* 22, 350, 1976.
29. **Rodbard, D., Faden, V. B., Hutt, D. M., and Huston, J. C., Jr.,** SIGMOID: Four-parameter Logistic Curve-fitting Program, NICHD, NIH, Bethesda (Previously referred to as BCTIC Computer Code Collection, MED-29, Vanderbilt Medical Center, Nashville, TN, 1980).
30. **Guardabasso, V., Munson, P. J., and Rodbard, D.,** A versatile method for simultaneous analysis of families of curves, *FASEB J.,* 2, 209, 1988.
31. **Guardabasso, V., Rodbard, D., and Munson, P. J.,** A model-free approach to estimation of relative potency in dose-response curve analysis, *Am. J. Physiol.,* 252 (*Endocrin. Metab.* 15), E357, 1987.
32. **Rodbard, D.,** Statistical estimation of the minimal detectable concentration ("sensitivity") for radioligand assays, *Analyt. Biochem.,* 90, 1, 1978.
33. **Oppenheimer, L., Capizzi, T. P., Weppelman, R. M., and Mehta, H.,** Determining the lowest limit of reliable assay measurement, *Clin. Chim. Acta,* 55, 638, 1983.
34. **Rodbard, D.,** Statistical quality control and routine data processing for radioimmunoassays and immunoradiometric assays, *Clin. Chem.,* 20, 1255, 1974.
35. **McDonagh, B. F., Munson, P. J., and Rodbard, D.,** A computerized approach to statistical quality control for radioimmunoassays in the clinical chemistry laboratory, *Comput. Progr. Biomed.,* 7, 179, 1977.
36. **Ayers, G., Burnett, D., Griffiths, A., and Richens, A.,** Quality control of drug assays, *Clin. Pharmacokin.,* 6, 106, 1981.
37. **Raab, G. M.,** Estimation of variance function, with application to radioimmunoassay, *J. R. Stat. Soc.,* Series C (*Appl. Stat.*), 30, 32, 1981.

38. **Ekins, R. P. and Edwards, P. R.,** The precision profile: its use in assay design, assessment and quality control, in *Immunoassays for Clinical Chemistry,* Hunter, W. M. and Corrie, J. E. T., Eds., Churchill Livingstone, Edinburgh, 1983, 106.

39. **Thakur, A. K., Listwak, S. J., and Rodbard, D.,** Quality Control for Radioimmunoassay, Paper IAE-CN-45/108, in Proc. Conf. Radiopharmaceuticals and Labelled Compounds, Vienna, 1985.

40. **Dudley, R. A., Edwards, P., Ekins, R. P., Finney, D. J., McKenzie, I. G. M., Raab, G. M., Rodbard, D., and Rodgers, R. P. C.,** Guidelines for immunoassay data processing, *Clin. Chem.,* 31, 1264, 1985.

41. **Neter, J. and Wasserman, W.,** *Applied Linear Statistical Models,* Irwin, Homewood, IL, 1974.

Chapter 16

ORGANIZATION OF THE *IN VITRO* FERTILIZATION/EMBRYO TRANSFER LABORATORY

Jeffrey V. May and Kelly Hanshew

TABLE OF CONTENTS

I. INTRODUCTION

The assisted reproductive technologies of *In Vitro* Fertilization/Embryo Transfer (IVF/ET) and Gamete Intrafallopian Transfer (GIFT) have forever altered the treatment of infertility by the direct isolation, characterization, and manipulation of gametes and embryos. The number of procedures performed and the number of centers involved in these technologies has increased dramatically. At the heart of these "high tech" procedures is the IVF/ET laboratory in which all gamete and embryo work occurs. As part of this handboodk dedicated to the laboratory diagnosis of infertility, we have attempted to develop a comprehensive description of the IVF/ET laboratory. Accordingly, many of the procedures described herein are detailed and are derived from the IVF/ET laboratory handbook developed within our program. This chapter is presented in a "hands-on" manner for direct use in an IVF/ET lab.

Many of the procedures and techniques utilized in the IVF/ET lab, such as the mouse embryo system and embryo cryopreservation, are presented in greater detail in other chapters of this handbook. Wherever possible, reference to these are noted in this chapter.

The methods and procedures described in this chapter are by no means the only ones, the most popular, nor perhaps the most recent. However, we have found them to be reproduceable and successful.

II. PHYSICAL LAYOUT OF THE IVF LABORATORY

When considering an organizational layout for an IVF lab it must always be remembered that the primary function of the facility is to provide an optimal environment for: (1) the retrieval and preparation of gametes; (2) the insemination and fertilization of oocytes; (3) embryo development *in vitro*; and (4) embryo transfer and/or cryopreservation. With this in mind, the laboratory can be organized to allow efficient and reproduceable performance of the procedures necessary for a successful program. At the University of Kansas School of Medicine-Wichita (Department of Obstetrics and Gynecology, HCA/Wesley Medical Center), the IVF Laboratory is subdivided into four components: the Embryo Lab; the Support Lab; an Office/Consultation Room; and a Semen Collection Room. For reference purposes, a schemetac diagram of the IVF Lab is illustrated in Figure 1. Subdivision of the IVF Laboratory allows for designated "work areas" where specific laboratory procedures are performed. Additionally, it is most important that the IVF Lab be a dedicated facility for use in IVF-related work only.

A. THE EMBRYO LABORATORY
1. Function
It is within the Embryo Lab that all of the oocyte and embryo-related procedures are

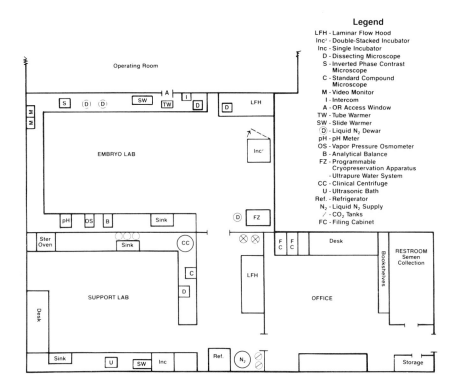

Legend

LFH - Laminar Flow Hood
Inc² - Double-Stacked Incubator
Inc - Single Incubator
D - Dissecting Microscope
S - Inverted Phase Contrast Microscope
C - Standard Compound Microscope
M - Video Monitor
I - Intercom
A - OR Access Window
TW - Tube Warmer
SW - Slide Warmer
Ⓓ - Liquid N_2 Dewar
pH - pH Meter
OS - Vapor Pressure Osmometer
B - Analytical Balance
FZ - Programmable Cryopreservation Apparatus
- Ultrapure Water System
CC - Clinical Centrifuge
U - Ultrasonic Bath
Ref. - Refrigerator
N_2 - Liquid N_2 Supply
╱ - CO₂ Tanks
FC - Filing Cabinet

FIGURE 1. Schematic diagram of the In Vitro Fertilization Laboratory illustrating the spatial relationships among the Embryo Lab, the Support Lab, the Office/Consultation Room, and the Semen Collection Room. The orientation of the equipment in the Embryo Lab and Support Lab is also illustrated.

performed including oocyte retrieval and grading, oocyte insemination, pronuclear-stage observation, embryo culture, embryo cryopreservation, and the initial stages of embryo transfer. Accordingly, *the Embryo Lab is considered an extension of the operating room (OR) and requires surgical attire and sterile procedure at all times.* This serves two purposes. As well as providing a mechanism for reducing potential contamination, it serves as a mental reminder to utilize sterile technique and maintain sterile conditions at all times. Access to the Embryo Lab is limited to the IVF team except for teaching purposes under the direction of the IVF team. To insure compliance of access, the single entry door into the Embryo Lab from the Support Lab (Figure 1) is equipped with a lock the combination of which is known only to the program director and the IVF team.

2. Communication

Communication between the reproductive endocrinologist in the OR and the laboratory personnel during oocyte retrieval and gamete (GIFT) or embryo (IVF) transfer is imperative. This is achieved via three independent mechanisms. First, there is physical contact between the OR and the Embryo Lab via an access window (Figure 1A and Figure 2) through which follicular aspirates obtained at laparoscopy or via transvaginal retrieval are passed from the OR to the Embryo Lab and where gametes (GIFT), embryos (IVF), or aspirate medium are passed from the lab to the OR. Secondly, there is visual communication in the form of video monitors (Figure 1M and Figure 3). Monitors are connected to the laparoscope or ultrasound scanner utilized by the reproductive endocrinologist to locate and aspirate follicles and also to the dissecting microscope used by the gamete physiologist to isolate and grade oocytes. Monitors are located in both the OR and the Embryo Lab to allow members of the IVF team to visually follow progress of the procedure. Lastly, there is audio communication

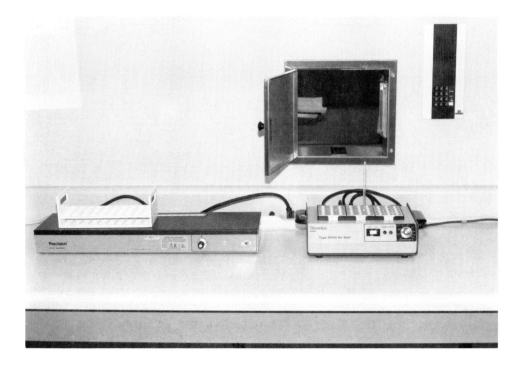

FIGURE 2.   Orientation of the OR/Embryo Lab access window, tube and slide warmers, and the intercom. Follicular aspirates are initially stored here where data concerning the aspirate is recorded.

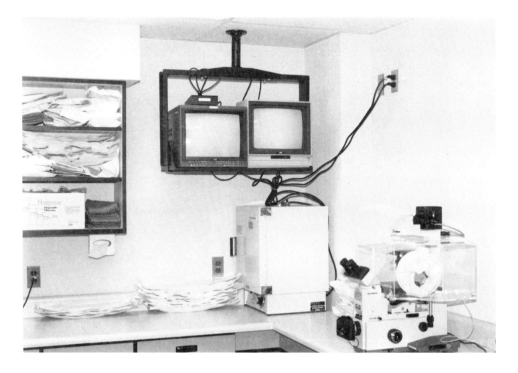

FIGURE 3.   Embryo Lab video monitors and the inverted phase contrast microscope used for photography. The left monitor is connected to the primary dissecting microscope used by the gamete physiologist to isolate oocytes and the right monitor is linked to either a laparoscope or to a scanning ultrasound.

between the OR and the Embryo Lab in the form of an intercom (Figure 1I and Figue 2). This allows the reproductive endocrinologist and the gamete physiologist to discuss directly any aspect of the procedure such as oocyte quality, granulosa cell appearance, etc.

3. Instrumentation for Oocyte Isolation and Embryo Manipulation

The most important aspects of the instrumentation and equipment used in an IVF lab is that it be adequate for the use intended and that it is acceptable to the personnel who will have to work with it. It is not the intent of this article to endorse any particular brand of instrument but rather describe the types of instrumentation necessary. It is, however, of benefit whenever possible, to utilize a single source of equipment. With microscopes for example, routine maintenance can be accomplished at one time and the optics and photographic equipment are interchangeable. Ultimately, the IVF Lab equipment configuration should be determined by the individuals who will have to utilize the equipment.

The Embryo Lab should be organized to facilitate rapid isolation of oocytes upon retrieval, to observe embryo development, and to prepare embryos (or gametes) for transfer or cryopreservation. This obviates a minimum of physical movement and a minimum exposure to changes in pH and temperature. Thus, a specific work area should be designed for this purpose such as that illustrated in Figure 1. Incoming follicle aspirates are received through the OR access window and placed into a 37C tube warmer (Thermolyne #16500 Dri-Bath, blocks with 20 mm holes, Figure 1, TW, and Figure 2). A slide warmer (Figure 1, SW, and Figure 2) is located adjacent to the tube warmer to keep large volume samples (i.e., cul-de-sac fluid) warm. Oocytes are located and isolated using a stereo dissecting microscope (Olympus SZH Zoom with SZH-ILCK transmitted illumination base, Figure 1D and Figure 4) equipped with a video camera (Javelin JE 3012/A Color). The microscope used should have an adequate working area at its base to accomodate several tissue culture dishes during oocyte isolation. During oocyte retrieval, the illuminated base becomes warm which helps keep the culture dishes and medium warm. The microscope should have easily adjustable magnification for locating, identifying, and finally, grading the oocytes.

The primary dissecting microscope should be located in a laminar flow console (Figure 1LFH and Figure 5). A second dissecting microscope is located adjacent to the primary microscope (Figure 1D and Figure 5) and is equipped with brightfield and darkfield illumination (Olympus SZH-ILLD illuminator). The laminar flow console is designed to provide a sterile environment for gamete and embryo work. We prefer a horizontal laminar flow cabinet rather than a conventional hood because of the easily accessable work area and the ability to place a microscope in the console (Figure 5). The horizontal air flow draws filtered air into the bottom of the unit and forces it from the back to the front of the console. Since the console is located in a ''clean room'' at our facility, we do not find it necessary to have the air flowing while working in the the console. If used in a general laboratory, however, work at the console should be performed with the air flow operational. When not in use the germicidal light should be turned on and the hood wiped clean with Milli-Q water and 70% ethanol.

Opposite and facing the console is a pair of stacked, water-jacketed, continuous flow, CO_2 incubators (Forma #3326, Figure 1, Inc.[2], and Figures 5 and 6.) The incubators are positioned to allow easy access from the primary dissecting microscope. The top incubator, the working incubator, is used to store pre-equilibrated medium, culture dishes, and semen for use during procedures, and the bottom incubator is used solely to culture oocytes and embryos. Both incubators are linked to a recording monitor (Forma #1565) which provides a hardcopy reading of incubator temperature and percent CO_2 every 2 h. The incubators are linked to supply CO_2 tanks located in the Support Lab. Arguments can be made for the use of a CO_2 guard device which engages a new CO_2 tank if the primary tank runs out. We have found that these units use an inordinate amount of CO_2 and have chosen not to use

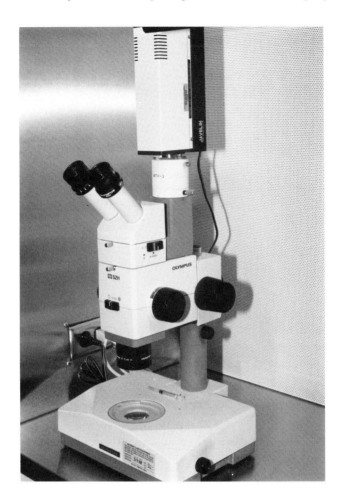

FIGURE 4.   The primary dissecting microscope used to isolate oocytes and monitor fertilization and embryo development. This microscope is located in the laminar flow console and is linked to video monitors in the Embryo Lab and the OR by a video camera.

one. A normal 5 ft CO_2 tank (approximately 1000 lbs/sq inch) should last 1 to 2 months in a closed incubator system. With proper quality control, running out of CO_2 should not be a problem.

For photography, an inverted phase contrast microscope equipped with a 35 mm camera is used (Olympus IMT-2 microscope and Olympus OM-2 camera, Figure 1S and Figures 3 and 7). The microscope is equipped with an environmental chamber to provide the necessary atmosphere for gamete/embryo maintenance when they are removed from the incubators for extended periods of time. *Generally speaking, we severely restrict photographing of gametes and embryos. We attempt to minimize, whenever possible, any unnecessary manipulation of the gametes and/or embryos.* In this laboratory, most photographs are taken of embryos during the cryoprotectant equilibration steps of cryopreservation when the embryos are contained in phosphate-buffered medium designed for use in room air.

As in most IVF/GIFT programs, embryos not transferred to the patient during the stimulation cycle are cryopreserved for future thaw and transfer. Embryos are maintained in liquid nitrogen dewars (Minnesota Valley Engineering, Apollo SX-35, 35 gallon capacity) located in the Embryo Lab (Figure 1D and Figure 8).

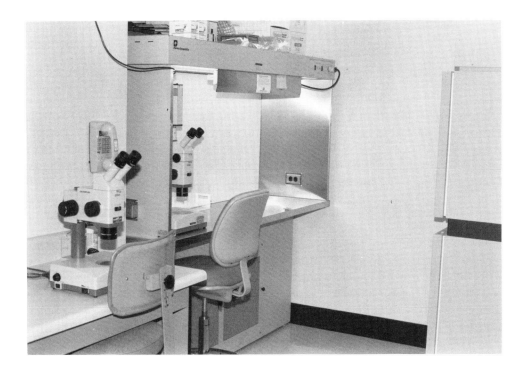

FIGURE 5. Orientation of the laminar flow console containing the primary dissecting microscope, the secondary dissecting microscope, and the double-stacked CO_2 incubators (to the right of the console).

4. Preparation of Embryo Culture Medium

Ham's F-10 nutrient medium (F-10) and Dulbecco's phosphate-buffered saline (DPBS) used for oocyte and embryo culture, oocyte retrieval, and sperm wash and rise, are prepared in the Embryo Lab. Unless they require refrigeration, medium and medium supplements are stored in the Embryo Lab. Reagents are measured using an analytical balance (Mettler AE 163, Figure 1B and Figure 9) and the pH and osmolarity of the medium are determined (Orion 701A pH meter and a Wescor #5500 vapor pressure osmometer, Figure 1, pH and OS, respectively, and Figure 9, see later sections for detailed protocols). As with the oocyte/embryo work area, a specified area containing all of the above equipment is located in a dedicated area for media preparation (Figures 1 and 9).

5. Embryo Lab Supplies

Supplies needed in the Embryo Lab are stored there in cabinets and shelves for easy access. This includes powdered nutrient medium and supplements, powdered DPBS, culture plasticware (culture dishes and tubes, pipettes, medium preparation and storage vessels), filters, laparoscopy needles, IVF and GIFT transfer catheters, pipette tips, syringes, etc. Additionally, surgical scrub, Milli-Q water, and 70 and 95% ethanol are available for cleaning hands.

B. THE SUPPORT LABORATORY

1. Function

Procedures and requisite equipment necessary to maintain a functioning Embryo Lab are performed and located in the Support Lab. These include the mouse embryo assay for quality control, semen preparation for IVF and GIFT procedures, cleaning and sterilizing of instruments and equipment, embryo cryopreservation, and media preparation. Additionally, the Support Lab houses the Milli-Q water system and bulk supplies such as liquid

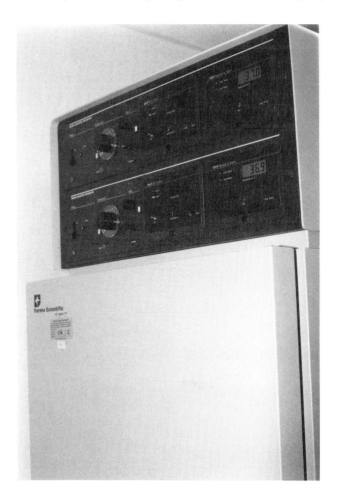

FIGURE 6.   Close-up photograph of one of the stacked CO_2 incubators (refer also to Figure 5).

nitrogen, CO_2, glassware etc., and houses refrigeration units. The Support Lab also contains office facilities for an IVF technician.

2. Ultra-Pure Water System

At the center of the IVF laboratory is the water system. *The need for high quality, pyrogen-free water cannot be overstated and has been recently reviewed.*[1] Initially, IVF laboratories utilized water distilled four to five times.[2,3] More recently, sophisticated cartridge filter systems consisting of prefiltration, reverse osmosis, carbon absorption, ion exchange, and 0.22 μm filtration steps have been utilized. The most recent systems include a final ultrafiltration step and automatic recirculation which continually polishes the water. Such a system is the Millipore-Q (Milli-Q) pyrogen-free system illustrated in Figures 10 and 11. This system is also known as the Milli-Q UF system. This system produces 18 megΩ water which exceeds the national standard for Type I reagent grade water (Table 1). Reverse osmosis water feeds into the system (Figure 11) and passes through: (a) a carbon adsorption cartridge (Super-C) to remove dissolved organics and residual chlorine; (b) two successive strong acid/base, mixed bed, deionizing cartridges to remove dissolved inorganics; (c) and an ultrafiltration cartridge to remove pyrogens, colloids, microorganisms and organics of 10,000 MW or greater. The final step is filtration through a pre-sterilized 0.22 μm filter

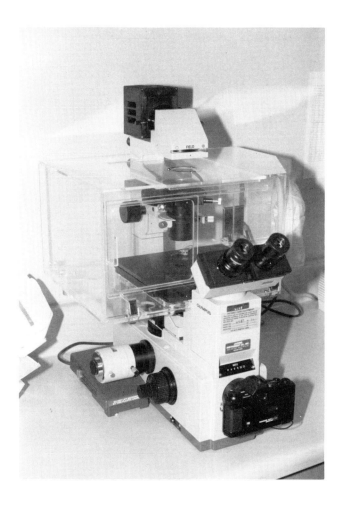

FIGURE 7. The inverted phase contrast microscope used for photography. The unit is equipped for temperature and environmental control and has a 35 mm camera attached for photography.

which removes microorganisms and microparticles. The system features an automatic re-circulation loop which activates every hour refiltering the water insuring its purity. The maintenance of this system is discussed in Section IV.B.

3. Semen Collection and Preparation

During IVF and GIFT procedures, the husband's semen sample is collected and prepared in the IVF Support Lab. The sample is collected in the Semen Collection Room adjacent to the Office and removed from the activity and noise of the Support Lab to allow a measure of privacy (Figure 1). The semen sample is prepared using a wash and rise method (see Section III. D) in a designated area within the Support Lab equipped with a laminar flow hood, CO_2 incubator, compound standard microscope, clinical centrifuge, and warming tray (Figure 1, LFH, Inc, C, CC, and SW, respectively, and Figures 12 to 14). Unlike the Embryo Lab, the Support Lab is not a "clean room", hence, work done in the Support Lab laminar flow hood is performed with the air flow on. Once prepared, the semen sample is moved into the Embryo Lab incubator until needed for transfer (GIFT) or oocyte insemination (IVF).

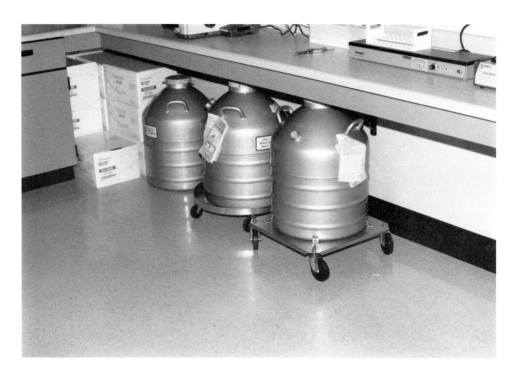

FIGURE 8. Liquid nitrogen dewars used to cryopreserve frozen embryos. Two units are actively used with a third held in reserve. The liquid nitrogen levels are checked weekly unless the dewars have been utilized significantly, then the levels are checked daily.

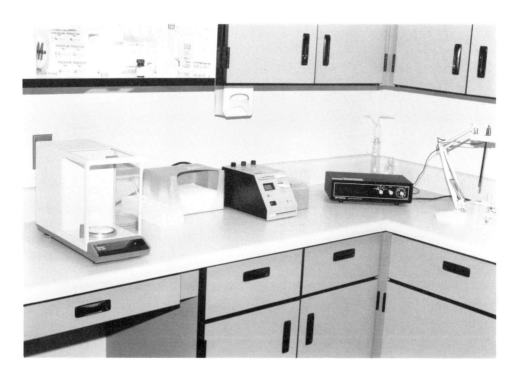

FIGURE 9. Orientation of the Embryo Lab equipment used in medium preparation. The pH meter, vapor pressure osmometer, and analytical balance are shown. Medium supplements not requiring refrigeration are stored on shelves above this equipment.

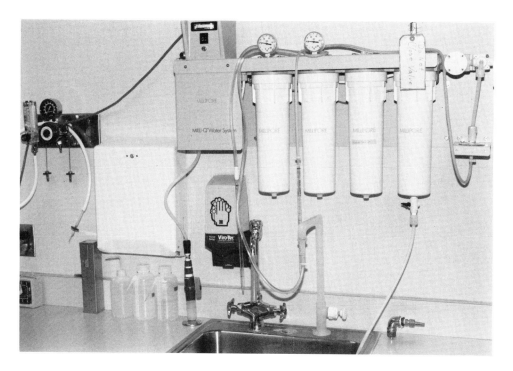

FIGURE 10. The Support Lab Milli-Q pyrogen-free, ultra-pure water system. Water generated by this unit is used in all phases of IVF/GIFT laboratory work. A description of the unit is presented in the text.

4. Mouse Embryo Quality Control System

It is standard procedure to test all reagents, media, plasticware, transfer catheters and other equipment for their ability to support embryo development prior to use with human gametes and embryos. The most common system is the two-cell mouse embryo system described in detail in Chapter 17. Mouse embryo retrieval is performed in the Support Lab and subsequent test cultures are established there. A designated work area containing a dissecting microscope is used for this purpose (Figure 1D and Figure 15). Once test cultures are established, they can be transfered into the Embryo Lab incubators. The use of the two-cell mouse embryo assay as a quality control measure is discussed further in Section III.C.

5. Cleaning and Sterilization of Equipment

The vast majority of supplies required for IVF and GIFT are disposable. However, certain pieces of equipment such as transfer catheters and laparoscopy needles may be re-used. These are cleaned and sterilized in the Support Lab. The requisite materials and equipment include Milli-Q pyrogen-free water, filtered air under pressure, sterilizing envelopes, a heat sealing unit (National Instruments #210, impulse sealer), an ultrasonic bath-type cleaner (Branson #5200), and a sterilizing oven (American Scientific Products DX-68 drying oven). This equipment is again located in one general area of the Support Lab (Figure 1).

6. Embryo Cryopreservation

The ability to cryopreserve extra embryos derived from IVF and GIFT procedures and obtain viable embryos after thawing offers great potential for enhancing the chances of obtaining a pregnancy from a given stimulation cycle. A detailed review of oocyte and embryo cryopreservation is presented in Chapter 18. Cryopreservation takes place in both the Embryo and Support Labs. The initial stages of cryopreservation including the cryopro-

MILLI-Q PYROGEN-FREE SYSTEM*

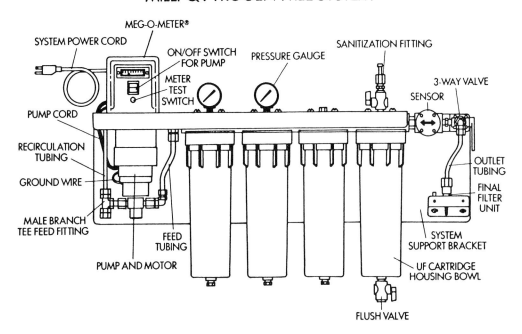

MILLI-Q PYROGEN-FREE SYSTEM

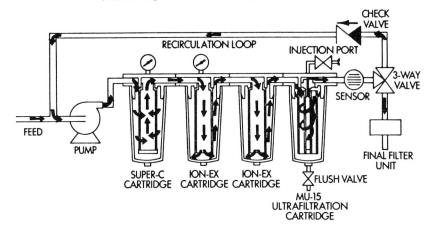

FIGURE 11. Schematic and flow diagram of the Millipore Milli-Q pyrogen-free water system. A description of the system is presented in the text. (Reprinted from the Millipore Milli-Q Operator's Manual OM-140, with permission from the Millipore Corporation, Bedford, MA)

tectant equilibration steps are performed in the Embryo Lab using the dissecting microscope. Once equilibrated with cryoprotectant, the embryos are loaded into straws (under the dissecting microscope) and frozen in the Support Lab. Currently we utilize a stepwise, slow cool procedure (detailed Section III.H) and a Planar R204 Programmable Freezer equipped with a Planar LNP4-A heater and a MVE Lab 20 liquid nitrogen dewar (Figure 16). This instrument, designed as a portable unit, has proven to be very reliable and doesn't require a great deal of space. Embryos are stored in liquid nitrogen dewars (MVE Cryogenics, Apollo SX-35) in the Embryo Lab (Figures 1 and 8). A supply of liquid nitrogen is maintained in the Support Lab (Figure 1, N2 and Figure 15).

TABLE 1
Comparison of Milli-Q Water Quality with Standards

	C.A.P.[a] Type			A.S.T.M.[b] Type				Milli-Q
	I	II	III	I	II	III	IV	
Conductance (microohm/cm)	0.1	0.5	10	0.06	1.0	1.0	5.0	0.056
Resistance (megohm/cm)	10	2.0	0.1	16.6	1.0	1.0	0.2	18 (with new expendables)
Silicates (mg/l)	0.05	0.1	1.0	—	—	—	—	<0.01
Heavy metals (mg/l)	.01	.01	.01	—	—	—	—	<0.01
Potassium permanganate reduction (min.)	60	60	60	60	60	10	10	—
Organics (ppb)	—	—	—	—	—	—	—	<50
Total dissolved solids (ppm)	—	—	—	—	—	—	—	<0.03
Sodium (mg/l)	0.1	0.1	0.1	—	—	—	—	<0.01
Hardness	Neg	Neg	Neg	—	—	—	—	—
Ammonia	0.1	0.1	0.1	—	—	—	—	<0.01
Bacterial growth (cfu/ml)	10	10^4	—	—	—	—	—	≤1.00
pH	—	—	5—8	—	6.2—7.5	5—8	—	—
CO_2 (mg/l)	3	3	3	—	—	—	—	—

[a] C.A.P. — College of American Pathologists.
[b] A.S.T.M. — American Society for Testing and Materials.

(Reprinted from the Millipore Milli-Q Operator's Manual OM-140, with permission of the Millipore Corporation, Bedford, MA.)

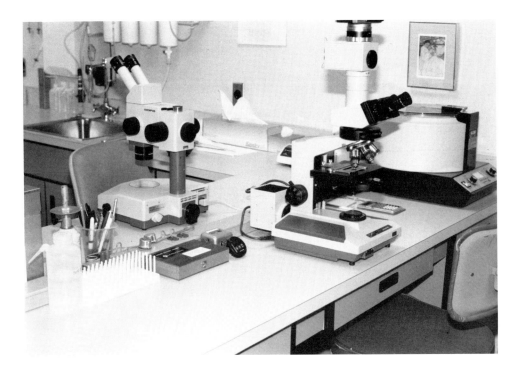

FIGURE 12.   Support Lab semen preparation area containing a standard compound microscope, clinical centrifuge, and Makler Counting Chamber.

C. OFFICE/CONSULTATION ROOM

Patient records, quality control records, forms, and other administrative items are housed in the IVF Lab Office (Figures 1 and 17). Additionally, it serves as a facility for patients wishing to consult with the IVF Lab Director. We encourage discussion of the IVF and/or GIFT procedures between the gamete physiologist and the patients. If possible, patients are permitted to view the Support and Embryo Labs.

D. SEMEN COLLECTION FACILITY

As mentioned earlier, this facility is a converted restroom designed to facilitate semen collection. It is removed from the laboratory as much as possible to reduce noise and congestion.

III. SPECIFIC LABORATORY PROCEDURES

A. PREPARATION OF HAM'S F-10 NUTRIENT MEDIUM

Numerous types of nutrient media have been utilized in IVF programs including modified Ham's F-10,[4] Eagle's,[5] Whittinghams T6,[6] and Whitten's.[7] Although each has been utilized successfully in IVF programs, in one long-term prospective study, there was no significant difference among them with respect to fertilization, cleavage, or pregnancy rates.[8] The pH of the culture media is very important and should be kept at 7.4. Media are generally buffered using a bicarbonate/CO_2 system requiring 5% CO_2 mixed with filtered air for oocyte and embryo culture, although medium buffered with Hepes and bicarbonate without CO_2 has been used for mouse embryo development.[9] The culture medium is routinely maintained at an osmolarity of 280 to 285 mOsm/kg. A controversial aspect of embryo culture medium is the addition of medium supplements. These include heat-inactivated maternal serum,[6,7] human umbilical cord serum,[10] and various serum albumins.[11] Whereas some studies suggest

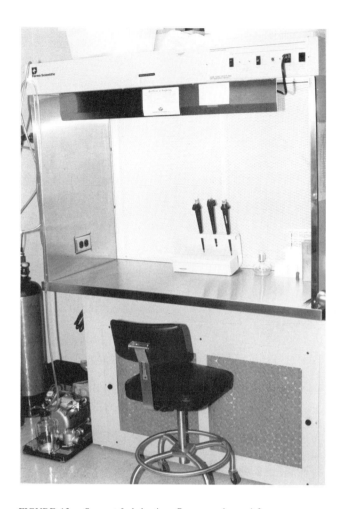

FIGURE 13. Support Lab laminar flow console used for semen preparation. The console is located directly opposite the semen preparation area illustrated in Figure 12. The console is also used to filter sterilize nutrient medium. A vacuum pump is located to the left of the console on the floor.

that serum-supplemented medium gives better cleavage rates relative to non-serum controls,[12] other studies suggest that medium supplemented with human serum albumin gives comparable results.[11] In one study, medium containing no protein supplement was compared to medium containing 10% maternal serum. There was no significant difference between the groups with respect to rates of fertilization, cleavage, pregnancy, or live births.[13]

It would appear that maternal or fetal cord serum, although used in many programs, is not necessary for IVF. Moreover, it represents a huge variable which cannot be controlled. Accordingly, we have chosen not to use serum-supplemented medium but rather a chemically defined medium (Ham's F-10) supplemented with highly purified human serum albumin (final concentration = 0.3%, Cutter Laboratories). This material is heat inactivated for 10 h at 56°C (personal communication) and thus, possesses little chance for transmission of viral diseases. The medium used in our program (Ham's F10 + 0.3% HSA) is utilized for oocyte and embryo culture and sperm preparation. The fertilization and cleavage rates for mature oocytes using the media for three independent cycles over a 9 month period, are 79.4 and 97.2%, respectively. Perhaps more importantly, the fertilization rates/cycle have steadily improved over the period (70.8 to 91.9%). Using this system, the mean stage of embryo development at 42 h postinsemination (48 h postretrieval) is 4.3 blastomeres per embryo.

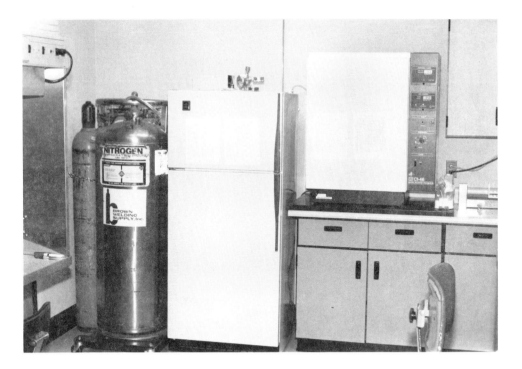

FIGURE 14.   Support Lab equipment and bulk storage. The incubator is used during semen preparation and to equilibrate medium for the sperm wash and rise. The refrigerator holds prepared and sterile nutrient medium, DPBS, and other reagents that require refrigeration.

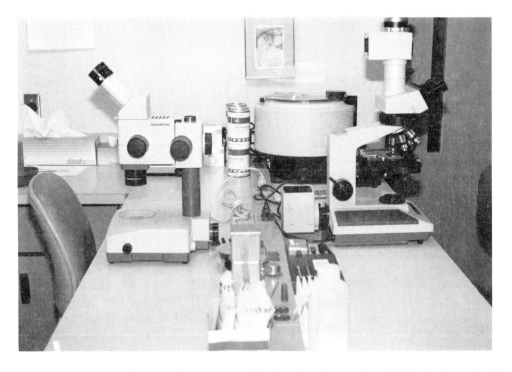

FIGURE 15.   Support Lab mouse embryo assay area. The dissecting microscope is used during the harvesting of mouse two-cell embryos and to monitor mouse embryo development for IVF/ET Lab quality conrol. Requisite supplies for the assay are located in drawers located under the workbench.

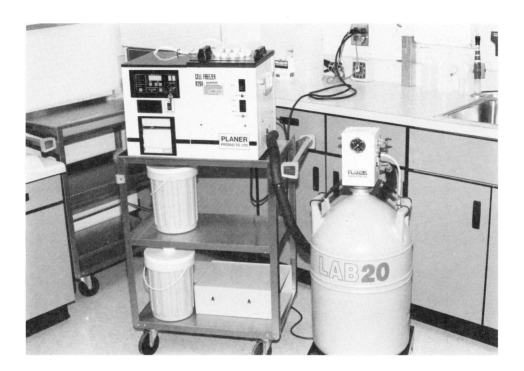

FIGURE 16. Equipment utilized for human embryo cryopreservation set up in the Support Lab. The Planar programmable unit is portable which facilitates easy storage of the unit when not in use.

The step-by-step procedure for making Ham's F-10 + 0.3% HSA is presented below.

1. Use a Ham's F-10 medium preparation sheet to record data (see Appendix VII A).
2. Mark tissue culture roller bottle (Falcon #3027) at approximate 1 liter area with a water resistant laboratory marker.
3. Fill roller bottle to approximately 750 ml with Milli-Q water.
4. Mark a sterile 50 ml graduated conical tube (Falcon #2093) for calcium lactate L(+) (Sigma L-4388) and add approximately 30 ml Milli-Q water to tube.
5. Weigh 0.050 g of streptomycin sulfate (Sigma S-9137) and place in roller bottle.
6. Weigh 0.254 g of calcium lactate L(+) and put in previously labeled 50 ml graduated conical tube. Cover and mix vigorously.
7. Carefully open bag of Ham's F-10 (Gibco 430-1200) medium and pour into roller bottle. Tear down side of media bag in order to free residual medium in the bottom of the bag and pour this into roller bottle. Shake vigorously to mix.
8. Weigh 0.075 g of Benzyl Penicillin G (Sigma P-3032) and transfer to roller bottle. Shake vigorously.
9. Weigh 1.68 g Sodium Bicarbonate (Sigma S-5761) and transfer to roller bottle. Shake vigorously. Media should turn pink/red.
10. Weigh 0.5076 g $KHCO_2$ (Sigma P-9144) and transfer to roller bottle. Shake and swirl vigorously.
11. Add calcium lactate in 50 ml graduated conical tube to media in roller bottle.
12. Add Milli-Q water to just below the liter mark on roller bottle.
13. Measure osmolarity of F-10 solution using a vapor pressure osmometer. Final osmolarity must be 280 to 285 mOsm. If the osmolarity is too high, adjust it. If it is too low, start over.

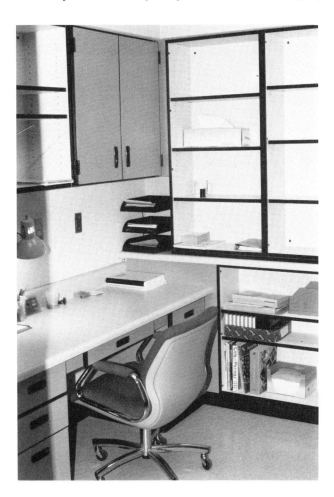

FIGURE 17.   IVF/ET Office/Consultation room.

14.   To adjust a high osmolarity, perform the following calculation:

$$\frac{\text{mOsm read} - 285 \text{ mOsm}}{\text{mOsm read}} \times \text{vol (ml) of media} = \text{ml to be adjusted}$$

15.   Take out of the roller bottle the volume to be adjusted rounding down to the nearest 10 ml. Example: 85 ml to be adjusted: remove 80 ml of media. This precaution will protect osmolarity from falling too low. Save extra media in a sterile tissue culture flask.

16.   Add the same volume of Milli-Q water to roller bottle as media extracted. Read osmolarity.

17.   Repeat steps 3 to 6 until osmolarity is 280 to 285 mOsm.

18.   Repeat steps 3 to 6 on accumulated extra media in the tissue culture flask until osmolarity is 280 to 285 mOsm. Add the adjusted extra media to the media in the roller bottle.

19.   pH the media using the dedicated pH meter. pH should be 7.4 +/- 0.1. If the pH is out of range, adjust with 1 *N* HCl if alkaline or 1 *N* NaOH if acidic.

20.   Filter sterilize media in Nalgene 250 ml disposable filterware (nylon filters). Filter 250 ml into each jar, using four filter units. Filter sterilize under laminar flow hood using vacuum pump.

21. The culture medium (F-10) is stored refrigerated without HSA. As required, add human serum albumin (HSA) to give a final concentration of 0.3%. F-10 + 0.3% HSA is prepared 24 h prior to use and equillibrated in the tissue culture incubation.

22. Test the medium (F-10 + 0.3% HSA) using the mouse embryo system and record results on the F-10 media preparation form (Appendix VII A). Discard media after 5 weeks.

B. PREPARATION OF DULBECCO'S PHOSPHATE-BUFFERED SALINE

Ham's F-10 based medium is intended for use in a 5% CO_2 atmosphere such as the tissue culture incubator. If removed from this environment, the medium rapidly becomes alkaline and begins to turn purple (due to phenol red indicator in the F-10 formulation). Accordingly, this medium or any HCO^-_3/CO_2 medium is inadquate for use in air unless buffered (such as with Hepes). For this purpose, an isotonic salt solution maintained at the proper osmolarity is used such as Dulbecco's phosphate-buffered saline (DPBS). This medium is used during oocyte retrieval and isolation and is also used in our laboratory as the basic medium for embryo cryopreservation. We further supplement the medium with 0.3% HSA as with Ham's F-10.

1. Fill out Dulbecco's Phosphate-Buffered Saline (DPBS) preparation form (Appendix VII B).

2. Mark tissue culture roller bottle (Falcon #3027) at approximate 1 liter volume.

3. Fill roller bottle to approximately 750 ml with Milli-Q water.

4. Mark a sterile graduated 50 ml conical tube (Falcon #2098) for $CaCl_2$ and fill with Milli-Q water to the 35 ml mark.

5. Carefully open a silver package of $CaCl_2$ with a razor blade and pour into graduated 50 ml conical tube. Tear down side of package to expel trapped $CaCl_2$ at bottom of pouch into conical tube.

6. Weigh 0.075 g of Benzyl Penicillin G (Sigma P-3032) and transfer to roller bottle.

7. Weigh 0.075 g of Streptomycin Sulfate (Sigma S-9137) and transfer to roller bottle.

8. Carefully open package of Dulbeccos (DPBS, Gibco 450-1300) saline with razor blade and transfer to roller bottle. Tear down side of package to expel residual medium and transfer to roller bottle. Shake roller bottle vigorously. Solution will be milky white then turn clear.

9. Weigh 0.001 g of phenol red (Sigma P-5530) and transfer to roller bottle. Shake vigorously. Solution will have a pink color.

10. Pour $CaCl_2$ solution from graduated 50 ml conical tube into roller bottle. Shake vigorously.

11. Add Milli-Q water to just under 1 liter mark on roller bottle.

12. Read osmolarity using vapor pressure osmometer. Final osmolarity must be 280 to 285 mOsm. If osmolarity is too high, adjust it. If osmolarity is too low, start over.

13. To adjust osmolarity, do the following calculation:

$$\frac{\text{mOsm read} - 285 \text{ mOsm}}{\text{mOsm read}} \times \text{vol (ml) of media} = \text{ml to be adjusted}$$

14. Take out volume to be adjusted, rounding down to the nearest 10 ml. Example: 85 ml to be adjusted: remove 80 ml media. This precaution will protect osmolarity from falling too low. Save extra media in tissue flask.

15. Add the same amount Milli-Q water as media taken out to roller bottle. Read osmolarity.

16. Repeat steps 11 to 14 until osmolarity is 280 to 285 mOsm.

17. Repeat steps 11 to 14 on accumulated extra media in tissue flask until osmolarity is 280 to 285 mOsm. Add the adjusted extra media to the media in roller bottle.
18. pH the medium using the pH probe and meter. pH should be 7.4 $+/- 0.1$. If pH is out of range, adjust with 1 *N* HCl if alkaline or 1 *N* NaOH if acidic.
19. Transfer 40 U/ml Heparin (Elkins-Sinn, 10,000 U/ml) into roller bottle and shake vigorously.
20. Filter sterilize media in Nalgene 1000 ml disposable filterware with nylon membrane. Filter all media into one unit in laminar flow hood using a vacuum pump.
21. Pour media from filter unit into sterile tissue flasks. Use 6 to 7 flasks with approximately 150 ml in each flask. Screw cap on tightly. Store at 4°C until used.
22. DPBS should be tested using the mouse embryo assay and the results recorded on the DPBS preparation form (Appendix VII.B).

C. MOUSE EMBRYO CULTURE ASSAY

Once batches of Ham's F-10 and DPBS have been made, they must be tested for use in human embryo culture. This is most often accomplished by testing the ability to support two-cell mouse embryo development to the blastocyst stage. A detailed review of this system is provided in Chapter 17 and hence, is not repeated here.

Studies have suggested that one-cell mouse embryos or mouse preimplantation embryos (zona-free blastocysts) are more sensitive than two-cell mouse embryos in detecting potential toxins in the culture media.[14,15] Whether other systems are indeed superior to the two-cell mouse embryo system is debatable. If one-cell mouse embryos fail to divide, how does one know if this is due to media effects or to lack of fertilization? At least with two-cell embryos, one can easily identify fertilized oocytes. It was reported that mouse preimplantation embryos were affected by media contaminants whereas zona-enclosed embryos were not. If the zona-enclosed embryos were not affected, are the so-called contaminants truly detrimental? Although intense screening of media is an important aspect of the IVF lab, one wonders if some of these tests introduce problems that are not evident realistically. In neither study mentioned above were the observations using mouse embryos extended to relate to rates of human fertilization, cleavage, or pregnancy.

It should be remembered that at best, any mouse embryo system truly only tests efficiency with respect to mouse embryo development. Correlation to human embryo development is inferred. Whereas poor mouse embryo development will likely yield poor human embryo development, good mouse embryo development does not guarantee good human embryo development.

Recently, mouse-tested medium for use in IVF and GIFT has become available commercially. It should be remembered that the nutrient medium is not the only item requiring testing prior to use for IVF. Virtually any item that will come in contact with human gametes or embryos, either directly or indirectly, should be tested for their ability to support mouse embryo development. These include tissue culture dishes (for oocyte isolation as well as embryo culture), culture tubes used to collect follicle aspirates, medium storage containers, pipettes, pipette tips, transfer catheters, disposables used for semen analysis, and finally, the tissue culture incubators themselves. Using the classic two-cell mouse embryo system, we screen all of these items extensively prior to an upcoming IVF cycle.

D. SEMEN PREPARATION FOR IVF AND GIFT

The semen sample utilized for IVF and GIFT protocols is prepared in the IVF lab on the day of oocyte retrieval. Standard semen analyses (Chapter 3) performed to detect potential male factor (count, motility, velocity, etc.) as well as more sophisticated analyses such as antisperm antibodies (Chapters 9 and 10) and hamster penetration tests (Chapter 7) are performed previously in a certified andrology lab. Detailed descriptions of the semen analysis are presented elsewhere in this monograph. For completeness, however, the protocol utilized in our laboratory is presented. We utilize a wash and rise protocol that takes approximately 3 h to perform.

Initially, sperm were processed using Ham's F-10 containing 10% maternal serum. At that time, maternal serum was utilized in the oocyte and embryo culture medium as well. We have subsequently changed to using F-10 containing 0.3% highly purified human serum albumin (HSA) for oocyte and embryo culture. Accordingly, F-10 + 0.3% HSA is used to process the semen sample. In our program, IVF procedures and GIFT procedures are initiated at 7:30 a.m. and 12:00 p.m., respectively, due to slightly different stimulation protocols and patient consideration. For IVF, the semen sample is obtained and processed after oocyte retrieval whereas for GIFT, it is obtained and processed prior to oocyte retrieval. As in most IVF programs, oocytes are cultured individually in organ culture dishes (Falcon #3037) containing 2.0 ml of Ham's F-10 medium in the center well and another 2.0 ml in the surrounding moat. Routinely, each mature oocyte is inseminated with 100,000 motile, hyperactive sperm in 25 μl obtained after the rise assuming the patient is normospermic. For those judged as having male factor, $2-5 \times 10^5$ sperm are used to inseminate oocytes.

1. Pre-equilibrate approximately 50 ml of F-10/0.3% HSA in the Support Lab incubator for 24 h.
2. Record data using an IVF/GIFT Semenology form (Appendix VII.F).
3. Patient will arrive to donate sample the morning of the procedure (after 9:00 for IVF, 11:00 for GIFT).
4. Sample is collected in a sterile collection cup by masturbation. Allow sample to liquify 10 to 30 min on a warming tray (37°C). Record time of collection.
5. After liquifaction, record time on form and transfer sample to sterile, 15 ml graduated conical tube (Falcon #2099).
6. Note viscosity and volume of sample on form. If semen pours in single droplets, it is classified as normal. If it flows in a solid mass or "strings out," the viscosity is rated on a scale from slight to gross viscosity.
7. Place 8 μl of semen sample on the glass stage of the Makler counting chamber (Sefi-Medical Instruments, Israel) with Eppendorf pipette and place Makler chamber on the microscope stage.
8. Split the specimen sample equally between two labeled sterile 15 ml conical tubes and add 1 to 2 volumes of F-10 + 0.3% HSA (equilibrated overnight) to the semen in the conical tubes; mix completely using a sterile pasteur pipette.
9. Centrifuge diluted semen for 10 min at 1100 rpm (clinical centrifuge). If count is low, spin sample 15 to 20 min at 1100 rpm. The sperm will form a pellet at the bottom of the tube.
10. Meanwhile, using the sample from step 7, do a pre-count, morphology, and kinetics estimate under the microscope at 20× magnification. Record data.
11. Following centrifugation, gently extract supernatant from the 15 ml conical tubes in step 8, leaving a small amount of medium above pellet. Save aspirated supernatant in a separate sterile 15 ml conical tube labeled with patient name and "wash 1", in case count is very low.
12. Add the same volume of fresh F-10 + 0.3% HSA to the 15 ml conical tubes as in step 8 and resuspend the sperm pellet completely in the medium. Centrifuge as in step 9.
13. Gently aspirate supernatant from 15 ml conical tubes, leaving a very small amount above pellet (~300 μl). Save supernatant in a separate 15 ml conical tube labeled with patient name and "wash 2".
14. Pipette 1 ml of equilibrated F-10 + 0.3% HSA into two labeled, sterile, capped polystyrene test tubes (Falcon #2058) and label with patient's name and "rise".

15.   Resuspend sperm in the small amount of media above the pellet with a sterile 5 $^3/_4''$ pipette. Be careful not to introduce air bubbles. A very concentrated but resuspended sample is required.

16.   Carefully aspirate resuspended sperm and underlay the 1.0 ml of F-10 + 0.3% HSA in the "rise" tube, being careful not to disturb media nor dilute concentrated semen. Repeat with the other semen fraction. Allow sperm to rise in the tissue culture incubator (5% CO_2) for 2 h. The "rise" tubes should incubate in a rack set at a 60° angle for optimal rise results.

17.   After 2 h carefully take off top portion of media containing hyperactive sperm without disturbing bottom layer of slower and dead sperm. Transfer and combine this fraction from both tubes in a new sterile capped test tube labeled with patient name and "combined rise".

18.   Take 8 μl of the "rise" and do a post-rise count and motility using the Makler chamber.

19.   Using this count, determine the dilution/concentration factor to make a final count of 100,000 sperm/25 μl media (i.e., 10^4/ml).

20.   Make dilution for insemination using correct amounts derived from the dilution equation in step 17 and check the dilution. Pipette 8 μl on a slide, under a coverslip and observe. There should be 4 to 8 sperm per 20× field if the dilution is correct.

21.   Store semen in embryo lab incubator until use.

22.   If the count after the rise is <1 × 10^6/ml, concentrate the sample by centrifugation. Reduce the volume by aspirating medium, resuspend sample, and recount.

E. OOCYTE RETRIEVAL FOR IVF, INSEMINATION, AND PRONUCLEAR STAGE OBSERVATION

It is the responsibility of the IVF Lab personnel to identify, isolate, and grade oocytes during retrieval. This must be done rapidly but with precision. The identification and characterization of oocytes is elegantly presented in Chapter 19 of this handbook and will not be detailed here. The general procedures utilized at our facility are presented.

The Day Prior to Retrieval

1.   Prepare sufficient F-10 + 0.3% human serum albumin (HSA) based upon the expected number of follicles to be aspirated.

2.   Prepare a sufficient number of oocyte organ culture dishes containing 2 ml of F-10/ 0.3% HSA in both the moat and the center well. Number the dishes consecutively and with the patient's name. If more than one procedure is anticipated, color code the dishes. Place the oocyte dishes and any extra medium in the Embryo Lab incubator to equilibrate.

3.   Place 2 to 3 150-ml flasks of Dulbecco's phosphate-buffered saline (DPBS) in the Embryo Lab incubator to temperature equilibrate. Tighten the caps securely to prevent CO_2 equilibration.

4.   Wipe the dissecting microscope and laminar flow console with 70% ethanol and turn on UV light.

5.   Turn on the slide and both tube warmers (one for the Embryo Lab and one to be used in the OR).

The Day of Retrieval

1.   Lab personnel dress in surgical attire including scrubs, head cover, face mask, and shoe covers. Wash and rinse hands thoroughly using Embryo Lab sink.

2.   Check the temperature of the tube and slide warmers (37°C) and assemble a unipette

capillary pipette (Becton/Dickinson #5878) on a 0.5 cc glaspak syringe (Becton/Dickinson #5878) using a short piece of amber rubber tubing.

3. Transfer to the OR, a sterile laparoscopic aspirating needle (if appropriate), temperature-adjusted tube warmer (tube blocks sterilized via the OR), a sterile container for DPBS transfer, and 150 ml of warm DPBS. The OR nursing staff aliquots 1.0 ml of DPBS into follicle aspiration tubes.

4. While the patient is being prepared, turn on monitors, focus microscopes, and make a last check that everything is in order. Fill out oocyte retrieval record (Appendix VII.G).

5. Upon aspiration of the follicle into the tube, the nursing personnel labels the tube with the following information: (1) left (L) or right (R) ovary; (2) follicle number; and (3) tube contents, i.e., 1 = follicular fluid, 2 = follicular wash, 3 = apparatus wash, etc.

6. Follicular aspirates are passed to the IVF Lab via the access window and the following data are recorded (refer to oocyte retrieval form):

   a. Left or right ovary
   b. Follicle number
   c. Tube contents: follicular fluid (1) or wash (2), etc.
   d. Volume of fluid in tube
   e. Appearance of fluid, i.e., straw colored, slightly bloody, or bloody

7. Mix contents of aspirate tube and pour into a 100 or 60 mm sterile plastic petri dish (greater or less than 1.5 ml volume, respectively). If the volume is excessive, the aspirate may have to be divided into two or more dishes. Jar the top of the aspirate tube on bottom of dish several times to completely expel all fluid. Swirl the dish to uniformly distribute the aspirate on the dish. *It is important to achieve as thin a layer of media covering the dish as possible. This will facilitate easy identification and classification of oocytes since they tend to "flatten out".*

8. The aspirates are examined for the presence of oocytes. *Since more than one follicle can be punctured during aspiration, particularly during ultrasound-guided transvaginal retrieval, it is not uncommon to find more than one oocyte per dish. This is especially true if the aspirate volume is very large (>5 ml).* Therefore, aspirates should be examined carefully even if one oocyte has been found. Typically, mature oocytes are surrounded by mucus inundated with cumulus cells, has an expanded and often radiant corona, and is accompanied by many mural granulosa cells. An intermediate oocyte (polar body not extruded) often has less mucus, a less expanded corona, and fewer granulosa cells. An immature oocyte will often present without mucus or granulosa cells, and a very tight corona. (Refer to Chapter 19).

9. Oocytes are graded for maturity and the following data are recorded on the oocyte retreival form:

   a. Oocyte number: each oocyte is numbered consecutively.
   b. Cumulus: appearance; tight to expanded to radiant.
   c. Corona: appearance; tight to expanded.
   d. Mucus: quantity; a little to a lot.
   e. Granulosa cells: quantity; few to many and appearance; sheets, clumps, grainy, etc.
   f. Maturity: immature, intermediate, or mature.
   g. Incubation time: oocyte first placed in incubator.

10. Information concerning the oocyte (originating follicle, tube number, and maturity level) is passed on to the OR.

11. The oocyte/mucus/cumulus mass is carefully pipetted from the aspirate dish, deposited into the moat of a numbered culture dish and briefly agitated to remove red cells, then transferred to the center well. The dish is covered and returned to the incubator until insemination.

12. Repeat steps 6 to 11 until all aspirates have been examined. Also examine any apparatus washes and cul-de-sac fluid.

13. Shortly after oocyte retrieval, the husband is brought to the IVF Lab for semen collection. The sample is prepared using a wash and rise procedure as previously described (see Section III.D).

14. Six hours postretrieval, the oocytes are re-evaluated and the data recorded on an oocyte/embryo observation form (Appendix VII.H). The status of the mucus, cumulus, and corona are noted. If mature, the oocyte is inseminated with 100,000 sperm in 25 μl medium. If intermediate, the oocyte is allowed to mature for 12 to 24 h upon which it is re-evaluated. Immature oocytes are incubated at least 24 h before they are re-evaluated.

15. At 15 to 20 h postinsemination, the oocytes are observed for fertilization. Using a finely drawn, fire-polished, sterile pasteur pipette connected to a mouthpiece using latex rubber tubing, the oocyte is lifted off the bottom of the dish (usually connected to cumulus cells which have begun to attach to the dish) and gently aspirated in and out to dislodge the oocyte from the somatic cells. This is usually accomplished easily if the oocytes are fertilized. The oocytes are observed *carefully* for the presence of two pronulcei, one derived from the oocyte and one from the sperm. This indicates normal fertilization. *The oocyte should be moved around with gentle swirling of the dish to allow for observation at different angles to insure that two and only two pronuclei are present.* Normally fertilized oocytes are transferred to a new culture dish containing fresh F-10/0.3% HSA (pre-equilibrated overnight). The labeled lid of the original dish can be transferred to the new one thus, avoiding potential confusion.

16. If the oocyte has not been fertilized but has expressed a polar body, the oocyte is reinseminated and the above procedures repeated.

17. If more than two pronuclei are identified, the oocyte is classified a polypronuclear and immediately culled from the group and discarded. Polypronuclear oocytes contain more genetic material than normal and thus, represent nonviable entities. *They are not transferred to the patient.* Pronuclear stage observation is extremely important and must be performed during a specific time interval (15 to 20 h). Pronuclei eventually fuse making it virtually impossible to distinguish between normal and polypronuclear zygotes. Additionally, polypronuclear oocytes can develop into normal-looking embryos. Thus, the pronuclear stage observation is critical step in the IVF procedure.

18. Normally fertilized oocytes are returned to the incubator for 24 h to allow for embryo development and are not disturbed further until embryo transfer.

19. At ~48 to 50 h postretrieval, embryos are transferred to the patient. Embryos are chosen based upon their appearance including eveness of blastomeres, number of blastomeres, and uniformity of blastomere cytoplasm. Routinely, four to five embryos are transferred to the patient 48 to 50 h postretrieval.

20. Embryos not utilized for immediate transfer are prepared for cryopreservation

21. Oocytes that have not matured and/or fertilized are discarded.

F. EMBRYO TRANSFER FOR IVF

Once embryos have been selected for transfer, they must be combined and loaded into a catheter for intrauterine transfer. The amount of medium transfered along with the embryos should be kept to a minimum. The loading of the transfer catheter should be done rapidly to minimize exposure of the embryos to the environment.

1. Lab personnel dress in surgical attire including scrubs, head cover, face mask and shoe covers.
2. The laminar flow console and primary dissecting microscope should be rinsed with Milli-Q water and 70% ethanol (the console UV light should be turned on overnight).
3. Approximately 30 min prior to transfer, the selected embryos should be combined in a single culture dish and held in the upper incubator. For ease of catheter loading, the embryos should be kept close together.
4. The primary dissecting microscope used to load the embryos should be adjusted to the satisfaction of the person loading the transfer catheter.
5. The gamete physiologist performs a surgical scrub of hands and forearms and rinses thoroughly including a final rinse of sterile water.
6. Sterile towels are used to dry hands, drape the OR access window, and drape a work area in the laminar flow console.
7. A sterile IVF transfer catheter (coaxial side hole catheter set, #KMETS-852100, Cook Ob/Gyn, Spencer, IN) is aseptically removed from its packaging onto the draped console followed by a sterile 1 ml tuberculin syringe. The outer sheath of the catheter is removed and the catheter connected to the syringe. Approximately 300 μl of air is drawn into the syringe.
8. An IVF technician retrieves the organ culture dish containing the transfer embryos and places it on the stage of the primary dissecting microscope so the embryos are readily apparent to the transfer person. If the embryos have moved apart, reassemble them together using a finally drawn, sterile pasteur pipette.
9. The transfer catheter should be wetted by drawing and releasing equilibrated but fresh F-10/0.3% HSA using the syringe.
10. 10 μl of F-10/HSA followed by 10 μl of air are drawn into the catheter. With an IVF technician holding the culture dish firmly onto the microscope stage, the side hole of the IVF transfer catheter is aligned directly over the nested embryos. The catheter is depressed slightly over the embryos using one hand and the plunger of the syringe is withdrawn slightly but quickly with the other hand. We have found that this technique brings the embryos into the catheter in a tight group with a minimum of medium (usually 25 to 30 μl).
11. After aspiration of the embryos, 10 μl of air then medium then air are brought into the catheter.
12. Before transfer of the loaded catheter to the OR, the IVF technician examines the culture dish to ensure that no embryos remain.
13. The outer sheath of the transfer catheter is gently slid over the embryo-containing catheter and the complete catheter still connected to the syringe is passed to the reproductive endocrinologist through the OR access window for uterine transfer.
14. Once transfer has been completed, the catheter is passed back to the IVF Lab and the catheter is rinsed thoroughly in an organ culture dish containing fresh F-10/HSA. The dish is scanned for the presence of embryos. If none are found the procedure is complete. If embryos are found, the endocrinologist is informed and the process described above is repeated using a new catheter.
15. Once the procedure is complete, clean the lab of surgical and disposable items, rinse catheters with Milli-Q water and place all sterile towels in the port hole for disposal by the surgical staff.
16. Complete the embryo transfer form (see Appendix VII.I). This form is completed by both IVF Lab Director and reproductive endocrinologist. The following is completed by IVF director:

  a. Date
  b. Patient name
  c. Insemination date and time
  d. Embryo transfer
     (1) Time of removal from incubator
     (2) Transfer time (when catheter is passed to surgeon)
     (3) Difference (time difference between removal and transfer)
  e. Amount of media
  f. Type of media
  g. Number of embryos transferred
  h. Cell stage of embryos (how many transferred at each stage of development)

The reproductive endocrinologist will complete the balance of the form.

G. Oocyte Retrieval for GIFT and Gamete Transfer

The laboratory aspects of GIFT are very similar to those for IVF except that gametes (sperm and oocytes) are transferred to the fallopian tubes of the patients rather than embryos to the uterus. Additionally, the gamete transfer is performed immediately after oocyte aspiration. Because the transfer occurs through the laparascope into the peritoneal cavity, extra precautions are taken to prevent the introduction of contaminants and possible infection.

The major objective of the IVF laboratory during GIFT is to identify and isolate four mature oocytes for transfer back to the patient along with an appropriate number of capacitated sperm. Any extra oocytes found are inseminated identically to that for IVF for eventual cryopreservation providing the couple has consented to cryopreservation.

The Day Prior to Retrieval

1. Prepare an adequate supply of F-10/0.3% HSA (100 to 150 ml) and equilibrate for 24 h in the Embryo Lab incubator (made up in and contained in Falcon conical culture tubes). Place two 150 ml flasks of DPBS in the incubator to temperature equilibrate.
2. If the patient has consented to embryo cryopreservation, prepare 8 to 12 organ tissue dishes (Falcon #3037) as described for IVF using the above F-10/0.3% HSA. Allow the dishes to equilibrate in the incubator for 24 h.
3. Wipe down the laminar flow console and other work areas with Milli-Q water and 70% ethanol and turn on UV light in the console. Check the temperature of the tube warmers and slide warmers

The Day of Oocyte Retrieval

1. Prior to the beginning of the procedure the spouse's semen sample should have been prepared (100,000 highly motile sperm/25 μl) and maintained in the Embryo Lab incubator.
2. Laboratory personnel should dress in surgical attire including scrubs, head cover, face mask, and shoe covers. The hands and forearms should be scrubbed thoroughly.
3. Pipette 2 ml of F-10/0.3% HSA into each of two 35 mm culture dishes, label A and B, and return them to the incubator. These dishes will be used to hold oocytes during the oocyte retrieval procedure.
4. Pipet ~5 ml of DPBS into 60 mm culture dish (Falcon #1007), cover and place on the stage of the primary dissecting microscope. This will be used to wash the oocytes free of contaminating red cells.

5. Obtain from the OR the following sterile items: surgical gown, drape, towels, gloves, and microscope cover to be used prior to transferring gametes back to the OR. Place these on a small cart at the far end of the embryo lab.

6. Pass to the OR a sterile laparoscopy needle and an IVF or GIFT transfer catheter. The catheter is used to probe the fallopian tube orafice while the IVF Lab is preparing for gamete transfer.

7. Oocyte retrieval, isolation, and characterization are as per steps 3 to 13 for IVF with the following exceptions:

   a. Oocytes graded as mature, type 3 (refer to oocyte retrieval form, Appendix VII. G) are rinsed in DPBS and transferred to either the ''A'' or ''B'' 35 mm dish containing F-10/0.3% HSA. The most mature oocytes are placed in A and those of lesser quality are placed in B as backup.

   b. When four mature oocytes have been isolated, the OR is informed. The IVF Lab personnel begin preparation for transfer while the reproductive endocrinologist aspirates any remaining follicles and begins preparation for transfer. Aspirate tubes not yet examined for oocytes are kept at 37°C in tube warmers until gamete intra-fallopian transfer is completed. Since the aspirates are diluted in DPBS they don't require maintenance in the CO_2 incubator.

Gamete Transfer

1. In preparation for gamete transfer, the IVF Lab personnel remove oocyte aspirate dishes from the laminar flow console and wipe it down with Milli-Q water and 70% ethanol.

2. The transfer procedure requires two people, the gamete physiologist and an IVF technician. The procedural elements are divided between these individuals as described below.

3. In the laminar flow console, 4×25 μl aliquots of semen (100,000 each) and 8 to 10×10 μl aliquots of F-10/0.3% HSA are placed in a 100 mm culture dish (Falcon #1029) by the physiologist.

4. The technician carefully unwraps the sterile drape, covers the cart, unwraps the package of sterile towels and the outer wrappings of the gown, gloves, and microscope cover.

5. The gamete physiologist is aseptically gowned and gloved for loading and transferring of gametes. The gloved hands are rinsed with sterile water. From this point until the procedure is completed, this individual must remain sterile.

6. The gamete physiologist places a sterile towel in the OR access window and on the console adjacent to the microscope. An open-ended sterile GIFT transfer catheter (KMETS 852100, 5 FR, Cook Ob/Gyn) and 1 cc tuberculin syringe are deposited on the console towel. A section of the sterile microscope cover is placed on the stage of the primary dissecting microscope.

7. The technician fills a 35 mm culture dish with F-10/0.3% HSA while the gamete physiologist assembles the transfer catheter and the syringe and aspirates this medium to wet the catheter.

8. Approximately 300 μl of air is loaded into the syringe (to facilitate emptying of the catheter into the fallopian tube) and the transfer catheter is filled with consecutively:

   (a) 10 μl of medium (F-10/0.3% HSA)
   (b) 10 μl of air
   (c) 25 μl of semen (normally 100,000 sperm)
   (d) 10 μl of air

(e)   25 μl of medium containing two oocytes
(f)   10 μl of air
(g)   10 μl of medium
(h)   10 μl of air

9. The catheter is carefully given to the OR via the access window for intrafallopian transfer.

10. When transfer is complete, the catheter is given back to the IVF Lab where it is aspirated with fresh medium and the rinse examined for the presence of oocytes. If none are found, the catheter is reloaded as described above for transfer to the second tube. If oocytes are found, they are reloaded for transfer to the first tube.

11. Typically, two mature oocytes and 100,000 motile sperm/fallopian tube are transferred for patients with two patent tubes. For patients with only one tube, three oocytes + 100,000 sperm are transferred.

12. When the procedure is completed the IVF Lab team unglove, degown, clean the lab of surgical paper and disposable items, and wipe down the console with Milli-Q water and 70% ethanol.

13. If patients have not consented to embryo cryopreservation, the remaining oocytes and aspirates are discarded and the procedure is complete. If the patients have consented to embryo cryopreservation, the remaining oocytes must be isolated and inseminated as for an IVF.

14. Oocytes not selected for gamete transfer and residing in dishes "A and B" are placed in individual organ culture dishes containing equilibrated F-10/0.3% HSA. Follicle aspirates not yet examined are examined for oocytes and those found are graded and placed into organ culture dishes.

15. Six hours postretrieval, the oocytes are observed (comments recorded on an oocyte observation form, Appendix VII.H) and mature oocytes are inseminated (100,000 sperm/25 μl). Intermediate and immature oocytes are treated as described for IVF.

16. From this point on the procedure is identical to that for IVF except that embryos are not transferred to the patient. Rather, all embryos are prepared for cryopreservation.

H. CRYOPRESERVATION OF HUMAN EMBRYOS

Cryopreservation of human embryos has proven to be an important new aspect of IVF technology for it facilitates multiple chances of obtaining a pregnancy from a single stimulation cycle and oocyte retrieval. The techniques and media used for cryopreservation are numerous and are the subject of a review in this handbook (see Chapter 18). The major problem associated with cryopreservation is the formation of intracellular ice crystals which can irreparably damage the cell.[16] Cryoprotectants minimize the injury to cells during freezing, although the exact mechanism by which this occurs is unknown. Three cryoprotectants are commonly used including glycerol, dimethylsulfoxide (DMSO), and 1,2 propanediol, each a small molecular weight substance which readily penetrates the cell plasma membrane. Each cryoprotectant has been used successfully although 1,2 propanediol has been reported to be less toxic than DMSO or glycerol.[17,18] At sufficiently high concentrations (generally $>2 M$), any cryoprotectant can be potentially toxic if utilized for extended periods of time.

When cells are placed in cryoprotectant an osmotic imbalance is created causing the cell to shrink. This can cause potential cellular damage. To minimize this, cryoprotectant is often introduced to cells in a stepwise manner gradually increasing the concentration.[17] The rate of freezing embryos varies from slow, stepwise cooling to ultrarapid cooling and vitrification. Each type of cooling introduces different physical, chemical, and osmotic conditions and requires different concentrations of cryoprotectant and exposure times.

Likewise, both slow and rapid thawing rates have been utilized. Generally speaking, rapid thaw rates avoid potential recrystalization of ice which can be damaging to cells. Removal of the cryoprotectant must be done carefully. Subjecting embryos frozen in high concentrations of cryoprotectant to medium devoid of cryoprotectant can again create an osmotic imbalance causing water to rapidly penetrate the cell and increasing the likelihood of cell disruption. To prevent this, cells are exposed to an osmotic buffer such as sucrose prior to freezing (since the cells are already sufficiently dehydrated, this does not damage the cells). Upon thawing, the sucrose is removed subsequent to the gradual, stepwise removal of cryoprotectant.

Of the many procedures available, we utilize one that involves stepwise equilibration of cryoprotectant (1,2, propanediol and sucrose), slow stepwise cooling, rapid thawing, and stepwise removal of cryoprotectant and sucrose. The method is that reported by Quinn[17] adapted from previous methods.[17-20] This procedure has proven to be effective for the cryopreservation of smaller embryos (two to four cell) which thus far, makeup the majority of embryos cryopreserved.[16] The step-by-step procedures for embryo cryopreservation, embryo thaw, and transfer are presented below.

1. Medium Preparation

1. Have prepared, 1 liter of sterile DPBS made without phenol red and heparin (see procedure for DPBS preparation) and stock 1,2 propanediol (Sigma, P-1009). Use 250 ml Falcon (#3023) tissue culture flasks to prepare and store media stocks and Nalgene 150 ml filter sterilizing units (nylon filters).
2. Prepare a cryopreservation media preparation form (Appendix VII.J)
3. Prepare 100 ml each of the following stock reagents and filter sterilize:

    #1. **1.5 M PDiol/0.2 M Sucrose/DPBS**—Dissolve 6.85 g sucrose in 50 ml of DPBS and add 11.0 ml PDiol, q.s. to 100 ml with DPBS.
    #2. **0.2 M Sucrose/DPBS**—Dissolve 6.85 g of sucrose in 100 ml of DPBS.
    #3. **1.5 M PDiol/DPBS**—Add 11 ml of PDiol to DPBS, q.s. to 100 ml.

4. Prepare the following working solutions from the above stocks:

    a. **1.5 M PDiol/0.2 M Sucrose/0.3% HSA/DPBS**—45 ml solution #1 + 0.54 ml HSA (25% stock)
    b. **1.0 M PDiol/0.2 M Sucrose/0.3% HSA/DPBS**—30 ml solution #1 + 15 ml solution #2 + 0.54 ml HSA
    c. **0.5 M PDiol/0.2 M Sucrose/0.3% HSA/DPBS**—15 ml solution #1 + 30 ml solution #2 + 0.54 ml HSA
    d. **0.0 M PDiol/0.2 M Sucrose/0.3% HSA/DPBS**—45 ml solution #2 + 0.54 ml HSA
    e. **1.5 M PDiol/0.3% HSA/DPBS**—45 ml solution #3 + 0.54 ml HSA
    f. **1.0 M PDiol/0.3% HSA/DPBS**—30 ml solution #3 + 15 ml DPBS + 0.54 ml HSA
    g. **0.5 M PDiol/0.3% HSA/DPBS**—15 ml solution #3 + 30 ml DPBS + 0.54 ml HSA
    h. **0.0 M PDiol/0.3% HSA/DPBS**—45 ml DPBS + 0.54 ml HSA

Store these working reagents at 4°C in sterile 50 ml conical culture tubes (Falcon #2098) sealed with Parafilm M.

2. Equilibration of Cryoprotectant
Prior to freezing, the cellular water must be displaced by cryoprotectant to prevent the

formation of intracellular ice crystals which can irreparably damage the embryo. This is accomplished in a stepwise manner to gradually introduce the cryoprotectant. The equilibration process occurs at room temperature and in room air since the media are made in DPBS. Embryos are handled using sterile, finely drawn, fire-polished pasteur pipettes.

1. The four freezing media (a, e—g above) are allowed to reach room temperature. 2.0 ml of each is pipetted into a labeled 35 mm culture dish (Falcon #1008) and placed adjacent to the dissecting microscope.

2. Recording the data on an Frozen Embryo Form (Appendix VII.L), embryos to be frozen are evaluated (number and uniformity of blastomeres, cytoplasmic consistancy, blebbing, etc.) and combined in a single organ culture dish. Embryos are frozen in variable sized groups depending upon the total number of embryos available. Generally, we cryopreseve in groups of two to four.

3. The embryos are transferred sequentially to the following media for the times indicated:

0.5 *M* PDiol/0.3% HSA/DPBS	sol'n	"g"	5 min
1.0 *M* PDiol/0.3% HSA/DPBS	sol'n	"f"	5 min
1.5 *M* PDiol/0.3% HSA/DPBS	sol'n	"e"	10 min
1.5 *M* PDiol/0.2 *M* Sucrose/0.3% HSA/DPBS	sol'n	"a"	5 min

4. It is within the last medium that the embryos are frozen; 250 μl plugged straws are used for cryopreservation. Using a mouth pipette approximately 25 μl of medium (1.5 *M* PDiol/0.2 *M* sucrose/0.3% HSA/DPBS) are drawn into the pipette followed by an equal volume of air and 150 μl of medium.

5. Under the dissecting microscope, the embryos are collected in a finely drawn pipette and deposited into the 150 μl volume of medium in the straw. This must be done carefully to avoid depositing the embryos on the side of the straw. Verify that the embryos are located in the straw by rotating the straw slowly while viewing it under the microscope.

6. Very carefully draw 50 μl of medium into the straw followed by air such that the first volume of medium brought into the straw wicks into the plug at the top.

7. Heat seal the bottom of straw (National Instruments, Model 210 impulse sealer). The embryos are now ready for cryopreservation.

3. Embryo Cryopreservation

The actual cryopreservation of human embryos involves a stepwise slow cooling procedure which takes 2 to 2.5 h. We utilize a Planar portable R204 freezer coupled with a Planar LNP-1-A heater and an MVE Lab 20 liquid nitrogen dewar. This instrument has proven to be reliable and the fact that it is portable allows it to be moved and stored when not in use.

1. Embryos are pre-equilibrated with cryprotectant as described above and the straws are placed into the freezing chamber.

2. The embryos are cooled from room temperature to −7°C at a rate of −2°C/min.

3. The embryos are held at this temperature for 20 min, during which time the straws are seeded for ice formation by touching the straw with a pair of large forceps chilled in liquid nitrogen. Just prior to the next step, the straws are examined briefly for complete freezing.

4. The frozen embryos are cooled from −7°C to −30°C at a rate of −0.3°C/min.

5. The embryos are removed rapidly using a pair of large forceps cooled in liquid nitrogen vapor and the straw is held in the liquid nitrogen vapor in a cryocontainer (just above the liquid meniscus) for 40 s.

6. The straw is then dropped into liquid nitrogen.
7. The straws are placed into polypropylene holders for use with canes and cardboard covers. These items are placed in liquid nitrogen prior to the addition of the straws to the holders.
8. The assembled cane and cover containing the straws of embryos are transferred to liquid nitrogen dewars for storage.
9. An IVF/GIFT summary form (Appendix VII.K) is filled out to reflect the disposition of embryos, either transferred or frozen.

4. Embryo Thawing for Transfer

The major concerns when thawing embryos are the potential recrystallization of ice particles and osmotic shock due to the rapid influx of water if the cryoprotectant is removed too rapidly. These factors can be minimized by rapidly thawing the embryos and a stepwise removal of the cryoprotectant over time.

1. A 1 liter beaker is filled with warm tap water, placed on a 37°C warming tray, and the temperature adjusted to 37°C.
2. Thaw media are removed from the refrigerator and allowed to reach ambient temperature.
3. The following thaw solutions described above are poured into either 35 or 60 mm culture dishes (Falcon #1008 or 1007) and placed adjacent to the dissecting microscope in the laminar flow console:

Solution "b"	—	60 mm
Solution "c"	—	35 mm
Solution "d"	—	35 mm
Solution "h"	—	60 mm

4. The embryo-containing straw is removed from liquid nitrogen and plunged directly into the 37°C water bath for 30 to 40 s and is then rinsed with Milli-Q water and wiped with a sterile gauze.
5. With one hand the straw is held next to the open 60 mm dish containing solution "b". The bottom end of the straw (that containing the heat seal) is snipped using a sharp pair of scissors and the end of the straw is *immediately placed over the dish in case any straw contents leaks out*. Keeping the top end of the straw outside of the dish (so it won't fall in) the top of the straw is cut. The contents of the straw should rapidly disperse into the dish. The embryos are maintained in this solution for 5 min (1.0 *M* PDiol/0.2 *M* Sucrose/0.3% HSA/DPBS).
6. During this initial period the embryos are located, moved together, and examined for viability. An embryo is considered viable if 50% or more of the blastomeres are intact. It has been our experience that the blastomeres will look either very good or very bad. It has not been difficult to judge the viability of the embryos. For further discussion, the reader is urged to consult the chapter on cryopreservation in this monograph.
7. Using finely drawn pasteur pipettes, viable embryos are transferred to the following solutions maintained at room temperature as indicated:

0.5 M PDiol/0.2 M Sucrose/0.3% HSA/DPBS	—	Solution "c"	—	5 min
0.0 M PDiol/0.2 M Sucrose/0.3% HSA/DPBS	—	Solution "d"	—	5 min
0.3% HSA/DPBS	—	Solution "h"	—	5 min

8. Embryos are equilibrated in F-10/0.3% HSA at 37°C (CO_2 incubator) for at least 60 min prior to transfer

5. Transfer of Cryopreserved Embryos

Following the thaw, removal of cryoprotectant, and equilibration, the viable embryos are transferred to the uterine cavity exactly as described for embryos for an IVF procedure. Embryos not surviving the freeze/thaw cycle are discarded.

IV. QUALITY CONTROL

As with any clinical laboratory, intense IVF Laboratory quality control is an absolute requisite for a successful program. Of all the components comprising an IVF program, it is the laboratory which often receives the most scrutiny. Accordingly, a quality control program should be established, documented, and incorporated into laboratory policy. Rigorous quality control assures that equipment is functional and accurate, that procedures are performed consistently, and that a high standard of performance is maintained.

Despite the fact that it has been 11 years since the birth of the first IVF baby, many of the assisted reproductive technologies including IVF and GIFT are still considered to be experimental procedures despite the fact that >14,000 transfer cycles were performed in 1987 according to the IVF Registry.[21] This yearly rate has no doubt increased significantly during the intervening period. With the increased number of procedures and centers performing these and other assisted reproductive procedures has come increased scrutiny from the media and government with respect to the qualifications of key personnel and to the actual procedures taking place in these programs. Among the prime targets for potential government regulation of IVF programs is the IVF Lab. This is due, in part, to precedent in that clinical laboratories are licensed and regulated, and that laboratories lend themselves to regulation due to the use of standard procedures which can be documented. The concept of certification and regulation of the IVF Lab was a topic for workshop entitled "IVF: Laboratory Update" held at the annual meeting of the American Fertility Society (October 12, 1988, Atlanta, GA). The consensus opinion of attendees was that certification and regulation are inevitable and that IVF Labs should begin preparing for this.

In this section many of the quality control measures in force in our program will be reviewed. Of particular importance is the need for documentation and record keeping to provide evidence of quality control measures in force.

Table 2 illustrates equipment and reagent quality control schedules for the IVF Lab. Many of the items are straightforward such as routine monitoring. Examples of records and forms are provided in Appendices VII. N—T. Other items such as sterilization of the Milli-Q water system and tissue culture incubators are detailed in the sections to follow.

A. IVF/ET LABORATORY QUALITY CONTROL

During IVF/GIFT cycles, equipment and apparatus are monitored for performance as indicated in Table 2. These data are recorded and the forms maintained as part of the permanent record of the laboratory. Temperature logs (Appendix VII.N) are kept for each tube and slide warmer and the refrigerator. A temperature and CO_2 log (Appendix VII.O) is maintained for each incubator. Logs are maintained for pH meter and osmometer standardization (Appendices VII.P and Q, respectively). Logs are maintained for dewar liquid nitrogen levels (Appendix VII.R) and CO_2 tank levels (Appendix VII.S). The logs are located near their respective pieces of equipment for ease of data entry.

Maintenance records (Appendix VII.T) are kept to document service to equipment. This includes inhouse maintenance such as Milli-Q water system sterilization, CO_2 incubator cleaning, and pipette calibration as well as professional maintenance such as servicing the laminar flow hoods, microscopes, centrifuges, and water system.

B. STERILIZATION OF THE MILLI-Q SYSTEM

The Milli-Q system should be cleaned weekly. This essentially consists of sterilization

TABLE 2
IVF Lab Quality Control Schedule

Frequency

Equipment/reagents	Daily	Weekly	Monthly	Quarterly	Other (comment)
1. CO$_2$ incubator					
a. % CO$_2$/temp.	X				
b. Mouse embryo assay					As required
c. Fyrite CO$_2$ check		X			
d. Clean and sterilize					3—4 weeks prior to new cycle
e. Temp. check: supplemental thermometer		X			
f. Replace sterile water in pan		X			
2. Microscopes					
a. Check bulbs, clean, inspect				X	
b. Professionally clean, adjust					Annually
3. Slide warmers	X				
4. Tube warmers	X				
5. Referigerator: temperature	X				
6. Sterilizing oven: temperature	X				
7. CO$_2$ tanks: pressure	X				
8. Milli-Q water system					
a. Conductivity	X				
b. Sterilize		X			
c. Change cartridges					As required
9. Liquid nitrogen Dewars: check and fill		X			
10. pH Meter					
a. Standardize		X			
b. Replace probe					As required
11. Osmometer					
a. Standardize		X			
b. Clean		X			
12. Automatic pipettes: calibrate					New cycle
13. Programmable freezer					
a. Temperature check					Prior to use
b. Mouse embryo bioassay					New cycle
c. Mechanical calibration					Annually
14. Culture medium: F-10, DPBS					
a. pH adjustment					When prepared
b. Osmolarity					When prepared
c. Mouse embryo bioassay					When prepared
d. CO$_2$ equil.					24 h prior to use
14. Timers					Annually
15. Centrifuges					Annually
16. Ultrasonic cleaner					Annually
17. Laminar flow hood					
a. Change filters					Biannually
b. Air flow check					Biannually
18. Plasticware: mouse embryo bioassay					New cycle
19. Transfer catheters: mouse embryo bioassay					New cycle
20. Freeze/thaw medium: mouse embryo bioassay					New cycle

of the final ultrafiltration cartridge. The procedure described is adapted from the technical manual for the system. The reader should refer to the diagrams of the system contained in Figure 11.

1. Before cleaning the system, collect 1 liter of water for use in cleaning the system.
2. Unplug the Milli-Q unit and turn off the feed water supply.
3. Prepare 100 ml of cleaning solution (3 to 4 ml of 5.25% sodium hypochlorite, i.e., Clorox, in Milli-Q water).
4. Open the three-way valve until no more water exists. This valve remains open throughout the cleaning procedure. *Slowly* open and leave open the flush valve at the bottom of the UF filter cartridge. Water will drain until the pressure in the system is zero.
5. With a 60 cc plastic syringe fitted to the sanitation fitting at the top of the UF cartridge, fill with cleaning solution. Open the sanitation fitting valve and inject the cleaning solution into the cartridge. Inject the remaining cleaning solution followed by 100 ml of Milli-Q water. Some liquid will drip out of the open flush valve at the bottom of the cartridge.
6. Close the sanitation fitting valve but keep the three-way valve open to prevent bleach from getting upstream to the other filters.
7. Open the feed water valve.
8. Immediately turn on the pump for 15 s, then simultaneously turn off the pump and turn off the feed water supply.
9. Allow the system to stand for 30 to 45 min.
10. Open the feed water valve while keeping the flush valve open. Flush the cartridge for 10 min to flush out bleach.
11. Close the flush valve, turn on the pump and continue to flush the final filter for 15 min. This step sanitizes the 0.22 μm final filter with very dilute bleach.
12. Reopen the flush valve and flush for 5 min.
13. Check the chlorine level in water taken from both the flush and three-way valve using a Hatch test kit. The level should be <0.1 ppm.
14. If the levels are >0.1 ppm, repeat steps 11 to 13. If the levels are <0.1 ppm, close the three-way and flush valves, turn on the pump and recirculate water through the system until the resistivity meter reads 18 Megohms.

Notes

1. The Super-C, both ion exchange cartridges, and the 0.22 μm final filter should be replaced every 4 months to insure optimal water quality.
2. The pump should never be turned on while the feed water supply is off.
3. If the chlorine cleaning solution exceeds 200 ppm, damage to the ultrafiltration membrane can occur.

C. PREPARATION AND STERILIZATION OF THE CO_2 TISSUE CULTURE INCUBATORS

Tissue culture incubators provide an optimal environment for oocyte maintenance and embryo development. Since all IVF work is performed aseptically, it is important that the incubators, potential sources of contamination, be clean and sterile. In between IVF cycles, the incubators are broken down, cleaned, reassembled, sterilized, and tested for their ability to support mouse embryo development. The procedures described below are for the Embryo Lab (Forma #3326) and the Support Lab (American Scientific Products CI-46) incubators.

1. Two to four weeks prior to the initiation of an IVF cycle, the incubators are sterilized.

2. Turn off incubators and CO_2 supply.
3. Remove water pan, shelves, and brackets and place in Support Lab sink.
4. Prepare a dilute solution of Roccal II (5 ml/l Milli-Q water)
5. Using rubber gloves and a sterile laparoscopy sponge, disinfect all interior surfaces of the incubator, the CO_2 sensor, and the blower wheel with dilute Roccal II.
6. Using fresh Milli-Q water and a fresh laparoscopy sponge each time, rinse all surfaces three times. Dry interior with a fresh laparoscopy sponge.
7. At the sink, scrub all shelves, water pan, and brackets with dilute Roccal II using a lap sponge. Rinse each piece with (1) tap water; (2) deionized water; and (3) Milli-Q water.
8. Heat sterilize shelves, water pan and brackets in the Support Lab sterilizing oven (2 h at 120°C).
9. When the incubator parts have cooled, reassemble in the incubator.
10. Fill the pan with Milli-Q water and change water every week.
11. Re-equilibrate the CO_2 as per the users manual and set the temperature to 37°C.

D. FYRITE MEASUREMENT OF INCUBATOR CO_2

The incubator CO_2 level should be checked weekly using an independent measurement. This can be accomplished using a Fyrite CO_2 Monitoring Kit.

1. Holding the unit upright and away from one's face, depress the plunger at the top to vent gases. With the plunger intact, invert the unit to drain the Fyrite solution into the top of the unit.
2. Return the unit to the upright position and allow the solution to drain to the bottom.
3. Loosen the lock nut retaining the sliding scale and move the scale such that the "O" aligns with the meniscus of the Fyrite solution. Tighten the lock nut. The unit is now zeroed.
4. Attach the open end of the rubber gas sampler hose to the sample port on the incubator. Pump the aspirator bulb approximately ten times to clear the line of residual gas.
5. Place the connector end of the tubing over the Fyrite plunger valve, depress the valve with the connector, and pump the aspirator bulb 18 times thus moving incubator air into the unit.
6. Release the connector end of the tubing and release the Fyrite plunger valve.
7. Invert the Fyrite unit allowing the soloution to enter the top of the unit, then right the unit allow solution to enter the bottom. Repeat one time.
8. Holding the unit upright, allow the solution to stabilize. Read the percent CO_2 from the scale zeroed earlier. Repeat the process to verify the initial measurement.

E. CLEANING AND STERILIZING TRANSFER CATHETERS AND LAPAROSCOPY NEEDLES

IVF and GIFT transfer catheters, guides, and laparoscopy needles are reused until there is evidence of wear or they become difficult to clean. Transvaginal retrieval needles are disposable. All cleaning and sterilization is performed in the Support Lab. After cleaning, the catheters are examined under the dissecting microscope for discoloration, damage, and/ or build up of any foreign material. If warranted, the catheters are discarded. Laparoscopy needles are discarded if they become dull.

1. As soon as possible after use, catheters, guides, and needles are connected to the Milli-Q water supply and rinsed under pressure for 5 min.
2. Catheters etc. are immersed in Milli-Q water contained in a bath-type ultrasonic cleaner (Branson #5200) and flushed with a syringe containing Milli-Q water. The catheters are cleaned for 2 to 3 h.

3. Each item is rinsed as in step 1 and dried by introducing 0.22 micron-filtered air through it.
4. Each catheter etc. is placed in 4 × 22 in. Optipeel sterilization tubing (Baxter #97004), double-heat sealed, and the excess packaging trimmed away (leave ~0.5 in. of pouch above seal). Heat sterilization tape is placed in the package.
5. This package is in turn placed in a 6 inch Optipeel sterilization tubing (Baxter #97006), double-heat sealed, trimmed of excess packaging, and heat tape placed on the outer package.
6. Place the double-wrapped packages in the sterilizing oven and sterilize 2 to 4 h (125°C).
7. Remove and transfer to the embryo lab.

F. PREPARATION OF EMBRYO TRANSFER PIPETTES

Fifteen to eighteen hours post insemination of oocytes, the oocytes must be examined for the presence of pronuclei. The oocytes are often located on the bottom of the culture dish surround by cumulus cells which have begun to attach and spread. It is necessary to free the oocyte in order to adequately assess fertilization and identify polypronuclear eggs. This is accomplished by using finely drawn, fire polished pasteur pipettes. These can be made at widely varying diameters for use in teasing the cumulus cells away from the oocytes. Additionally, these ''micropipettes'' are extremely useful for embryo manipulation such as routine movement from dish to dish and during cryopreservation. They are prepared as follows:

1. Standard 9″ borosilicate pipettes are used.
2. Quantities of these are placed in 2 liter beakers and washed extensively in Milli-Q water.
3. Washed pipettes are loaded into metal sterilizing cans with sterile gauze in the bottom and heat sterilized (2 to 4 h at 125°C).
4. Twenty-four hours prior to use, finely drawn, hand-made pipettes are made.
5. Individual pipettes are heated using a bunsen or propane burner at the point where the pipette begins to narrow and while rotating the pipette. When the glass become male-able, the pipette is drawn apart in a linear fashion. The longer the draw, the narrower the diameter of the pipette.
6. The tip of each pipette is fire polished by rapidly thrusting the tip of the pipette into the flame. After each thrust, the tip is examined under the dissecting microscope to ensure that there are no jagged or sharp edges which could damage oocytes or embryos.
7. Acceptable pipettes are placed inverted in a test tube rack and placed in the laminar flow console under UV light until used.
8. Fifteen to twenty pipettes having many different diameters are made.

ACKNOWLEDGMENTS

The authors wish to acknowledge the Department of Obstetrics and Gynecology, the University of Kansas School of Medicine-Wichita, and HCA/Wesley Hospital for establishing and maintaining a quality IVF/ET facility. The authors wish to acknowledge the Wesley Foundation, Wichita, KS, for its support of the Women's Research Institute. This facilitates intellectual and scientific support for clinical programs of the Department of Obstetrics and Gynecology such as In Vitro Fertilization. Finally, the authors wish to thank Charles A. Torbit, Ph.D. for his instructional assistance in learning IVF-related procedures and his contribution in designing the IVF/ET laboratory.

REFERENCES

1. **Danforth, R. A., Piana, S. D., and Smith, M.,** High purity water: an important component for success in in vitro fertilization, *Am. Biotech. Lab.,* 5, 58, 1987.
2. **Jones, H. W., Jones, G. S., Andrews, M. C., Acosta, A., Bundren, C., Garcia, J., Sandow, B., Veeck, L., Wilkes, C., Witmyer, J., Wortham, J. E., and Wright, G.,** The program for in vitro fertilization at Norfolk, *Fertil. Steril.,* 38, 14, 1982.
3. **Quinn, P., Warner, G. M., Klein, J. F., and Kirby, C.,** Culture factors affecting the success rate of in vitro fertilization and embryo transfer, *Ann. N.Y. Acad. Sci.,* 442, 195, 1985.
4. **Lopata, A., Johnston, I. W. H., Hoult, I. J., and Speins, A. L.,** Pregnancy following intrauterine implantation of an embryo obtained by in vitro fertilization of a preovulatory egg, *Fertil. Steril.,* 33, 117, 1980.
5. **Purdy, J. M.,** Methods for fertilization and embryo culture in vitro, in *Human Conception In Vitro,* Edwards, R. G. and Purdy, J. M., Eds., Academic Press, London, 1983, 135.
6. **Wood, C. and Kovacs, G.,** Extracorporeal fertilization, in *Progress in Obstetrics and Gynecology,* Vol. 3, Studd, J., Ed., Churchill Livingstone, London, 1983, 267.
7. **Trounson, A. O., Teeton, J. F., Wood, C., Webb, J., and Kovacs, G.,** The investigation of idiopathic infertility by in vitro fertilization, *Fertil. Steril.,* 34, 432, 1980.
8. **Trounson, A. O.,** In vitro fertilization and embryo preservation, in *In Vitro Fertilization and Embryo Transfer,* Trounson, A. V. and Wood, C., Eds., Churchill Livingstone, London, 1984, 111.
9. **Mahadevan, M. M., Fleetham, J., Church, R. B., and Taylor, P. J.,** Growth of mouse embryos in bicarbonate media buffered by carbon dioxide, hepes, and phosphate, *J. In Vitro Fertil. Embryo Trans.,* 3, 304, 1986.
10. **Leung, P. C. S., Gronow, M. J., Kellow, G. N., Lopata, A., Speirs, A. L., McBain, J. C., du Plersis, Y. P., and Johnston, I.,** Serum supplement in human in vitro fertilization and embryo development, *Fertil. Steril.,* 41, 36, 1984.
11. **Menezo, Y., Testart, J., and Perrone, D.,** Serum is not necessary in human in vitro fertilization, early embryo culture, and transfer, *Fertil. Steril.,* 42, 750, 1984.
12. **Kruger, T. F., Stander, F. S. H., Smith, K., Van Der Merue, J. P., and Lombard, C. J.,** The effect of serum supplementation on the cleavage of human embryos, *J. In Vitro Fertil. Embryo Trans.,* 4, 10, 1987.
13. **Caro, C. M. and Trounson, A.,** Successful fertilization, embryo development, and pregnancy in human in vitro fertilization (IVF) using a chemically defined culture medium containing no protein, *J. In Vitro Fertil. Embryo Trans.,* 3, 215, 1986.
14. **Davidson, A., Vermesh, M., Lobo, R. A., and Paulsen, R. J.,** Mouse embryo culture as quality control for human in vitro fertilization: the one-cell versus two-cell model, *Fertil. Steril.,* 49, 516, 1988.
15. **Fleming, T. P., Pratt, H. P. M., and Braude, P. R.,** The use of mouse preimplantation embryos for quality control of culture reagents in human in vitro fertilization programs: a cautionary note, *Fertil. Steril.,* 47, 858, 1987.
16. **Friedler, S., Giudice, L. C., and Lamb, E. J.,** Cryopreservation of embryos and ova, *Fertil. Steril.,* 49, 743, 1988.
17. **Quinn, P.,** Cryoprotectants and media for cooling cells, *Proc. Freezing Embryos — A Hands-On Course in Laboratory Technique,* Soules, M. R., (Chmn.), July 23—25 (1987), Seattle, WA, published by The American Fertility Society.
18. **Lassalle, B., Testart, J., and Renard, J.-P.,** Human embryo features that influence the success of cryopreservation with the use of 1,2 propanediol, *Fertil. Steril.,* 44, 645, 1985.
19. **Renard, J.-P., Nguyen, B.-X., and Garnier, V.,** Two-step freezing of two-cell rabbit embryos after partial dehydration at room temperature, *J. Reprod. Fertil.,* 71, 573, 1984.
20. **Testart, J., Lassalle, B., Belaisch-Allart, J., Hazout, A., Forman, R., Rainhorn, J. D., and Frydman, R.,** High pregnancy rate after early human embryo freezing, *Fertil. Steril.,* 46, 268, 1986.
21. Medical Research International and the Society of Assisted Reproductive Technology, The American Fertility Society. In vitro fertilization/embryo transfer in the United States: 1987 results from the National IVF-ET Registry, *Fertil. Steril.,* 51, 13, 1989.

Chapter 17

MOUSE PRE-EMBRYO CULTURE AS AN EVALUATION FOR HUMAN PRE-EMBRYO REQUIREMENTS

William E. Findley and William E. Gibbons

TABLE OF CONTENTS

INTRODUCTION

Among the various causes of infertility are those conditions which may prevent (a) the formation of a zygote from viable gametes (i.e., fertilization), (b) the continued development of zygotes to blastocysts capable of implantation and (c) the transport of the developing pre-embryo to the uterus. The *in vitro* culture of preimplantation mouse pre-embryos has been used both in the diagnosis and, to a larger extent, in the treatment of infertility arising from such conditions in the human. With respect to the diagnosis of potential *in vivo* inhibitors of pre-embryo development, embryotoxic effects have been noted when two-cell mouse pre-embryos[1] were cultured in the presence of substances such as peritoneal fluid from patients with endometriosis,[2,3] the supernatant from cultures of peritoneal fluid leukocytes from women with endometriosis,[4] and the psychoactive ingredient of marijuana.[5] With respect to treatment, infertility due to suboptimal fertilization or impaired pre-embryo transport to the uterus may be alleviated with *in vitro* fertilization (IVF), and when at least one fallopian tube is functional, associated procedures such as zygote intrafallopian transfer (ZIFT) and gamete intrafallopian transfer (GIFT). All such procedures require the short term (0.5 to 12 + h) culture of gametes while the first two also require the culture of the pre-embryos. Consequently, it is necessary to evaluate the culture conditions for their ability to support fertilization and continued embryonic development. As described by Edwards et al.[6] in 1980, the first technique to be used for such evaluations was the culture of washed human spermatozoa for 3 days. If the motility was maintained during this period, the medium was judged suitable for use with IVF. However, with the large increase in the number of IVF programs after Steptoe and Edwards' initial report in 1978, the use of mouse pre-embryo cultures has become the primary technique for evaluating the culture conditions.

This chapter describes the use of mouse pre-embryo culture as an evaluation of culture conditions for human IVF and related assisted reproductive technologies. A brief description of the various assays and the results obtained with their use is presented in the first section. The second section contains a detailed description of the assay based on the blastulation of mouse zygotes. The third and final section includes a discussion of the various factors, including assay conditions and equipment, which may effect the results of such assays.

II. EVALUATIONS USING THE CULTURE OF MOUSE PRE-EMBRYOS

A. EVALUATIONS BASED ON THE CULTURE OF TWO-CELL MOUSE PRE-EMBRYOS

Although some groups used *in vitro* fertilization of mouse eggs for evaluating culture conditions, the results tended to be quite variable even within the same strain. In addition, less than 50% of the resulting zygotes progressed past the four-cell stage.[8] Consequently, the continued development of two-cell mouse pre-embryos to the blastocyst stage became the most widely used quality control parameter.[8,10] Such pre-embryos are easily obtained by flushing the oviducts of superovulated mice approximately 34 to 40 h after mating. In addition, well over 50% of two-cell pre-embryos derived from any of several hybrid matings (F_1 offspring) will develop to blastocysts within 72 h.

Given its relative ease of performance along with its fairly reproducible results, the two-cell mouse assay has been widely used to evaluate a number of components used for IVF and related procedures. Items known to be toxic to two-cell mouse pre-embryos and, therefore, presumably to human pre-embryos, include several types of gloves,[11,12] ultrasound coupling gels,[13] some types of catheters,[14,15] serum exposed to several types of blood collection tubes,[10] and the anesthetic Lidocaine.[16,17] By far, the most common use of the assay is for the evaluation of culture media to be used for human IVF-related procedures.[11,18] The quality of the water used to prepare media has been extensively examined. In 1971 Whittingham[19] reported that three-times glass-distilled water resulted in the highest blastulation rate of two-cell mouse embryos. Although others have similarly discussed the importance of water, Fukuda et al.[20] were the first to correlate the chemical composition of several sources of water with mouse embryogenesis in media containing such water. Blastulation rates increased with the reduction of hydrophilic organic compounds with the best results being obtained with Milli-Q water (Nihon Millipore Ltd., Tokyo, Japan, marketed in the U.S. by Millipore Corporation, Bedford, MA). However, Silverman et al.[22] have a lack of sensitivity with a similar two-cell assay. In their study, identical blastulation rates were observed for two-cell mouse pre-embryos cultured in medium constituted with either highly purified water or untreated tap water.

Other media components have also been evaluated with the two-cell mouse culture system. Heparin is often included in the media which is added to follicular aspirates to prevent clotting. In 1984, (after several years of routine use) heparin was shown to exert no inhibition of the blastulation of two-cell pre-embryos even at doses several fold higher than that used to inhibit clotting in follicular aspirates.[22] More recently a parallel lack of effect has been confirmed for human IVF.[23]

Most IVF and related programs add a protein supplement to the medium. The two-cell mouse assay has been widely used to evaluate the potentially embryotropic response to such supplements. Saito et al.[18] reported that a minimum of 10% fetal cord serum resulted in the highest rate of blastulation of two-cell mouse embryos. Others, however, have noted that human serum proteins inhibit mouse embryogenesis. Caro and Trounson[24] reported that fewer two-cell mouse pre-embryos developed to blastocysts when cultured in the presence of human serum or purified human serum albumin compared to those cultured in the presence of fetal calf serum or bovine serum albumin (BSA) or in medium containing no protein supplement. We (unpublished data) and others[25,26] have also observed inhibition of mouse embryogenesis by human serum including that collected from patients one day prior to IVF. However, in these studies no correlation was observed between the ability of serum to support mouse blastulation and its ability to support human embryogenesis in associated IVF procedures.

B. EVALUATIONS BASED ON THE CULTURE OF MOUSE ZYGOTES

The lack of correlation between the two-cell mouse assay and human IVF results has also been noted by us and others.[27] Consequently, the culture of one-cell zygotes has been examined as a more sensitive assay. Compared to two-cell pre-embryos, mouse zygotes are known to have more stringent growth requirements. For an energy source they primarily utilize pyruvate and, to a lesser extent, oxaloacetate.[28] In addition, optimal development occurs within a relatively narrow concentration range of pyruvate.[29] In contrast, two-cell pre-embryos are able to utilize lactate, pyruvate, phosphoenol pyruvate and oxaloacetate.[30] Likewise, optimum development occurs at a more restricted oxygen concentration of approximately 5% and at an osmolality between approximately 250 and 280 mOsm.[29] It has also been reported that zygotes are more sensitive to the absence of fatty acids than are two-cell pre-embryos.[31] More recently, Davidson et al.[32] performed simultaneous cultures of one- and two-cell pre-embryos under various culture conditions and noted a greater sensitivity of the one-cell zygotes to suboptimal conditions. Specifically, the rate of development of the zygotes, compared to that of the two-cell pre-embryos, was inhibited by smaller deviations of pH and osmolality from optimum and also by more dilute concentrations of the sterilizing solution, Cidex.

The first extensive evaluation of human IVF conditions using the development of mouse zygotes was made by Quinn et al.[15] These authors reported that the continued development of zygotes was inhibited by exposure to such items as unrinsed Tomcat catheters and pipettes.

TABLE 1
Development of Zygotes in an Atmosphere Containing 5% O_2
without and with an Initial 1-H Exposure to 20% O_2

Culture atmosphere	Morulae (at 72 h)	Blastocysts (at 96 h)	Blastocysts (at 120 h)
Continuous 5% O_2	80%	56%	71%
Initial 1 h, 20% O_2 followed by continuous 5% O_2	58%	36%	44%

Note: Early zygotes were cultured continuously in 5% CO_2 at 37°C for 120 h. In one group (n = 145) the atmosphere also contained 5% O_2 for the entire culture period. In the other group (n = 113), the atmosphere contained 20% O_2 for the first hour and then 5% O_2 for the remainder of the culture period. The differences between the two groups were significant at all times examined (*p* <0.005).

Adapted from Pabon, J. E., Jr., Findley, W. E., and Gibbons, W. E., *Fertil. Steril.*, 51, 896, 1989.

However, there was no correlation observed between the mouse blastulation rates in the various batches of medium and the pregnancy rate in the IVF patients for which the respective batches were used. It should be noted, however, that of 30 batches of medium tested, only 2 supported a blastulation rate of less than 60%. In a later study, however, these authors did observe a correlation between mouse zygote blastulation and pregnancy in an associated human IVF program. The zygote culture assay was used to evalutate two different culture media, one of which supported a statistically greater blastulation rate of mouse zygotes. This same medium was also associated with a three-fold greater pregnancy rate (33 vs. 11%).[33]

The presence of a protein source such as serum or albumin can mask potential insufficiencies of culture media. Serum contains a variety of hormones and growth factors which may possibly influence embryogenesis.[2,24-26] Moreover, albumin alone may be contaminated with embryotropic substances.[34,35] We therefore initiated studies on completely defined, protein-free media for the culture of pre-embryos. After confirming that two-cell pre-embryos could blastulate *in vitro* equally well in the presence and absence of any added protein,[2,22] we initiated cultures of zygotes in the same protein-free medium. A retrospective analysis was performed on ten batches of culture medium which had been used for the culture of 132 IVF zygotes obtained from 31 patients. These batches had all passed our quality control, then in use, by supporting the blastulation of at least 75% of two-cell mouse pre-embryos within 72 h of culture. The results indicated that (1) the blastulation rate of mouse zygotes, but not that of the two-cell pre-embryos, was correlated with the quality (number of cells and grade) of the human pre-embryos cultured in the same batch of media, and (2) none of the 13 pregnancies occurred with media having a zygote blastulation rate (ZBR) of less than 46% (n = 6) with only one occurring with media having a ZBR of less than 58% (n = 14).[36]

The results discussed above indicate that, compared to the two-cell embryo culture assay, the blastulation of zygotes, especially in the absence of added protein, is a much more sensitive test for suboptimal culture conditions. In further support of this, we have observed that, unlike two-cell mouse pre-embryos, mouse zygotes are adversely affected by media exposed to light[37] and even short durations of atmospheric oxygen concentrations (Table 1).[38] Thus, the ability of culture conditions, including the culture medium, to support the blastulation of early mouse zygotes appears to be a necessary (but, of course, not sufficient) condition for successful human IVF and pre-embryo development.

III. DESCRIPTION OF THE ZYGOTE CULTURE ASSAY

The following is a description of the techniques used for the mouse zygote culture assay including the superovulation of the mice, the collection of the zygotes, the culture of zygotes, and the evaluation of their development.

A. SUPEROVULATION AND COLLECTION OF ZYGOTES

Day 1 — Inject sexually mature female mice (donors) with 10 IU pregnant mare serum gonadotropin (PMSG) intraperitoneally (i.p.) within 1 to 2 h preceeding the time the lights turn off.

Day 3 — Inject donors with 10 IU human chorionic gonadotropin (hCG) i.p. 30 to 60 min before the lights turn off. Thirty minutes later, transfer each donor to a cage containing a cage-conditioned male. Prepare culture dishes and leave in the incubator overnight. The incubator should be equilibrated with an atmosphere of 5% CO_2 and 5 to 7% O_2 at 37°C.

Day 4 — Examine the donor for the presence of a vaginal plug to confirm that mating has occurred. (The lack of a plug, especially at later times, may be observed in females which have, in fact, mated.) Sacrifice the donor within 14 to 17 h after the time the lights have turned off on the previous day. Swab the ventral and lateral surfaces with alcohol. This not only sterilizes the area to be opened but also prevents loose hair from entering the abdominal cavity. Open the abdominal cavity by grasping the ventral skin with a pair of forceps and, beginning at the midline, cut through the body wall laterally from a point approximately two thirds of the distance from the sternum to the vaginal orifice. Continue to cut in an anterior direction of both sides to a point adjacent to the rib cage. Then, still holding the skin fold with the forceps, pull the resulting flap anteriorly folding it over onto the body over the sternum. It should remain there if both surfaces are moist and the lateral cuts were extended sufficiently to the anterior.

Using forceps, pull the intestines out of the body cavity to an anterior position. With small forceps grasp the anterior end of a uterine horn about 1 to 2 mm from its junction with the oviduct. Lifting up on the uterus will reveal the mesosalpinx which should be trimmed to release the grasped portion of the uterus and the attached oviduct. By gently pulling up on the uterus, the oviduct will be slightly separated from the ovary. Completely sever it from the ovary by slipping the open points of small scissors around its juncture with the ovary and, gently pressing on the ovary, cutting the bursa. (See Figure 1.) The uterus is then also severed on the other side of the forceps and the resulting oviduct with the tip of the uterus attached is placed in a 35 mm culture dish containing 2 ml of equilibrated media. The other oviduct is collected in a similar manner and the dish is taken to a dissecting microscope.

At this time, any remaining fat may be trimmed off by using jewelers forceps and iridectomy scissors. The zygotes enclosed in cumulus can be observed in the swollen ampulla of the oviduct (Figure 2). The oviduct is then transferred to another 35 mm dish freshly removed from the incubator. The ampulla is cut or torn open at which time the cumulus mass will be extruded (Figure 3). If some still remains in the oviduct it can be easily expelled by gently sliding the tip of the scissors over the oviduct forcing the cumulus mass out the opening.

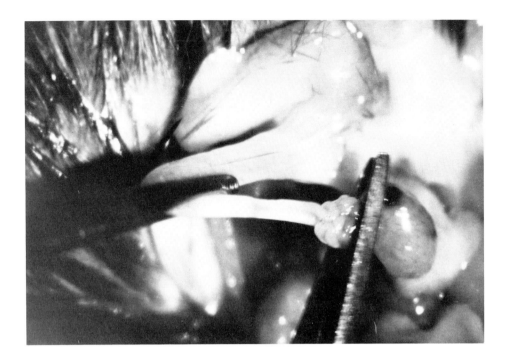

FIGURE 1.   Separation of the coiled oviduct from the mouse ovary. Note the stigmata where an ovulation has occurred at the top of the ovary, just below the tips of the scissors. (Magnification × 10.6.)

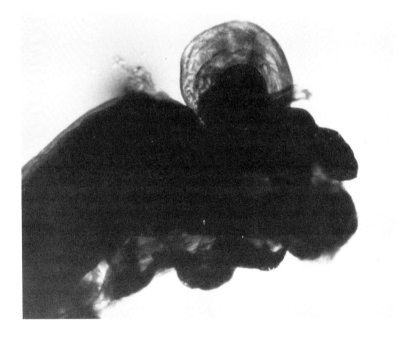

FIGURE 2.   Swollen ampulla viewed with transmitted light through a dissecting microscope (Nikon SMZ-10). The cumulus-enclosed zygotes appear as dark masses filling the center two-thirds of the translucent ampulla. The tightly coiled oviduct is still closely attached to the tip of the uterus which extends from the center to the lower left. (Magnification × 48.)

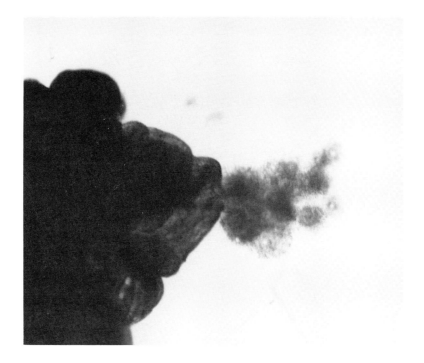

FIGURE 3.   Mass of cumulus-enclosed zygotes extruded from the ampulla of the oviduct immediately after the ampulla has been punctured. (Transmitted light, magnification × 48.)

The mass may be divided into smaller groups of cumulus-enclosed zygotes by gently teasing apart the cumulus. Such separations are facilitated by partially dispersing the mass and then allowing the dish to stand in the incubator 10 to 15 min. During this time, the cumulus enclosed zygotes will often become completely separated from each other (Figure 4).

For the routine evaluation of culture media, at least 15 zygotes from each of two donors are cultured in separate dishes.

B. CULTURE OF ZYGOTES

As stated above, all culture dishes should be incubated overnight to equilibrate with the atmosphere in the incubator. An alternative to this is bubbling a mixture of 5% CO_2, 5% O_2, 90% N_2 through the medium. It is necessary to first humidify such a gas by bubbling it through purified water (e.g., in a side arm flask), followed by a 0.2 μm filter. Otherwise, the osmolality will rise as the medium evaporates. The duration of this bubbling will depend on the flow rate and the volume of medium and will have to be determined experimentally. A minimum duration for the displacement of sufficient amounts of oxygen is probably about twice as long as the time required to add sufficient CO_2 to lower the pH to 7.4.

The zygotes are transferred to the appropriate culture dishes by carefully drawing them into a drawn-out pasteur pipette. It is important to have a column of medium extending at least 10 mm into the tip before drawing any zygotes into the pipette. This will help prevent the cumulus masses from sticking to the meniscus and to the walls of the pipette when no protein is present in the medium. Such losses are also minimized by transferring only a few zygotes at a time in a minimum volume so that they do not have time to rest on the edge of the pipette and adhere.

Only cumulus-enclosed presumptive zygotes should be used. The occasional oocytes

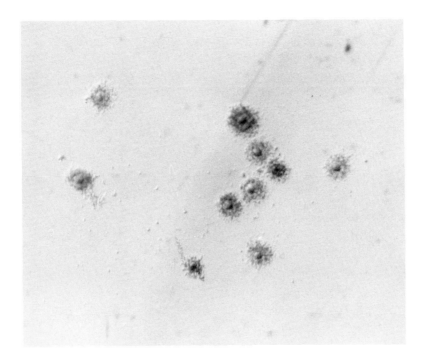

FIGURE 4.   Cumulus-enclosed zygotes viewed as in Figure 2. The individual zygotes have dispersed from the mass shown in Figure 3 after a 15 min incubation in the incubator as described in the text. (Transmitted light, magnification × 48.)

without a cumulus at these early times are seldom fertilized. It has also been noted that tightly enclosed cumulus masses, especially those which do not tend to separate after the 15 min incubation described above, are often not fertilized.

After 24 h of culture, the number of two-cell pre-embryos in each dish is counted. Given that an occasional unfertilized oocyte will be transferred to a dish, this number, which is generally 80 to 100% of the number of presumptive zygotes originally placed in the dish, is assumed to be the actual number of zygotes. At this time, most, if not all, of the cumulus cells will have been dispersed from the pre-embryo (Figure 5). If desired, any remaining cumulus cells may be removed from the zona pellucida by repeated aspiration with a pasteur pipette (Figure 6). An oocyte-cumulus-complex which has not been exposed to sperm will often be largely intact at this time.

The cultures may be examined after 48 and 72 h of culture for differences in rates of development, especially in experimental protocols. However, after 96 and 120 h of culture the number and stage of the pre-embryos is evaluated for all cultures.

C. EVALUATION OF RESULTS

For the quality control of culture media for IVF, our program requires that each individual batch of medium support the blastulation of greater than 60% of the zygotes in the absence of any added protein (e.g., serum or albumin) or other macromolecules (e.g., polyvinyl-pyrrolidone). Although this endpoint may be reached by 96 h of culture, more often less than 50% have formed blastocysts by this time. Consequently, the cultures are often continued through 120 h (5 days). Examples of early and late blastocysts are shown in Figure 7. Those with a thin layer of cells around the periphery and a larger diameter are the mature (late) expanded blastocysts, some of which are beginning to hatch as indicated by the small blebs on their surfaces.

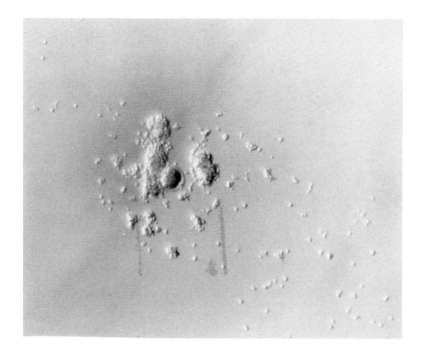

FIGURE 5.   A two-cell pre-embryo collected as a cumulus-enclosed zygote 24 h earlier. The individual blastomeres are arranged with the one toward the bottom of the photograph covering approximately $^2/_3$ of the other. The cumulus cells have detached from most of the surface of the zona pellucida and have begun to plate out on the surface of the dish. (Transmitted light, magnification × 128.)

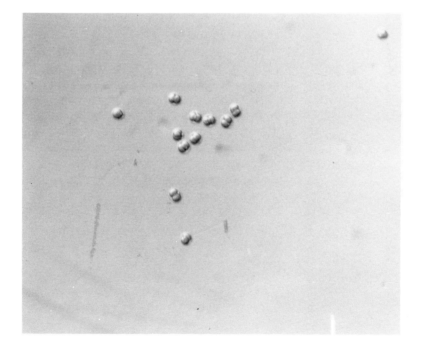

FIGURE 6.   Two cell pre-embryos. A polar body can be seen at the right juncture of the two blastomeres of the pre-embryo located between the main group of eight and the lower most pre-embryo. (Transmitted light, magnification × 64.)

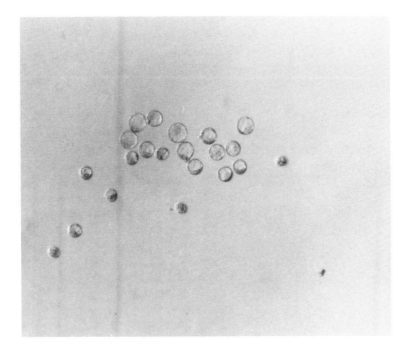

FIGURE 7.   Blastocysts developed from zygotes after 120 h of culture. The less mature blastocysts are generally located more toward the bottom of the photograph. Notice the smaller diameter, and smaller incomplete blastocoel in these compared to the more mature expanding blastocysts located toward the upper portion of the photograph. Some of the expanded blastocysts have small blebs indicating they are beginning to hatch from their zonae pellucidae. (Transmitted light, magnification × 64.)

IV. FACTORS INFLUENCING THE RESULTS OF THE ASSAY

Other authors have reported the use of other assay conditions and endpoints but these are generally less stringent and, as previously discussed, have been reported to not correlate well with the results in associated human IVF programs.

A. PROTEIN SUPPLEMENTATION OF MEDIA

The most common variation from the protocol described above is the addition of a protein source, usually albumin, to the medium.[15,20,32,39] Such additives facilitate the manipulation of the embryos by preventing the sticky cumulus masses from adhering to the pipettes or dishes from which they are transferred during the initiation of the culture. However, as discussed above, the addition of albumin or serum may mask insufficiencies in the medium itself, and albumin, as well as serum, may be embryotropic. In keeping with these observations, the blastulation rate of zygotes has been reported to be higher in media containing protein than in protein-free media.[40]

B. DONORS AND SUPEROVULATION

It has often been observed that embryos from different strains of mice develop at different rates and to different stages. Jackson and Kiessling[39] have reported that such differences are a primary factor in determining the rate of development of zygotes exposed to different culture media and conditions. Thus, the actual blastulation rates will depend on the strain of mouse used and comparisons with the work of others should take this factor into account.

Another important factor influencing the quantity and quality of the zygotes is the gonadotropin used to stimulate superovulation. Although most investigators use PMSG for the stimulation of increased follicular development, the source and the dose are known to have an influence on the the outcome. The most widely used preparation in the U.S. is the PMSG obtained from Sigma (St. Louis, MO). Using this preparation, we have had consistent ovarian stimulation with respect to the number of viable zygotes produced by sexually mature donors.

The dose of PMSG reported by the groups using Sigma PMSG has ranged from 5 to 10 IU for superovulation of both immature and mature mice. The upper portion of this range has generally been reserved for older, sexually mature mice.[2,10,12,18,21,25,32,41] If low numbers of zygotes/oocytes are consistently retrieved, a dose-response curve should be generated with at least two mice per dose per stimulation with at least two stimulations performed at least 1 week apart and with doses differing by 5 IU. The source and dose of hCG is much less critical with 5 to 10 IU being the range administered by most investigators. At this time we are not aware of any commercial source of hCG having been reported to be unsatisfactory.

The housing conditions of the mice should also be examined. In addition to irregular light cycles and poor temperature control, the presence of certain insecticides and the use of some cleaning agents will reduce the mating efficiency and the ability of the pre-embryos to develop.[41] The sensitivity of the assay may also be influenced by the time of sacrifice of the animal. During some of our preliminary studies on oxidative damage, it was observed that zygotes collected later in the day tended to be less sensitive to suboptimal culture condition. Therefore for maximum sensitivity, zygotes are collected within 14 to 17 h after the lights go off.

C. INCUBATORS

The choice of the incubation system is much more important for the growth of zygotes than it is for the growth of two-cell pre-embryos. As previously described, few mouse zygotes (from most strains) will form blastocysts when cultured continuously in atmospheric oxygen concentrations.[29,38,42] We have extended these observations to short exposures as might be encountered in an IVF laboratory.[38] As shown in Table 1, under the culture conditions used in our laboratory, an exposure of mouse zygotes to as little as 1 h of atmospheric oxygen (20%) results in reduced numbers of morulae as well as a reduced number of blastocysts.

A partial exception to these observations are those of Ogawa and Marrs[40] who reported a zygote blastulation rate exceeding 70% in an atmosphere of 5% CO_2 in air. Their system will be interesting to study with respect to oxygen toxicity in that the culture medium (TYH-280 containing BSA) and the strain of mouse ($B_6 C_3 F_1$ hybrid) were different from those used in previous studies of this phenomenon. Likewise, their data indicated that the relatively high concentration of BSA (8 mg/ml) had a protective effect. If the initial culture was carried out in the absence of BSA, the blastulation rate was greatly reduced.

Therefore, for the culture of mouse zygotes, particularly in protein-free medium, the incubation system should have an atmosphere with a reduced oxygen concentration, generally 5 to 7%. Incubators which control only CO_2 may be adapted to this system by placing a gas-tight container in the interior into which is introduced a premixed source of gas containing 5% CO_2, 5% O_2, and 90% N_2. This gas must first be humidified by bubbling it through a flask containing water. This is best done with the flask in the incubator so that the gas is warmed before entering the chamber. If the chamber has an exit port and the gas is turned off after the chamber is judged to be equilibrated, the port should have a piece of tubing attached to it with the other end submerged in a beaker of water. This will prevent the incubator's atmosphere from entering the chamber. Chambers which have been used for culturing embryos include dessicators and the Modular Incubator Chamber produced by Billups-Rothenberg (Del Mar, CA). The latter device is particularly useful in that it has two hose connectors on the base, three stacking trays in its interior, and an easily removed lid which is clamped tightly when closed.

Incubators which control the O_2 concentration are available from a number of manufactures. The gas control is generally by one of two systems. One system maintains a given O_2 concentration by proportioning the amount of O_2 and/or N_2 which is injected into the system to replace the O_2 from the atmosphere. In these systems there is either a continuous, low volume flow or a timed, intermittent pulse of gas. In either case the proper gas concentration must be set by trial and error although rough approximations of the settings are usually supplied by manufacturer. Purging the system after a door opening is generally accomplished by an increased flow of N_2 and CO_2 of a preset duration.

The second type of gas control involves the actual measurement of the oxygen concentration and an injection of N_2 when such a measurement indicates the need to reduce the oxygen concentration to a preset value. This type of system is more accurate in its control especially following a purge. (The gas content of the incubator should be frequently confirmed with a Fyrite or similar instrument as some detectors will drift.) The feedback system also has the advantage of using less gas. In addition to being more economical, this system will tend to have less evaporation of the culture media because less dry gas is introduced to the system.

The humidification of the atmosphere is much more important when culturing zygotes for 4 to 5 days than when culturing two-cell pre-embryos for 3 days or human pre-embryos for 1 to 2 days before changing the medium. A slow evaporation of the medium may become quite significant after only 3 days in some types of incubators. This will lead to reduced blastulation rates which are independent of the initial quality of the culture medium. Some types of incubators have a passive evaporative humidification system which relies on water evaporating from a reservoir on the floor of the incubator. Following a purge in which a large amount (approximately 2 incubator volumes) of absolutely dry N_2 and CO_2 is introduced to the chamber atmosphere, a significant amount of evaporation will take place, especially at 37°C. Other manufacturers use some form of active humidification in which the gases are bubbled through the water reservoir as they enter the chamber (semiactive system) or in which the humidity is actually controlled with a sensor which causes water vapor to be injected when the humidity falls below a setpoint (active system).

The effects of an evaporative and a semi-active system on the osmolality of medium in two types of culture dishes are shown in Figure 8. With the evaporative humidification (Figure 8A), osmolalities may exceed 300 mOsm by day 3 of incubation. Development of zygotes in our system is adversely affected by osmolalities of 300 mOsm or greater. This limit for hyperosmolality has also been observed by Davidson et al.[32] using the same culture medium but which also contained albumin. Therefore, pre-embryos cultured in an evaporative humidification system must be maintained in a vessel which minimizes evaporation. As shown in Figure 8, the Falcon 3037 culture dish is effective in reducing evaporation from the culture chamber, due to the moat which surrounds the center well containing the pre-embryos. If petri dishes or other containers with a large surface to volume ratio are used, the surface may be overlaid with paraffin oil as described by Purdy.[43] It should be emphasized that the increases in osmolality shown in Figure 8 are the minimum to be expected because the door to the incubator was only opened once each day. As discussed above, more frequent door openings will introduce more dry gas with each purge.

The semiactive humidification system, Figure 8B, maintains safe levels of osmolalities in both types of culture dishes until day 5. Gas introduced during the purge is at least partially, if not completely, saturated with water. Therefore, unlike the evaporative system, more frequent door openings probably do not cause a further increase in the osmolality in this system.

The above discussion indicates that if mouse zygotes fail to blastulate sufficiently, there

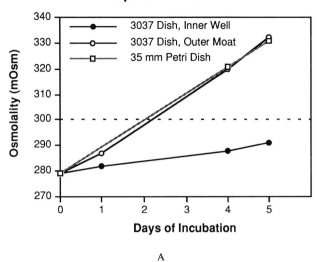

Evaporative Humidification

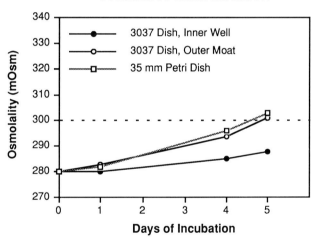

Semiactive Humidification

B

FIGURE 8. Effect of incubator humidification system on the osmolality during a 5 day incubation. The dotted line extending from 300 mOsm indicates the osmolality below which mouse pre-embryos must be maintained for optimal development. On day 0 six 35 mm petri dishes and each chamber of six Falcon 3037 mm culture dishes were filled with 2.0 ml of modified Ham's F-10 with no added protein. Three of each type of dish were placed in one of the incubators. At the times indicated, one of each dish was removed from each incubator and the osmolality determined on a freezing point depression osmometer.

are two factors associated with the incubator which should be examined. First, the total duration of exposure to high O_2 concentrations should be determined. If the incubator does not have an O_2 sensor and associated display, a Fyrite (Bacharach, Inc., Pittsburgh, PA) may be used to measure the O_2 concentrations at various intervals after the door is closed. Second, the osmolality of the medium should be measured on the last day of culture to determine if it is still under 300 mOsm.

D. MEDIA

Several media used for human IVF have been simultaneously evaluated using mouse zygote blastulation. Quinn et al.[15] used a modified Tyrode's solution which supported at least 60% blastulation in 28 batches in the presence of 5 mg/ml BSA. Although they observed no correlation with the quality of the human pre-embryos or pregnancy after IVF, there were no pregnancies in the patients whose embryos were cultured in the two batches with less than 39% blastulation (N = 8).

A medium reflecting the potassium content of human tubal fluid has also been evaluated using the blastulation of mouse zygotes. Compared to the modified Tyrode's discussed above, this medium, designated HTF, resulted in a higher zygote blastulation rate (88 vs. 77%, $p < 0.025$).[33] Although in the associated IVF program, there was not a consistent difference in the fertilization rate or the percent cleaved with the two different media, the pregnancy rate was significantly higher with HTF (33 vs. 11%, $p < 0.025$).

Modified Ham's F-10 medium (which has a potassium content similar to HTF) is widely used by a number of programs in the U.S.[21,25,44-47] As discussed in Section II.B, we performed a retrospective analysis of the ability of 10 batches of this medium to support mouse zygote and two-cell pre-embryo blastulation. These results were correlated with the results of IVF and the pre-embryo development in 31 patients. Although no correlation was observed between the results of the two-cell assay and the patients' outcomes, the results of the one-cell zygote assay were correlated both the quality of the pre-embryos and the pregnancy rate.[36]

V. SUMMARY

Compared to the *in vitro* blastulation of two-cell pre-embryos, the blastulation of zygotes is a much more sensitive evaluation of culture condition. Unlike those of the two-cell system, results of the evaluation of media using mouse zygotes have been shown to correlate with the results of human IVF results. Because of the increased sensitivity of the zygote blastulation assay, the culture conditions must be more rigidly controlled. In addition to its value for quality control, this system with its use of protein-free chemically defined media will also allow a more systematic evaluation of the nutritional requirements of pre-embryos.

ACKNOWLEDGMENTS

The authors wish to thank Julia Findley for her expert word processing, especially during the several revisions of the text. In addition, we thank Lori Esparcia for her detailed proof-reading and suggestions.

REFERENCES

1. The term "preembryo" refers to the organism which develops during the first 4 to 5 days after fertilization. During this time there is little embryonic development. Instead, by the end of this time period, there has begun to form the extraembryonic trophoblast in preparation for implantation. For a more complete discussion see, The biologic characteristics of the preembryo, *Fertil. Steril.*, 46(Suppl. 1), 26S, 1986.
2. **Morcos, R., Gibbons, W. E., and Findley, W. E.,** Effect of peritoneal fluid on in vitro cleavage of 2-cell mouse embryos: Possible role in infertility associated with endometriosis, *Fertil. Steril.*, 44, 678, 1985.
3. **Stuyt, E. B., Ulsun, O. E., DeLeon, F. D., Word, A., Word, L., Dorsett, M., and Heine, M. W.,** Effect of human peritoneal macrophages and fluid from fertile and infertile patients on the development of 2-cell mouse embryos in vitro, presented at the 43rd Annual Meeting, American Fertility Society, Reno, September 28—30, 1987, 108.

4. **Hill, J. A., Haimovici, F., Schiff, I., and Anderson, D. J.,** Supernatants of cultured peritoneal fluid leukocytes from women with endometriosis inhibit mouse embryo development in vitro, presented at the 43rd Annual Meeting, American Fertility Society, Reno, September 28—30, 1987, 083.

5. **Findley, W. E., Berenson, A., Huang, N. H., Gitlin, S., and Gibbons, W. E.,** The influence of serum components on the toxicity of delta 9-tetrahydrocannabinol in early embryonic growth, presented at the 40th Annual Meeting, American Fertility Society, New Orleans, April 2—7, 1984, 24S.

6. **Edwards, R. G., Steptoe, P. C., and Purdy, J. M.,** Establishing full term human pregnancies using cleaving embryos grown in vitro, *Br. J. Obstet, Gynaecol., 87*, 737, 1980.

7. **Steptoe, P. C. and Edwards, R. G.,** Birth after the reimplantation of a human embryo, *Lancet, 2*, 366, 1978.

8. **Ackerman, S. B., Swanson, R. J., Adams, P. J., and Wortham, J. W. E., Jr.,** Comparison of strains and culture media used for mouse in vitro fertilization, *Gamete Res., 7*, 103, 1983.

9. **Trounson, A. and Conti, A.,** Research in human in vitro fertilization and embryo transfer, *Br. Med. J., 285*, 244, 1982.

10. **Ackerman, S. B., Taylor, S. P., Swanson, R. J., and Laurell, L. H.,** Mouse embryo culture for screening in human IVF, *Arch. Androl., 12*(Suppl.), 129, 1984.

11. **Ackerman, S. B., Stokes, G. L., Swanson, R. J., Taylor, S. P., and Fenwick, L.,** Toxicity testing for human in vitro fertilization programs, *JIVFET, 2*, 132, 1985.

12. **Naz, R. K., Janousek, J. T., Moody, T., and Stillman, R. J.,** Factors influencing murine embryo bioassay: effects of proteins, aging of medium, and surgical glove coatings, *Fertil. Steril., 46*, 914, 1986.

13. **Sheean, L. A., Goldfarb, J. J., Kiwi, R., and Utian, W. H.,** Arrest of embyro development by ultrasound coupling gels, *Fertil. Steril., 45*, 568, 1986.

14. **Parinaud, J., Reme, J.-M., Monrozies, X., Favrin, S., Sarramon, M.-F., and Pontonnier, G.,** Mouse system quality control is necessary before the use of new material for in vitro fertilization and embryo transfer, *JIVFET, 4*, 56, 1987.

15. **Quinn, P., Warnes, G. M., Kerin, J. F., and Kirby, C.,** Culture factors in relation to the success of human in vitro fertilization and embryo transfer, *Fertil. Steril., 41*, 202, 1984.

16. **Schnell, V., Ataya, K., Sacco, A., and Moore, R.,** Lidocaine decreases mouse in vitro fertilization and embryo cleavage presented at the 44th Annual Meeting, American Fertility Society, Atlanta, October 10—13, 1988, S94.

17. **Thorneycroft, I. H., Wun, W-S. A., Ewell, M., Wheeler, C., and McFarland, C.,** Lidocaine effects on mouse embryo development in vitro, presented at the 44th Annual Meeting, American Fertility Society, Atlanta, October 10—13, 1988, S119.

18. **Saito, H., Berger, T., Mischell, D. R., and Marrs, R. P.,** Effect of variable concentrations of serum on mouse embryo development, *Fertil. Steril., 41*, 460, 1984.

19. **Whittingham, D. G.,** Culture of mouse ova, *J. Reprod. Fertil., 14*(Suppl.) 7, 1971.

20. **Fukuda, A., Noda, Y., Tsukui, S., Matsumoto, H., Yano, J., and Mori, T.,** Influence of water quality on in vitro fertilization and embryo development for the mouse, *JIVFET, 4*, 40, 1987.

21. **Silverman, I. H., Cook, C. L., Sanfilippo, J. S., Yussman, M. A., Schultz, G. S., and Hilton, F. H.,** Ham's F-10 constituted with tap water supports mouse conceptus development in vitro, *JIVFET, 4*, 185, 1987.

22. **Findley, W. E., Syms, A., and Gibbons, W. E.,** Effect of heparin on in vitro fertilization and early embryonic development, presented at the 40th Annual Meeting, American Fertility Society, New Orleans, April 2—7, 1984, 59S.

23. **Boyers, S. P., Tarlatsis, B. C., Stronk, J. N., and DeCherney, A. H.,** Fertilization and cleavage rates of heparin-exposed human oocytes in vitro, and the effect of heparin on the acrosome reaction, *Fertil. Steril., 48*, 628, 1987.

24. **Caro, C. M. and Trounson, A.,** The effect of protein on preimplantation mouse embryo development in vitro, *JIVFET, 1*, 183, 1984.

25. **Shirley, B., Wortham, Jr., J. W. E., Witmyer, J., Condon-Mahony, M., and Fort, G.,** Effects of human serum and plasma on development of mouse embryos in culture media, *Fertil. Steril., 43*, 129, 1985.

26. **Shirley, B., Wortham, J. W. E., Jr., Peoples, D., White, S., and Condon-Mahony, M.,** Inhibition of embryo development by some maternal sera, *JIVFET, 4*, 93, 1987.

27. **Ackerman, S. B., Swanson, R. J., Stokes, G. K., and Veeck, L. L.,** Culture of mouse preimplantation embryos as a quality control assay for human in vitro fertilization, *Gamete Res., 9*, 145, 1984.

28. **Biggers, J. D., Whittingham, D. G., and Donahue, R. P.,** The pattern of energy metabolism in the mouse oocyte and zygote, *Proc. Natl. Acad. Sci. U.S.A., 58*, 560, 1967.

29. **Whitten, W. K.,** Nutrient requirements for the culture of preimplantation embryos in vitro, in *Advances in the Biosciences*, Vol. 6, Raspé, G., Ed., Pergamon Press, New York, 1970, 129.

30. **Brinster, R. L.,** Studies on the development of mouse embryos in vitro. II. The effect of energy source, *J. Exp. Zool., 148*, 59, 165.

31. **Quinn, P. and Whittingham, D. G.,** Effect of fatty acids on fertilization and development of mouse embryos in vitro, *J. Androl.,* 3, 440, 1982.

32. **Davidson, A., Vermesh, M., Lobo, R. A., and Paulson, R. J.,** Mouse embryo culture as quality control for human in vitro fertilization: the one-cell versus the two-cell model, *Fertil. Steril.,* 49, 516, 1988.

33. **Quinn, P., Kerin, J. F., and Warnes, G. M.,** Improved pregnancy rate in human in vitro fertilization with the use of a medium based on the composition of human tubal fluid, *Fertil. Steril.,* 44, 493, 1985.

34. **Kane, M. T. and Headon, D. R.,** The role of commercial bovine serum albumin preparations in the culture of one-cell rabbit embryos to blastocysts, *J. Reprod. Fertil.,* 60, 469, 1980.

35. **Kane, M. T.,** Variability in different lots of commercial bovine serum albumin affects cell multiplication and hatching of rabbit blastocysts in culture, *J. Reprod. Fertil.,* 69, 555, 1983.

36. **Findley, W. E., Pabon, J., and Besch, P. K.,** The efficacy of mouse zygote blastulation rates in evaluating media for embryo culture, presented at the 43rd Annual Meeting, American Fertility Society, Reno, September 28—30, 1987, P280.

37. **Findley, W. E. and Besch, P. K.,** Inhibition of embryogenesis by culture media exposed to fluorescent light, presented at the 43rd annual Meeting, American Fertility Society, Reno, September 28—30, 1987, P149.

38. **Pabon, J. E., Jr., Findley, W. E., and Gibbons, W. E.,** The toxic effect of short exposures to the atmospheric oxygen concentration on early mouse embryonic development, *Fertil. Steril.,* 51, 896, 1989.

39. **Jackson, K. V. and Kiessling, A. A.,** Fertilization and cleavage of mouse oocytes exposed to the conditions of human oocyte retrieval for in vitro fertilization, *Fertil. Steril.,* 51, 675, 1989.

40. **Ogawa, T. and Marrs, R.,** The effect of protein supplementation on single-cell mouse embryos in vitro, *Fertil. Steril.,* 47, 156, 1986.

41. **Cheung, S. W., Strickler, R. C., Yang, V. C., deVera, M., and Spitznagal, E. L.,** A mouse embryo culture system for quality control testing of human in vitro fertilization and embryo transfer media and fetal cord sera, *Gamete Res.,* 11, 411, 1985.

42. **Quinn, P. and Harlow, G.,** The effect of oxygen on the development of preimplantation mouse embryos in vitro, *J. Exp. Zool.,* 206, 73, 1978.

43. **Purdy, J. M.,** Methods for fertilization and embryo culture in vitro, in *Human Conception in vitro,* Edwards, R. C. and Purdy, J. M., Eds., Academic Press, New York, 1982, 135.

44. **Jones, H. W., Jones, G. S., Andrews, M. C., Acosta, A., Bundren, C., Garcia, J., Sandow, B., Veek, L., Wiles, C., Witmyer, J., Wortham, J. F., and Wright, G.,** The program for in vitro fertilization at Norfolk, *Fertil. Steril.,* 38, 19, 1982.

45. **Laufer, N., DeCherney, A. H., Haseltine, F. P., Polan, M. L., Mezer, M. C., Dlugi, A. M., Sweeney, D., Nero, F., and Naftolin, F.,** The use of high-dose human menopausal gonadotropins in an in vitro fertilization program, *Fertil. Steril.,* 40, 734, 1983.

46. **Chetkowski, R. J., Nass, T. E., Matt, D. W., Hamilton, F., Steingold, K. A., Randle, D., and Meldrum, D. R.,** Optimization of hydrogen-ion concentration during aspiration of oocytes and culture and transfer of embryos, *J IVFET,* 2, 207, 1985.

47. **Dandekar, P. V. and Quigley, M. M.,** Laboratory setup for human in vitro fertilization, *Fertil. Steril.,* 42, 1, 1984.

Chapter 18

OOCYTE AND EMBRYO CRYOPRESERVATION TECHNIQUES AND RESULTS

Richard P. Marrs and Patrick Quinn

TABLE OF CONTENTS

I. INTRODUCTION

The use of cryobiology for the preservation of human cells has had a relatively short history. In 1949 the first human cells were successfully cryopreserved. The cells that were preserved in that original study were human spermatozoa.[1] Following that, Burge et al. reported the clinical use of frozen semen in a series of patients in 1954.[2] It was not until 1983 that Trounson reported successful freezing and thawing of a human embryo resulting in an ongoing pregnancy.[3] The most recent accomplishment with cryobiology, in the human, was reported in 1986 when Chen reported a successful twin pregnancy from cryopreserved human unfertilized oocytes that were subsequently thawed, fertilized and produced ongoing pregnancy and delivery after *in vitro* fertilization and embryo transfer.[4] The use of various animal models has provided the basic knowledge and technology that has been carried over to human oocyte and human embryo freezing. In the past decade, with the advent of the assisted reproductive technologies, the necessity for cryopreservation of gametes and human oocyte has become extremely important. With the ability to stimulate multiple oocytes in a single ovulatory cycle in the human female, the requirement for safe storage of either the unfertilized oocyte or the developing embryo has become paramount and an ancillary part of cycles of *in vitro* fertilization and embryo transfer (IVF-ET) and gamete intrafallopian transfer (GIFT). The ability to safely store embryos from individual cycles allows an improvement of pregnancy outcome on a per patient basis as well as improving the cost efficiency of the assisted reproductive technologies. Moreover, with the improvement in survival and pregnancy outcome with donated embryos, the use of embryo storage in young females facing loss of ovarian function from various disease states can now be performed and thus allow these individuals to carry a genetically related pregnancy to term after treatment of the condition is completed. This has been a method in use for preserving male reproductive potential should testicular loss (or failure) be anticipated. With the ability to safely freeze and store the embryo, it is now an acceptable procedure for the reproductive age female. In the future, as oocyte cryopreservation becomes more commonplace and reproducible, the desire would be to store the unfertilized egg rather than store the fertilized embryo in a large majority of these cases.

This chapter will attempt to describe the various cryobiologic principles that are utilized in oocyte and embryo cryopreservation and storage as well as clinical outcome that has been the result of these techniques. The use of oocyte cryopreservation and human embryo cryopreservation will be discussed separately as each of these systems require a different type of handling and the clinical results have shown a wide variance in outcome.

II. CRYOBIOLOGIC PRINCIPLES

The basic steps required in cryopreservation of single or multicell systems include the use of a cryoprotectant which can be a permeating or nonpermeating chemical, and after the addition of the cryoprotectant an equilibration between the cryoprotectant and the intra and extra cellular mileau. Once this equilibration has occurred, slow or rapid cooling down to a seeding temperature is required, and after seeding or ice crystal formation, slow cooling down to the desired sub-zero temperature takes place. Storage with thawing after a period of time will result in a reverse dilution of the cryoprotectant from the cell to the medium preparation and thus return the cell or cell systems to the normal physiologic environment.

It appears from studies performed over several decades that the most difficult periods during freezing and thawing of cells occur during the phase of initial cooling to low temperature through the seeding process and later the return to a normal physiologic environment. Most cell systems and single cells are stored at $-196°C$ in liquid nitrogen. This level of sub-zero storage maintains the viability of the cell, and long term storage can take place.

TABLE 1
Summary of Pregnancies Resulting from
Cryopreserved Unfertilized Oocytes

Investigator	Oocytes thawed and fertilized	Pregnancy
Chen	1/12	0
Chen	27/50	3/27
Diedrich	23/93	2/23
Schuh	9/28	1/9

The actual events that the cells undergo during the cooling process and the interaction between the cryoprotectant is essentially a freeze-dried process. If a permeable cryoprotectant is used, the cryoprotectant permeates the cell membrane, displacing the intracellular water. As cooling takes place, the cell dehydrates. At the point of ice crystal formation, the extracellular environment will crystallize with total dehydration of the cell and no intracellular ice formation thereby protecting the intracellular matrix.

The cryoprotectants fall into two broad categories: permeating cryoprotectants and nonpermeating agents. The most commonly used permeating agents are glycerol, dimethol sulfoxide (DMSO) and propanediol. The more commonly used nonpermeating agents that have been used in human work include monosaccharides and disaccharides such as glucose and sucrose.

With the knowledge gained from animal studies using animal oocytes, spermatozoa, and early and late stage embryos, the methodology for the use in human cell systems has been developed. The human embryo is generally cryopreserved with the use of a permeating cryoprotectant, and in some cases a combination of a nonpermeating and a permeating cryoprotectant. Unfertilized oocyte freezing and thawing is in such an early stage, definitive methodology for freezing, storage, and thawing of the unfertilized oocyte is still uncertain.

III. OOCYTE CRYOPRESERVATION

There have been six successful human pregnancies following cryopreservation of the unfertilized human egg. The success rate with oocyte freezing compared to embryo freezing is quite low. However, in time it is expected that utilization of the unfertilized egg may be a better alternative than human embryo freezing. At the present time, there is concern of an increased risk in aneuploidy in embryos that are produced from eggs that have been exposed to cryoprotectants and freezing and thawing.[5] This theoretical concern stems from the fact that the preovulatory oocyte is arrested in metaphase of the second meiotic division, and therefore the chromosomes are still attached to the meiotic spindle. It is thought that the meiotic spindle is temperature sensitive and thus during cooling for cryopreservation, there could be polarization which could interfere with the separation of the sister chromatids when fertilization occurs. This polarization could result in chromatid nondisjunction and aneuploidy after the extrusion of the second polar body. There has been a report utilizing mouse oocytes in which polyploidy was seen in an increased rate in frozen/thawed eggs, but the degree of aneuploidy was the same as that in fresh oocytes, and after transfer into pseudo-pregnant mice, the embryos from frozen/thawed eggs resulted in normal fetal development in the same proportion as nonfrozen oocytes.[6]

A standard methodology for cryopreservation of the unfertilized oocyte has not yet been accepted. The current results with human oocyte cryopreservation have been obtained with the use of DMSO with various combinations of cooling and thawing rates (Table 1). The first reported human pregnancies occurred with the use of DMSO, $1.5\,M$, with a slow cooling rate down to $-36°C$ and then a rapid thawing.[4] Dietrich et al. reported fertilization and

TABLE 2
Embryo Cryopreservation Protocol with DMSO

- Embryos loaded into freezing vial or straw
- Embryo cooled from $+23$ to $-6°C$ at $2°C/min$
- Seed and hold for 10 min at $-6°C$
- Embryo cooled at $-0.1°C/min$ to $-80°C$
- Plunge into liquid nitrogen
- DMSO added in 0.25 M increments at 10 min intervals to 1.5 M concentration at room temperature ($+23°C$)

human pregnancies also using DMSO with a slow cooling to $-30°C$ and a rapid thaw.[7] A relatively new technique has been reported by Trounson et al. utilizing a high concentraiton of DMSO, 3 M and a sucrose for a short period of time, 2 to 6 min, followed by a rapid freezing and thawing. No pregnancies have as yet been reported with this ultrarapid freezing technique.[5] Vitrification may offer a better method of storing and preserving oocytes, but the clinical experience with this technique in the human oocyte is limited and no pregnancies have been reported.

With the identification and analysis of data from five viable pregnancies resulting from human oocyte freezing, experience is limited and procedural steps for the most successful methodology are yet to be identified. In the future, the potential use of ultrarapid freezing and/or modification of the vitrification procedure could make oocyte preservation a clinical reality and a useful process for young women facing loss of ovarian function or women desiring to store and preserve oocytes before the effect of age becomes a problem with their overall fertility.

IV. EMBRYO CRYOPRESERVATION

The first human pregnancy resulting from a transfer of a human embryo that had been cryopreserved and thawed was reported by Trounson in 1983.[8] Since that time, the use of cryopreserved human embryos in assisted reproductive technologies has become widespread. Prior to 1987, 3577 embryos had been cryopreserved using various methods, and thawed for transfer. Approximately 50% of these embryos (1794) were viable after thawing and were involved in 1119 embryo transfers. One hundred sixty-three clinical pregnancies were established (13.4%) with spontaneous abortions occurring in 26% of the pregnancies, and ectopics in 4%. Thus far there have been two identified fetal abnormalities diagnosed in utero and terminated.[9]

The first human embryos that produced live offspring were cryopreserved using a quite different technique than that most widely employed today. In the original protocol, described by Trounson, embryos were cryopreserved using a 1.5 M DMSO concentration and the cryoprotectant was added in stepwise increments at 10 min intervals at room temperature. Initial concentrations of DMSO concentration was 0.25 M, progressing to 0.5, 1 and 1.5 M in PBS medium. After the equilibration of 1.5 M DMSO, the embryos were placed in a glass vial and the ampules were cooled from room temperature to -6 at $2°C/min$. A manual seeding was then performed and the ampules held at $-6°$ for 30 min. The ampules were then cooled at $0.3°C/min$ to $-80°C$, then plunged into liquid nitrogen ($-196°C$) where storage was carried out (Table 2). At the time of thawing, the embryos were transferred from liquid nitrogen to a controlled chamber at $-80°C$ and then were thawed at $8°C/min$ to $+4°C$. The DMSO was diluted out in a reverse fashion. With this original protocol utilizing DMSO and a four- or an eight-cell developed embryo, 68 of 136 embryos survived with half or more of their blastomeres intact. Sixty-eight embryos were transferred in 45 patients and resulted in nine clinical pregnancies.[10]

Shortly after the announcement of human clinical pregnancies from the use of cleaving

TABLE 3
Blastocyst Cryopreservation Protocol

- Blastocyst cooled from $+23$ to $-7°C$ at $2°C/min$
- Seed and hold for 10 min
- Cool at $0.3°C/min$ to $-30°C$
- Plunge into liquid nitrogen

Note: Glycerol added in five steps at 10 min intervals from 1% to an 8% final concentration at room temperature.

TABLE 4
Method of Embryo Cryopreservation with 1,2-propanediol (PROH)

- PROH added in $0.5\ M$ increments at 10 min intervals to $1.5\ M$ concentration at room temperature
- Embryo loaded in straws with 0.2 ml PROH in HEPES-HTF medium and $0.2\ M$ sucrose
- Embryo cooled at $2°C/min.$ to $-7°C$
- Seed and hold at $-7°C$ for 10 min.
- Embryo cooled at $0.3°C/min.$ to $-30°C$
- Plunge into liquid nitrogen

embryos frozen with DMSO as a cryoprotectant, Cohen et al. reported live births resulting from frozen/thawed human blastocysts.[11] In this report, embryos obtained at the time of *in vitro* fertilization were allowed to stay in the culture environment for 4 to 7 days after insemination. If blastocyst development occurred, the embryos were placed into Earl's solution, and glycerol was added at room temperature over six different incremental steps to a final concentration of 8 or 10% glycerol. The embryos were then placed into glass ampules and cooled from room temperature to $-7°C$ at $1°C/min$, and manual seeding was carried out. Thereafter, the ampules were cooled at a rate of $0.3°C/min$ down to $-36°C$ and then plunged into liquid nitrogen (Table 3). The embryos when thawed underwent a rapid thaw by removing the ampules from the liquid nitrogen container to a water bath at $30°C$. The glycerol cryoprotectant was then removed over a period of time diluting the media to 8% glycerol for 10 min, then 6% for 12 min, 5% for 14 min, 4% for 16 min, 3% for 18 min, 2% for 20 min, and 1% for 20 min. The embryos were then washed in fresh culture media and transferred. In this first series with human blastocysts, 11 patients had embryo transfer performed with two resulting in pregnancies. Testart et al. reported the use of propylene glycol (1,2-propanediol, PROH) as an efficient method to cryopreserve and store day 1 and day 2 *in vitro* cultured embryos. With the use of PROH as a cryoprotectant, embryos can be preserved at the pronuclear stage, two-cell stage, or four-cell stage of development[12] (Table 4). Most recently, Cohen et al. reported a series of 47 embryo transfer cycles resulting in 12 clinical pregnancies utilizing PROH as a cryoprotectant.[13] It was also demonstrated in this recent report that the timing of the replacement of the thawed embryo was important in establishing improved clinical outcomes. The data supported a synchronous thawing with the natural cycle. In other words, the LH surge indicated the onset of ovulation in the replacement cycle and the embryo was thawed in a synchronous fashion within 3 h of the natural cycle of ovulation. If synchrony went beyond 3 to 12 h later than what a synchronous thawing would have required, no pregnancies were established. Thus, when embryos that were thawed approximately at the same interval after ovulation were compared to the oocyte collection cycle up to 12 h earlier, the best pregnancy rates were demonstrated.

At our Institute, propanediol is the most commonly used cryoprotectant for early stage embryo freezing with a small percentage of embryos being allowed to advance to blastocyst for freezing with glycerol as a cryoprotectant.[14] By utilizing this method of embryo selection for freezing, embryos that do not appear perfectly regular at the two- or four-cell stage can be allowed to go to blastocyst formation and if they reach this developmental stage, embryo cryopreservation can be performed.

The best approach today in cryopreservation of embryos is storage of the embryos at the earliest stage possible if the embryos demonstrate normal developmental progress. The shorter the embryos are in the *in vitro* culture environment, the better the clinical outcome. However, in some cases when embryo development is irregular, development to the blastocyst stage before freezing is an alternative to identify a viable embryo prior to freezing and storage. Very recently a report from Trounson and Sjoblom demonstrated the feasibility of utilizing an ultrarapid freeze methodology for human embryos.[15] The embryos were placed in Dulbecco's phosphate buffered saline, containing 3 *M* DMSO and 0.25 *M* sucrose and placed in freezing straws. The straws were sealed, the embryos were left in the DMSO solution for 3 min at room temperature and then plunged directly into liquid nitrogen − 196°C. The embryos were thawed by placing them directly from liquid nitrogen to 37°C water bath. Of the 22 embryos frozen with ultrarapid freezing, 18 survived intact.

V. SUMMARY

In review of the clinical experience with human oocyte and embryo freezing, indeed the successful outcomes are relatively few. However, over the past 5 years, the use of cryopreservation for the unfertilized oocyte and the embryo has demonstrated remarkable improvement and reproducible pregnancy outcomes. Since 1985 the use of cryopreservation technology for excess or extra embryos produced by the *in vitro* fertilization process and/ or GIFT procedure has been a routine part of assisted reproductive technologies at The Institute for Reproductive Research in Los Angeles. In June 1986 the first live offspring resulting from a cryopreserved human embryo in the U.S. was reported.[14] Since that time, our policy for embryo freezing has changed, and now involves the use of two different types of freezing methodology. Early developed embryos are frozen with propanediol, and advanced embryo development (blastocyst) are cryopreserved utilizing glycerol. The selection of embryos for either of these freezing technologies is based on the quality of the embryo and the stage of development. If embryos at 24 h after inseminaiton have good clear cytoplasm and recognizable separate male and female pronuclei, propanediol is used to cryopreserve the embryo at the pronuclear stage. Remaining embryos are observed at 48 h after insemination. If they are found to be equally dividing three- to five-cell embryos with good clear blastomeres and clear cytoplasm, they are also cryopreserved using propanediol. If embryos appear irregular or slow in development, they are left in the *in vitro* culture environment up to 6 days after insemination. If blastocyst formation occurs with good clear expansion and blastocoel formation, glycerol is used for cryopreservation of the expanded blastocyst. By utilizing this dual approach, embryos that are questionable at the 24 to 48 h stage of development can be allowed to continue their development. If blastocyst development occurs, evidence of embryo viability and quality is then established. It is a policy in our Institute that if patients have embryos frozen at both the early and late stages, the early developing embryos are used first. If viability after thawing is not established, the same cycle of monitoring is utilized to thaw the blastocyst for transfer at 4 or 5 days after ovulation has been predicted. With the use of this approach, an ongoing and reproducible clinical pregnancy rate has been established with the use of cryopreserved embryos. (Table 5).

Overall, the addition of cryobiology to the assisted reproductive technologies has demonstrated an improvement in cost-effectiveness and clinical pregnancy outcome. When pregnancies from cycles of *in vitro* fertilization or GIFT are added to followup cycles where cryopreserved embryos have produced clinical pregnancies, the overall clinical pregnancy outcome improves significantly. As freezing becomes more feasible for human unfertilized oocytes, the use of this methodology to store the unfertilized gamete in women who are facing ovarian loss will become standard clinical practice. Until that time, the use of embryo freezing is the only alternative for a woman with impending ovarian loss due to chemotherapy

TABLE 5
Clinical Success with Human Embryo Cryopreservation at Institute for Reproductive Medicine, Los Angeles, CA

	Day 1	Day 2	Days 5—6
No. patients	37	50	17
No. embryos frozen	67	97	29
No. embryos viable after thaw	47	75	21
No. patients with ET	29	49	14
No. preg/ET	4/29 (14%)	4/49 (8%)	2/17 (12%)
No. preg/embryos frozen	4/67 (6%)	4/97 (4%)	2/29 (7%)
No. preg/viable embryos	4/47 (9%)	4/75 (5%)	2/21 (10%)

or surgical treatment. Even though early advancement has been seen with cryopreservation technology, increased knowledge about human gamete and embryo function during cryopreservation should provide for improved clinical outcomes.

REFERENCES

1. **Polge, C., Smith, A. U., and Parkes, A. S.,** Revival of spermatozoa after vitrification and dehydration at low temperatures, *Nature,* 164, 66, 1949.
2. **Burge, R. G., Keettal, W. C., and Sherman, J. K.,** Clinical use of frozen semen, *Fertil. Steril.,* 5, 520, 1954.
3. **Trounson, A. and Mohr, L.,** Human pregnancy following cryopreservation, thawing and transfer of an eight-cell embryo, *Nature,* 305, 707, 1983.
4. **Chen, C.,** Pregnancy after human oocyte cryopreservation, *Lancet,* I, 884, 1986.
5. **Trounson, A. O.,** Preservation of human eggs and embryos, *Fertil. Steril.,* 46, 1, 1986.
6. **Glenister, P. H., Wood, M. J., Kirby, C., and Whittingham, D. G.,** Incidence of chromosomal anomalies in first-cleavage mouse embryos obtained from frozen-thawed oocytes fertilized in vitro, *Gamete Res.,* 16, 205, 1987.
7. **Diedrich, K.,** Cryopreservation of rabbit and human oocytes, 5th World Congress on In Vitro Fertilization and Embryo Transfer, Norfolk, VA, April 5—10, 1987.
8. **Trounson, A. and Mohr, L.,** Human pregnancy following cryopreservation, thawing and transfer of an eight-cell embryo, *Nature,* 305, 707, 1983.
9. **Mohr, L. A., Trounson, A. O., and Freeman, L.,** Deep-freezing and transfer of human embryos, *J. In Vitro Fertil. Embryo Trans.,* 2, 1, 1985.
10. **Friedler, S., Giudie, L. C., and Lamb, E. J.,** Cryopreservation of embryos and ova, *Fertil. Steril.,* 49, 743, 1988.
11. **Cohen, J., Simons, R. F., Edwards, R. G., Fehilly, C. B., and Fishel, S. B.,** Pregnancies following the frozen storage of expanding human blastocysts, *J. In Vitro Fertil. Embryo Trans.,* 2, 59, 1985.
12. **Testart, J., LaSalle, B., Belaisch-Allart, J., Hazout, A., Forena, R., Rainhorn, J. D., and Frydman, R.,** High pregnancy rate after human embryo freezing, *Fertil. Steril.,* 46, 268, 1986.
13. **Cohen, J., DeVane, G. W., Elsner, C. W., Kort, H. I., Massey, J. B., and Norbury, S. E.,** Cryopreserved zygotes and embryos and endocrinologic factors in the replacement cycle, *Fertil. Steril.,* 50, 61, 1988.
14. **Marrs, R. P., Brown, J., Saito, F., Ogawa, T., Yee, B., Paulson, R., Serafini, P. C., and Vargyas, J. M.,** Successful pregnancies from cryopreserved human embryos produced by in vitro fertilization, *Am. J. Obstet. Gynecol.,* 156, 1503, 1987.
15. **Trounson, A. O. and Sjoblom, P.,** Cleavage and development of human embryos in vitro after ultrarapid freezing and thawing, *Fertil. Steril.,* 50, 373, 1988.

Chapter 19

THE MORPHOLOGICAL ASSESSMENT OF HUMAN OOCYTES AND EARLY CONCEPTI

Lucinda L. Veeck

TABLE OF CONTENTS

I. BACKGROUND

The correct assessment of oocyte maturity at the time of collection for *in vitro* fertilization (IVF) is an important prerequisite for ensuring normal development of the subsequent conceptus. Errors in assessing oocyte maturational status may lead to improper timing for insemination and often results in abnormal fertilization and/or poor developmental potential of the gamete. It has been observed by Sathananthan et al. that oocytes inseminated prior to reaching a metaphase II state may be penetrated by spermatozoa and yet fail to initiate events leading to sperm chromatin decondensation.[1] These oocytes ultimately lack functional male pronuclei. Assessment of nuclear maturation and understanding of cytoplasmic maturation has steadily been recognized as important to the IVF process. This author has previously stressed the importance of oocyte evaluation:

It is recognized that human oocytes may display abnormal fertilization (one pronucleus or three + pronuclei) when they are inseminated in either an immature or post-mature state. In immature oocytes the cortical granule numbers and response may be inadequate. In post-mature oocytes either cortical granule release after sperm penetration may be inhibited, or the zona reaction may be poorly functional. Therefore, it becomes very important to determine the correct timing for insemination. It is postulated that at least a brief period of time is required after extrusion of the first polar body for the oocyte to gain full cytoplasmic competence before insemination.[2]

Other authors have reached similar conclusions:

One of the salient prerequisites for successful *in vitro* fertilization is the completion of oocyte maturation. One must endeavour to obtain oocytes that are ripe, not immature or aging in culture. Both cytoplasmic and nuclear maturation are now considered important criteria in the assessment of oocytes for IVF.[1]

Examination of oocyte morphology under the light microscope enables the laboratory scientist to make sound judgments regarding subsequent handling and timing of laboratory events. To date, no biochemical assay or indirect testing method has proven as successful as the microscopic examination for determining oocyte viability and maturation. As methods for ovarian stimulation become more sophisticated, one finds more available oocytes which are collected at varying stages of meiotic maturation and which must be handled individually to achieve the best result. What methods may be used to ensure that meiotic maturation has been reached prior to clinical insemination?

II. METHODS OF OOCYTE ASSESSMENT

A. EVALUATION BASED UPON CELLULAR MORPHOLOGY

Historically, evaluation of oocyte maturity has been based upon the expansion and radiance of the cumulus/corona complex which surrounds the harvested oocyte. Using this method, one may quickly categorize oocytes as mature (preovulatory) when possessing an expanded and luteinized cumulus matrix and a radiant or "sun-burst" corona radiata (Figure 1). A less expanded cumulus/corona complex may be designated as intermediate in maturity (Figure 2), and absence of expanded cumulus might indicate oocyte immaturity (Figure 3). While this assessment provides a relatively close approximation of oocyte maturity, the method is often faulty and unreliable. Often, nuclear maturation of the oocyte and cellular maturation of the cumulus and corona are disparate, a situation which leads to erroneous handling and improper timing of insemination. With some ovarian stimulation protocols involving gonadotropins (especially purified FSH), most all of the oocytes collected will possess luteinized cellular characteristics, including oocytes at very immature stages. Besides the obvious fertilization failure which may occur when oocytes are poorly evaluated, other disadvantages become apparent: ovulation induction protocols may not be properly assessed and male factor infertility becomes difficult to interpret based upon fertilization results.

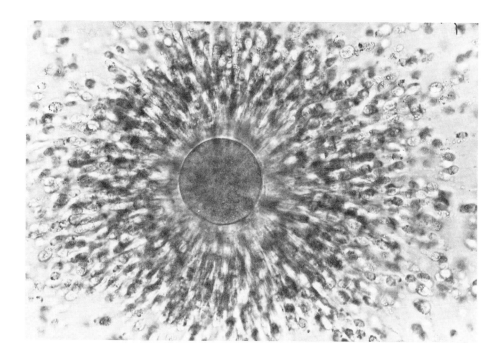

FIGURE 1. Expanded cumulus and radiant corona radiata which is typical of a mature human oocyte. (From Veeck, L. L., in *Atlas of the Human Oocyte and Early Conceptus,* Williams & Wilkins, Baltimore, 1986. With permission.)

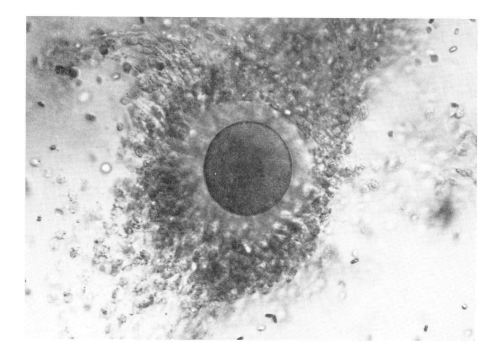

FIGURE 2. Dense cumulus mass and slightly compact corona radiata which usually indicates an intermediate stage of oocyte maturity when cytoplasm is clear. (From Veeck, L. L., in *Atlas of the Human Oocyte and Early Conceptus,* Williams & Wilkins, Baltimore, 1986. With permission.)

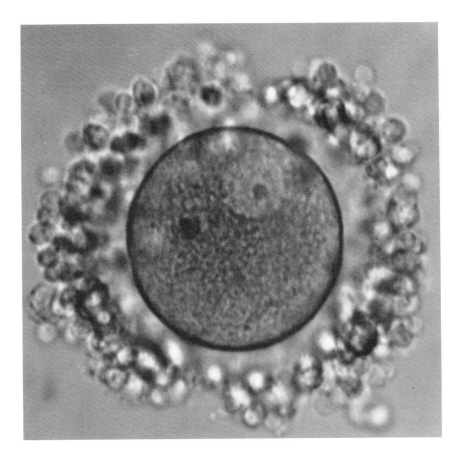

FIGURE 3.   Compact cumulus and corona cells typical of the immature human oocyte. (From Veeck, L. L., in *Atlas of the Human Oocyte and Early Conceptus,* Williams & Wilkins, Baltimore, 1986. With permission.)

Additionally, a treatment cycle yielding only a single oocyte may result in needless failure and without pre-embryo transfer simply because of unnecessary fertilization loss. Finally, the unscientific nature of cellular evaluation should discourage most academicians from utilizing these methods.

B. EVALUATION BASED UPON NUCLEAR ASSESSMENT

Newer techniques have been developed to more accurately assess the nuclear state of the oocyte collected for IVF. Various grading systems may be used which serve to produce a maturation ''score'',[3] or methods may be utilized which allow the direct visualization of the oocyte and its nuclear states. In Norfolk, direct visualization methods are used and are believed to best serve the morphological examination.[2]

In Norfolk, we began to assess the nuclear maturation of some oocytes in early 1985. By late 1986 we were evaluating each and every oocyte for its exact meiotic status. This was achieved by means of a cumulus spreading technique which involves the following steps:

1.   Placement of the oocyte/cumulus/corona complex in a small droplet of culture medium or follicular fluid (approximately 50 μl) on the flat surface of a sterile petri dish
2.   Jarring the dish with the palm of the hand to spread the droplet and to flatten the cumulus for better visualization of the ooplasm and the perivitelline space

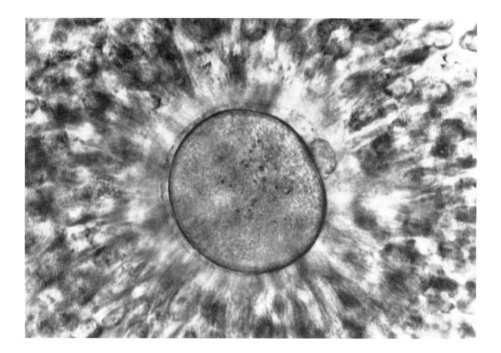

FIGURE 4. An oocyte at metaphase II stage of maturation which is characterized by the presence of a first polar body and clear cytoplasm.

3. Examination of the oocyte under an inverted high resolution microscope for identification of physical characteristics
4. Immediate flushing of the oocyte with equilibrated medium to restore pH and osmolality balance, and
5. Return to incubation and culture

Oocytes are classified according to the presence or absence of germinal vesicles and polar bodies as desscribed here:

a. Metaphase II (MII): first polar body present, no germinal vesicle (Figure 4)
b. Metaphase I (MI): no first polar body, no germinal vesicle (Figure 5)
c. Prophase I (PI): germinal vesicle present (Figure 6)

After initial evaluation of meiotic status, oocytes are inseminated according to their maturational development:

1. MII: inseminated 2 to 5 h after collection
2. MI: inseminated 1 to 3 h after extrusion of the first polar body (examined for polar body status every 2 to 3 h after collection)
3. PI: inseminated as for a MI oocyte or at a fixed time of 29 h after collection

Oocytes are incubated under conditions of 5% CO_2 in air at 37°C with full saturated humidity. Ham's F-10 culture medium is routinely used and supplemented with either 7.5 or 15% human fetal cord serum.[4] Oocytes are inseminated with 5×10^4 motile sperm per milliliter within a 3 ml volume of medium in organ culture dishes. Fertilization is assessed 12 to 18 h after insemination and cleaving concepti are transcervically transferred at 40 to 45 h

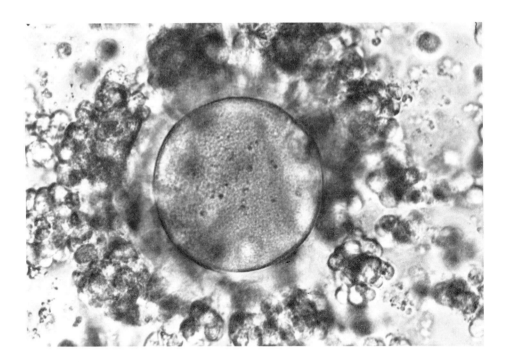

FIGURE 5. An oocyte at metaphase I stage of maturation which is characterized by the absence of either a first polar body or an intact germinal vesicle — cytoplasm is clear in late MI stages. (From Veeck, L. L., in *Atlas of the Human Oocyte and Early Conceptus*, Williams & Wilkins, Baltimore, 1986. With permission.)

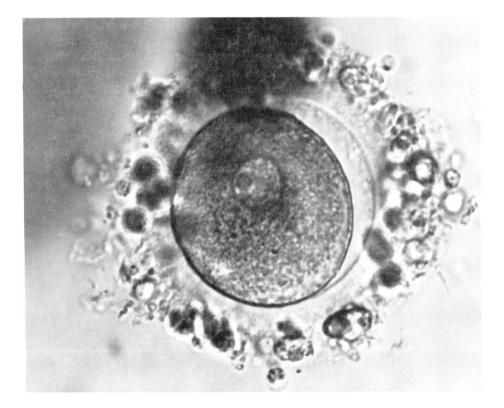

FIGURE 6. An oocyte at prophase I stage of maturation which is characterized by the presence of an intact germinal vesicle — cytoplasm is usually centrally granular in immature oocytes

TABLE 1
Atypical Oocyte Morphology of Oocytes at Metaphase II of
Maturation (Norfolk Series 24—26)

Observation	No.	% normal fert. (2 pronuclei)	% abnormal fert. (1 or 3+ pronuclei)
Fragmented 1st pb[a]	32	75	19
Very small 1st pb	8	75	13
Very large 1st pb	6	50	17
Detached 1st pb	3	$^2/_3$	$^1/_3$
Very granular ooplasm	65	80	8
Refractile body	47	2	—
Control MII oocytes	683	86	6

[a] pb, polar body.

postinsemination. Pregnancy is diagnosed by serum beta-hCG levels (radioimmunoassay) greater than 10 mIU/ml on luteal days 11 to 13, followed by subsequent higher levels and elevating estradiol and/or progesterone values.[5]

III. NON-NUCLEAR OOCYTE MORPHOLOGY

A. OOPLASMIC MORPHOLOGY AT COLLECTION

In an earlier study done in Norfolk, it was determined that certain characteristics of Metaphase II oocytes could be correlated with a reduced fertilization success.[2] Oocytes with atypically formed polar bodies (fragmented, very small, or overly large) demonstrated slight decreases in normal fertilization along with an increased incidence of abnormal fertilization as compared to controls (Table 1). A very granular ooplasm did not appear to affect the outcome of fertilization, but the existence of a refractile body in the ooplasm was significantly correlated with the inability to develop pronuclear structures.[7] The refractile body, so-called because of its refractile nature under bright field microscopy, is a structure which has only recently been described in the literature (Figure 7). When observed in the ooplasm of a human oocyte at collection, it indicates a poor prognosis for fertilization. Under electron microscopy it appears as a multivesicular body with lipid droplets (giving the refractile appearance), dense granules, small vesicles, and fibrillar material. The evolution of this structure and its relationship to oocyte maturity and viability are not yet understood. A strong tendency is observed for oocytes with refractile bodies to be recurrent for the same patient in repetitive treatment cycles.

B. DEGENERATIVE CHARACTERISTICS OF HARVESTED OOCYTES

Degenerating and atretic oocytes may be harvested during the course of oocyte collection for IVF. These oocytes are the simplest to identify because of their very darkened and unhealthy ooplasm (Figure 8). Usually, very few follicular cells are associated with these types of oocytes, but occasionally they can be observed.

Cytoplasmic vacuoles are occasionally observed within the ooplasm of some oocytes. While a single vacuole may not be prognostic of fertilization failure, multiple vacuoles and a darkened ooplasm most certainly indicate a poor prognosis for normal development (Figures 9 and 10).

Oocytes may be collected with breaks or "fractures" in the zona pellucida. These types of oocytes are commonly referred to as "fractured zona" oocytes (Figure 11). It is believed that degenerative changes in the zona, brought on by atresia, predispose these oocytes to mechanical damage at the time of follicular aspiration. One would expect such oocytes to

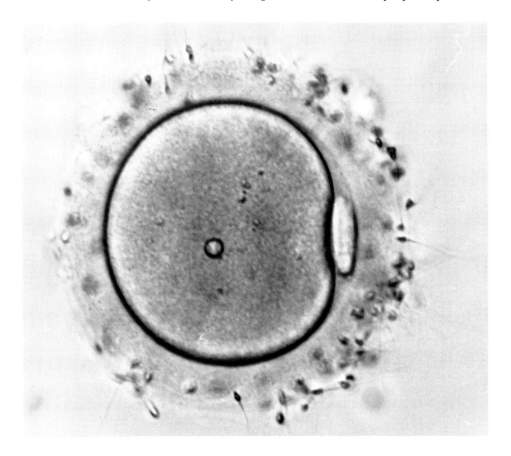

FIGURE 7. The "refractile body", visible at the center of the oocyte, is associated with a failure to give rise to pronuclear structures after insemination with sperm. (From Veeck, L. L., in *Atlas of the Human Oocyte and Early Conceptus,* Williams & Wilkins, Baltimore, 1986. With permission.)

display mature characteristics of the cumulus and corona cell matrix, an obvious break in the zona pellucida, and darkened ooplasm escaping the confines of the broken zona. Often, pure mechanical damage can result in a similar observation, but ooplasm appears light in color at the initial examination. Excessive negative or positive pressure during the collection process is almost always indicated in these situations.

Postmature oocytes may be observed in cycles with poor ovarian stimulation when oocytes have been held in follicles past the optimal time for retrieval and insemination. This stimulation problem is occasionally seen in patients under gonadotropin protocols where endogenous LH is suppressed. Postmature oocytes may or may not exhibit some darkness of the ooplasm, darkened and clumped corona cells, and darkened, clumped, and scanty cumulus (Figure 12). Incidence of triploid fertilization is high and resulting degeneration in culture is common with many of these oocytes.

IV. FERTILIZATION OUTCOME ACCORDING TO NUCLEAR MATURATION AT COLLECTION

Fertilization results are summarized in Table 2 for 8827 human oocytes collected during a 3-year period in Norfolk. Oocytes collected at more mature stages for IVF demonstrated the greatest ability to form two pronuclei after insemination. Fertilization rates dropped slightly when oocytes required a period of 5 to 15 h in culture before attaining meiotic

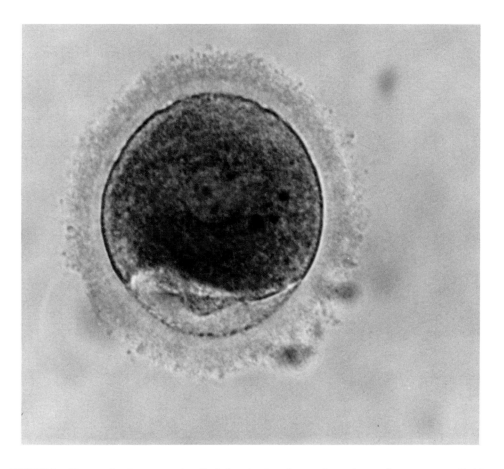

FIGURE 8. Degenerative human oocyte with dark and extremely granular ooplasm and porous zona pellucida. (From Veeck, L. L., in *Atlas of the Human Oocyte and Early Conceptus,* Williams & Wilkins, Baltimore, 1986. With permission.)

competence, and development of pronuclei was markedly reduced when more than 15 h was needed to complete the maturational process. It should be noted that semen samples were routinely collected soon after oocytes were harvested, thus, spermatozoa were also kept in culture for the ensuing hours until oocytes were ready for insemination. Under these circumstances, it cannot be stated that lowered fertilization potential is correlated solely with oocyte maturity - reduction in sperm quality may also be involved. Early MI oocytes which were incubated overnight before insemination and PI oocytes which were incubated for an average of 29 h before insemination exhibited the lowest fertilization rates in the study. Earlier studies done in Norfolk showed a much better fertilization rate for these less mature oocytes when fresh semen was collected on the second day (82%; Table 3).[6]

Rates of triploid fertilization were not statistically different for any groups except MII and PI (examples of oocytes with two and three pronuclei are shown in Figures 13 and 14).

V. INCIDENCE OF PREGNANCY IN RELATION TO OOCYTE NUCLEAR MATURATION AT COLLECTION

A total of 1804 transfer cycles have been divided into categories which reflect the original nuclear status of the transferred concepti. Of these cycles, exactly 1000 can be placed into one of five "pure" groups, groups denoting the transfer of one or more concepti

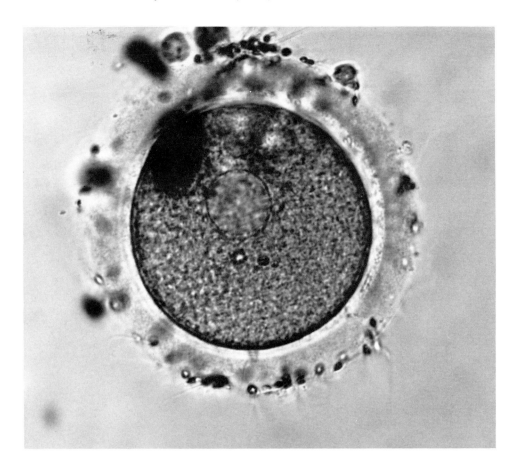

FIGURE 9.   Human oocyte with a single, large, and central vacoule.

of a single nuclear state at collection. For example, a MII pure group consists of transfer cycles where only pre-embryos developed from MII oocytes were transferred; MI-mature transfer cycles had only pre-embryos which developed from MI oocytes and which required less than 15 h in culture before attaining meiotic competence; MI-immature transfer cycles included only pre-embryos which developed from MI oocytes requiring longer than 15 h in culture; PI transfer cycles included those cycles which only replaced PI concepti. An additional group is included which is designated the "undetermined" maturational status group and includes those cycles with the transfer of unclassified oocytes (presumed mature by virtue of an expanded cumulus and corona radiata). These "pure" groups would be opposed to "mixed" transfer cycles where more than one conceptus was transferred, the concepti were of different maturational origins, and identification of the pre-embryo responsible for pregnancy was therefore impossible. Pregnancy rates have been examined for each of these pure groups and for each mixed group. Results are summarized in Tables 4 and 5. Pure groups of Metaphase II and Metaphase I concepti demonstrated similar pregnancy rates. Only cycles with the transfer of pre-embryos developed solely from PI oocytes showed any significant difference in pregnancy rate. Mixed transfer cycles represented an overall pregnancy rate of 32%. This somewhat higher rate can be attributed primarily to the larger number of pre-embryos transferred per cycle.

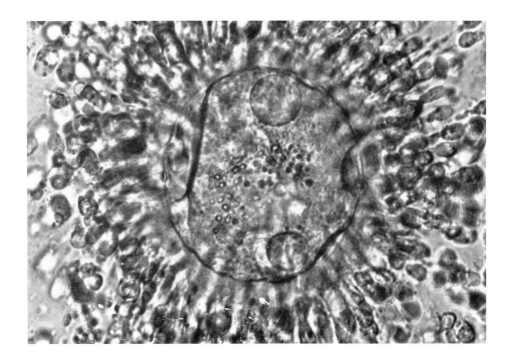

FIGURE 10. Human oocyte with degenerative features and multiple vacuoles.

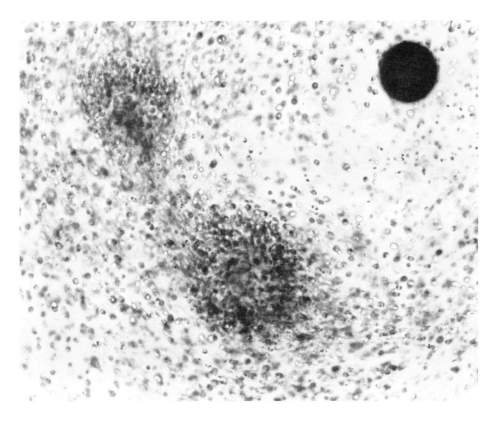

FIGURE 11. ''Fractured zona'' oocyte.

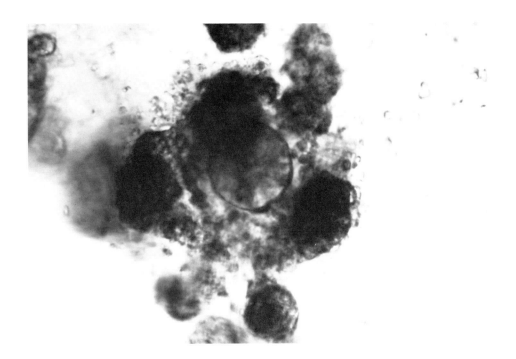

FIGURE 12. Oocyte with postmature characteristics of cumulus and corona cells (dark, clumped) at collection. (From Veeck, L. L., in *Atlas of the Human Oocyte and Early Conceptus,* Williams & Wilkins, Baltimore, 1986. With permission.)

TABLE 2
Fertilization Rate According to Nuclear Maturation at Collection (Norfolk, January 1985—June 1988)

Nuclear status at collection	No.	Avg. hours to insemination	% fert.	% triploid
MII	4010	4	90	8
Undetermined (mature cumulus)	579	6	89	7
MI-Mature	2136	8	84	6
MI-Immature	379	21	66[a]	4
PI	1723	29	48[a]	3

[a] All inseminated with day-old semen samples.

TABLE 3
In Vitro Maturation and Fertilization of Prophase I Oocytes

	Matured to MII		
	Total PI oocytes	(%)	% fert.
Norfolk Series 2—13 (freshly collected semen processed for insemination)	$\frac{565}{688}$	(82)	82
Norfolk Series 18—26 (day-old processed sperm used for insemination)	$\frac{1748}{2098}$	(83)	49

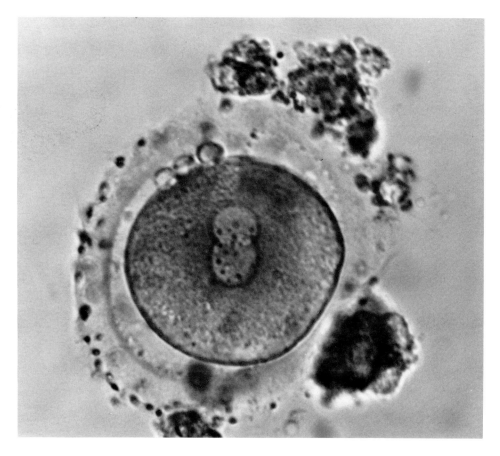

FIGURE 13. Human pre-zygote with two pronuclei. (From Veeck, L. L., in *Atlas of the Human Oocyte and Early Conceptus,* Williams & Wilkins, Baltimore, 1986. With permission.)

VI. PREGNANCY LOSS IN RELATIONSHIP TO OOCYTE MATURATION AT COLLECTION

Cycles which have ended in spontaneous abortion have been examined; results are summarized on Table 6. Pregnancy loss is noted to be higher with MII oocytes when compared to other pure transfer groups.

VII. PRE-EMBRYO GRADING

Attempts have been made to grade the morphology of cleaving concepti and to classify transfers according to the grade of the best looking pre-embryo which was transferred. The grading system which was used is as follows, with Grade 1 representing perfect morphology:

Grade 1 — Pre-embryo with blastomeres of equal size; no cytoplasmic fragments
Grade 2 — Pre-embryo with blastomeres of equal size; minor cytoplasmic fragments or blebs noted
Grade 3 — Pre-embryo with blastomeres of distinctly unequal size; no cytoplasmic fragments
Grade 4 — Pre-embryo with blastomeres of equal or unequal size; moderate to heavy fragmentation noted
Grade 5 — Pre-embryo with few blastomeres of any size; major or complete fragmentation noted

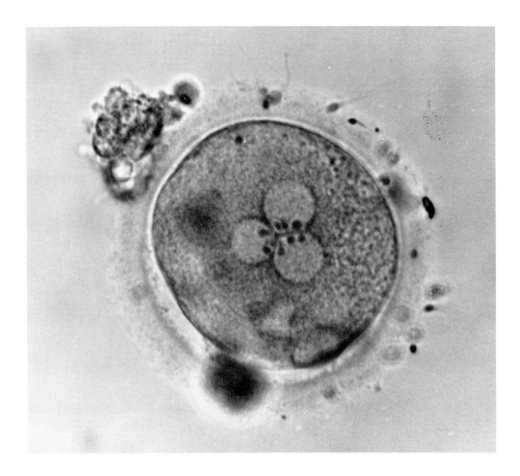

FIGURE 14.   Human pre-zygote with three pronuclei (third pronucleus presumed of male origin because of larger size).

TABLE 4
Incidence of Pregnancy in Relation to Oocyte Maturation at Collection (Norfolk, January 1985—June 1988)

Pure Transfer Groups

Pure transfer group	Avg. no. embryos transferred	Pregnancy/transfer	(%)
Metaphase II (MII)	2.6	167/624	27
Metaphase I-Mature (MI-M)	2.0	45/205	22
Unclassified Mature (?)	2.6	19/93	20
Metaphase I-Immature (MI-I)	2.0	5/29	17
Prophase I (PI)	2.1	3/49	6

Pregnancy results for each morphologic grade are given in Table 7. Only cycles with at least one pre-embryo of grade 1 quality demonstrated any significant difference in the establishment of pregnancy (Figure 15). However, pregnancy was possible even in cycles with grade 4 or 5 morphology which denoted moderate to severe cytoplasmic fragmentation.

TABLE 5
Incidence of Pregnancy in Relation to Oocyte Maturation at Collection (Norfolk, January 1985—June 1988)

Mixed Transfer Groups

Mixed transfer group	Avg. no. embryos transferred	Pregnancy/transfer	(%)
MII + ?	4.0	24/63	38
MII + MI-M	3.5	177/567	31
MII + MI-I	3.4	13/41	32
MII + MI-M + ?	4.5	8/24	33
MII + MI-I + ?	4.0	1/3	33
MII + MI-M + MI-I	4.5	18/52	35
MII + MI-M + MI-I + ?	4.0	0/2	
MI-M + ?	3.2	9/20	45
MI-M + MI-I	3.2	4/24	17
MI-M + MI-I + ?	3.5	2/2	
MI-I + ?	3.4	2/6	33

TABLE 6
Pregnancy Loss in Relation to Oocyte Maturation at Collection (Norfolk, January 1985—June 1988)

Pure Transfer Groups

Pure transfer group	Loss/clinical pregnancy	(%)
Unclassified Mature (?)	8/19	50
Metaphase II (MII)	65/167	39
Metaphase I-Mature (MI-M)	9/45	20
Metaphase I-Immature (MI-I)	1/5	20
Prophase I (PI)	0/3	0

TABLE 7
Pre-Embryo Grading of Morphology (Norfolk Series 26—31)

Morphology grade	Avg. no. transferred	Pregnancy Transfer	Live birth Transfer
1	3.2	127/283 (45%)	(33%)
2	2.8	84/310 (27%)	(17%)
3	2.5	6/55 (11%)	(7%)
4	2.7	45/210 (21%)	(13%)
5	2.4	6/90 (7%)	(3%)
Total		268/948 (28%)	(19%)

VIII. CONCLUSIONS

Correct evaluation of the maturational status of an oocyte collected for IVF leads to proper timing of insemination and correct handling. Various methods may be used to evaluate oocyte maturity, but direct examination of nuclear elements is recommended for best overall results. A "cumulus spreading" or "flattening" technique allows visualization of germinal vesicle and polar body status without apparent detriment to fertilization, development, establishment of pregnancy, or ongoing pregnancy rate. This technique does not increase the

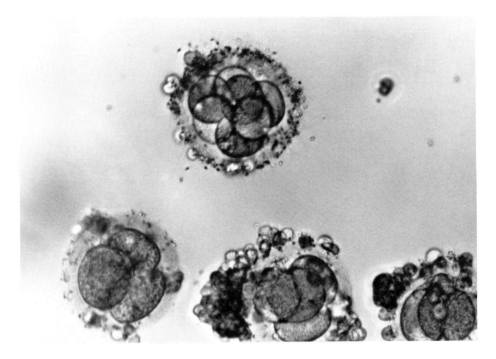

FIGURE 15.   Grade 1 transfer with pre-embryos of near perfect morphology.

incidence of triploid fertilization as evidenced by comparable triploidy rates associated with oocytes not evaluated in this manner (the undetermined nuclear status group).

The more advanced the nuclear maturation of an oocyte at the time of harvest and the shorter the interval is between sperm preparation and insemination, the higher the incidence of fertilization. A period of at least 2 to 3 h is recommended after extrusion of the first polar body for completion of cytoplasmic maturation of the oocyte. Oocytes inseminated too soon after observation of the first polar body display an increased rate of triploid fertilization and failed fertilization.[2]

Once fertilized and transferred, any pre-embryo developed from an oocyte of a maturation greater than PI may be fairly successful in implantation. Only pre-embryos developed from PI oocytes demonstrate any significant decrease in ability to produce pregnancy. Pregnancy loss after implantation may be somewhat higher with oocytes of more advance maturation at harvest.

Atypical morphology of first polar bodies (fragmentation, irregularity in size) is associated with a slight decrease in normal fertilization and increase in abnormal fertilization. This may be due to oocyte postmaturity. A homogeneously granular cytoplasm does not appear to have a negative impact upon fertilizing potential, but the appearance of a refractile body most certainly does reflect poorly on subsequent development.

Pregnancy can be established after the transfer of pre-embryos displaying unequal sized blastomeres or cytoplasmic fragments, but pregnancy and ongoing pregnancy is highly correlated with pre-embryos displaying perfect morphology.

REFERENCES

1. **Sathananthan, A. H. and Trounson, A. O.,** *Atlas of Fine Structure of Human Sperm Penetration, Eggs and Embryos Cultured In Vitro,* Praeger, New York, 1986, 2.
2. **Veeck, L. L.,** Oocyte assessment and biological performance, *In Vitro Fertilization and Embryo Transfer,* Annals of the New York Academy of Sciences, in press.
3. **Mahadevan, J. and Fleetham, J.,** Relationship of a human oocyte scoring system to oocyte maturity and fertilizing capacity, abstract (P-070) to the 44th annual meeting of the American Fertility Society, Atlanta, 1988, S67.
4. **Veeck, L. L.,** Insemination and fertilization, in *In Vitro Fertilization — Norfolk,* Jones, H. W., Jr., Jones, G. S., Hodgen, G. D., and Rosenwaks, Z., Eds., Williams & Wilkins, Baltimore, 1986, 183.
5. **Muasher, S. J. and Garcia, J.,** Pregnancy and its outcome, in *In Vitro Fertilization — Norfolk,* Jones, H. W., Jr., Jones, G. S., Hodgen, G. D., and Rosenwaks, Z., Eds., Williams & Wilkins, Baltimore, 1986, 238.
6. **Veeck, L. L.,** Extracorporeal maturation: Norfolk, 1984, in *In Vitro Fertilization and Embryo Transfer,* Annals of the New York Academy of Sciences, 442, 357, 1985.
7. **Veeck, L. L.,** *Atlas of the Human Oocyte and Early Conceptus,* Williams & Wilkins, Baltimore, 1986, 314.

APPENDIX I
Morphological Stains

IA Rapid Wrights-Gram Stain

1. Prepare semen smear, air dry.
2. Camco Quick Stain (0.4% Wrights stain in methanol, Scientific Products B4130): 5 — 30 min.
3. Rinse with running tap water, 15 sec.
4. Flood slide with gram crystal violet (DIFCO 3329-75), 3—5 sec.
5. Rinse with running tap water, 15—30 sec.
6. Air dry.

IB Crystal Violet-Rose Bengal Stain

1. Prepare semen smear, air dry.
2. Flood slide with 5% chloramine T in distilled water, 5 min.
3. Rinse with 95% ETOH.
4. 25% crystal violet in distilled water, 8 min.
5. Rinse with 95% ETOH.
6. 1% rose bengal in distilled water, 8 sec.
7. Rinse with distilled water.

IC Hematoxylin-Eosin Stain

1. Prepare semen smear, air dry.
2. Lithium carbonate solution: 1.5 ml saturated lithium carbonate in 650 ml 70% ETOH.
3. Acid alcohol: 1.5 ml concentrated HCl in 650 ml 70% ETOH.
4. 100% ETOH   15 dips × 2
5. 95%, 80%, 70% ETOH   15 dips each
6. Distilled water   15 dips
7. Harris hematoxylin (Fisher SH30)   2 min
8. Running tap water wash   1 min
9. Acid alcohol   2 dips
10. Running tap water wash   30 sec
11. Lithium carbonate solution   1 min
12. Distilled water   15 dips
13. 50% ETOH   15 dips
14. 1% Eosin Y solution (Fisher SE23)   20 sec
15. Running tap water wash   1 min
16. 95% ETOH   15 dips × 2
17. 100% ETOH   15 dips
18. 100% ETOH   1 min
19. Xylene   15 dips × 2
20. Xylene   5—10 min

ID Papanicolaou Stain

1. Prepare a thin semen smear and air dry
2. Formalin   5 min
3. Distilled water   8 to 10 dips
4. Harris hematoxylin (Fisher SH30)   5 min
5. Distilled water   8 to 10 dips
6. 0.5% HCl   1 quick dip
7. Distilled water   8 to 10 dips
8. 1.5% NH$_4$OH in 95% ETOH   5 dips
9. 95% ETOH   10 dips
10. OG-6 (Fisher SP5)   3 min
11. 95% ETOH   10 dips
12. EA-50 (Fisher SP11)   2 min
13. 95% ETOH   10 dips

14.	95% ETOH	10 dips
15.	100% ETOH	10 dips
16.	1:1 100% ETOH and Xylene	10 dips
17.	Xylene	5 min

IE Eosin Live-Dead Vital Stain

1. Prepare a 0.5% solution of blue eosin (Eosin B, Certified, Kodak #C5322; 0.5 g/100 ml distilled H_2O). Solution should be prepared fresh each day of use.
2. Mix one drop of well mixed semen with one drop of the eosin solution on a slide.
3. Cover with a coverslip and examine after 1—2 min.
4. Viable spermatozoa remain unstained against a pink background. Dead sperm are stained red ("red = dead").
5. Count at least 200 total sperm and calculate percent viable.

APPENDIX II
Buffers and Solutions

IIA Dulbecco's Phosphate Buffered Saline

Compound	g/final volume of			
	100 ml	250 ml	500 ml	1000 ml
NaCl	0.8	2.0	4.0	8.0
KCl	0.02	0.05	0.1	0.2
Na_2HPO_4	0.115	0.288	0.575	1.15
$CaCl_2$	0.01	0.025	0.05	0.10
$MgSO_4 \cdot 7H_2O$	0.012	0.03	0.06	0.12
pH 7.40				

IIB Tyrode's Solution

Compound	g/final volume of			
	100 ml	250 ml	500 ml	1000 ml
NaCl	0.8	2.0	4.0	8.0
KCl	0.02	0.05	0.1	0.2
$CaCl_2$ anhydrous	0.02	0.05	0.1	0.2
$NaHCO_3$	0.1	0.25	0.5	1.0
$MgCl_2 \cdot 6H_2O$	0.01	0.025	0.05	0.1
NaH_2PO_4	0.005	0.012	0.025	0.05
Glucose	0.1	0.25	0.5	0.1
pH 8.00				

IIC Phosphate Buffered Saline (0.01 M)

Compound	g/final volume of			
	100 ml	250 ml	500 ml	1000 ml
$NaH_2PO_4 \cdot H_2O$	0.0262	0.0655	0.131	0.262
$Na_2HPO_4 \cdot 7H_2O$	0.2173	0.5432	1.086	2.173
NaCl	0.85	2.125	4.25	8.5
pH 7.40				
	Normal saline (0.9%)			
NaCl	0.85	2.125	4.25	8.5

IID Locke's Solution

Compound	g/final volume of			
	100 ml	250 ml	500 ml	1000 ml
$CaCl_2$	0.024	0.06	0.12	0.24
KCl	0.042	0.105	0.21	0.42
$NaHCO_3$	0.01	0.025	0.05	0.1
NaCl	0.9	2.25	4.50	9.0
pH 7.20				

IIE Baker's Buffer

Compound	g/final volume of			
	100 ml	250 ml	500 ml	1000 ml
Glucose	3.0	7.5	15.0	30.0
Na_2HPO_4	0.6	1.5	3.0	6.0
KH_2PO_4	0.01	0.025	0.05	0.1
NaCl	0.2	0.5	1.0	2.0
pH 7.70—7.80				

IIF Biggers, Whitten and Wittingham (BWW)

Compound	g/final volume of			
	100 ml	250 ml	500 ml	1000 ml
NaCl	0.553	1.382	2.765	5.53
KCl	0.036	0.089	0.178	0.356
$CaCl_2$ anhydrous	0.019	0.048	0.095	0.19
KH_2PO_4	0.016	0.040	0.081	0.162
$MgSO_4 \cdot 7H_2O$	0.029	0.074	0.147	0.294
$NaHCO_3$	0.21	0.525	1.050	2.10
Glucose	0.1	0.25	0.5	1.0
Na pyruvate	0.003	0.007	0.014	0.028
Lactic acid syrup (60%)*	0.37 ml	0.925 ml	1.85 ml	3.7 ml
Pen/strep solution**	1.0 ml	2.5 ml	5.0 ml	10.0 ml
pH 7.40 with 2 *M* Hepes				

* Sodium lactate syrup (60%) obtained from Sigma (#L1375)

** Penicillin (10,000 IU/ml) — Streptomycin (10,000 µg/ml) solution obtained from GIBCO (#600-5140)

IIG TEST- Yolk Buffer

Compound	g/final volume of			
	100 ml	250 ml	500 ml	1000 ml
TES*	4.83	12.08	24.15	48.3
TRIS**	1.16	2.9	5.8	11.6
Dextrose	0.2	0.5	1.0	2.0
Egg yolk	20 ml	50 ml	100 ml	200 ml
pH 7.2 with TES				
320—327 mOsm with distilled water				

* TES = N-Tris (hydroxmethyl) methyl-2-aminoethane sulfonic acid

** TRIS = Tris (hydroxymethyl) aminomethane

From Jaskey, D. G. and Cohen, M. R., *Fertil. Steril.*, 35, 205, 1981. With permission.

APPENDIX III
Suppliers

Abbott Laboratories
1400 Sheridan Road
North Chicago, IL 60064
1-800-323-9100

Accumetric
P.O. Box 843
Elizabethtown, KY 42701
(502) 769-3385

American Scientific Products (Baxter Travenol Co.)
1430 Waukegan Road
McGraw Parks, IL 60085
(312) 689-8410

Apex Medical Technologies, Inc.
10064 Mesa Ridge Court, Suite 202
San Diego, CA 92121
(619) 535-0012

Arrow Glass Company
P.O.Box 2308
South Vineland, NJ 08360
(609) 691-1350

Bacharach, Inc.
625 Alpha Drive
Pittsburgh, PA 15238
(414) 963-2000

Baxter Healthcare Corporation
Dade Division
P.O. Box 520672
Miami, FL 33152-0672
(305) 948-5677

Bio-Rad Laboratories
2200 Wright Avenue
Richmond, CA 94804
(415) 234-4130

Calbiochem
P.O. Box 12087
San Diego, CA 92112
(800) 854-3417

Chartpak
1 River Road
Leeds, MA 01053
(413) 584-5446

Continental Plastic Corporation
P.O. Box C
Delavan, WI 53115
(414) 728-5501

Cook OB/Gyn
P.O. Box 271
Spencer, IN 47460
(812) 829-4891

Corning Glass Works
814 Busse Highway
Park Ridge, IL 60068
(312) 823-9066

Cozzoli Machine Company
401 East Third Street
Plainfield, NJ 07060
(201) 757-2040

CryoMed
51529 Birch Street
New Baltimore, MI 48047
(313) 725-4614

Cryo Resources, Ltd.
Sixth Floor Suite
701 Seventh Avenue
New York, NY 10036
(212) 840-1233

Curtin Matheson Scientific, Inc.
6111 Deramus Road
Kansas City, MO 64120
(800) 821-8491

Cutter Laboratories
P.O. Box 1986
Berkely, CA 94701
(415) 420-5000

DIFCO Laboratories
P.O. Box 1058
Detroit, MI 48232
(313) 961-0800

Drummond Scientific Company
500 Parkway
Bloomall, PA 19008
(215) 353-0200

Edwards Agricultural Supply
Box 65
Baraboo, WI 53913
(608) 356-6641

Elkins-Sinn
2 Esterbrook Lane
Cherry Hill, NJ 08003
(609) 424-3700

Fisher Scientific
Corporate Headquarters
711 Forbes Avenue
Pittsburgh, PA 15219
(412) 562-8300

GIBCO Life Technologies, Inc.
3175 Stayley Road
Grand Island, NY 14072
(800) 828-6686

Hamilton Company
P.O. Box 10030
Reno, NV 89520
(800) 648-5950

Hamilton-Thorn Research
30A Cherry Hill Drive
Danvers, MA 01923
(508) 777-9050

HDC Corporation
2551 Casey Avenue
Mountain View, CA 94043
(800) 227-8162

ICN Biomedicals
P.O. Box 19536
Irvine, CA 92714
1-800-854-0530

Interlab
2373 Teller Road, Suite 103
Newburg Park, CA 91320

Irvine Scientific
2511 Daimler Street
Santa Ana, CA 93705-5588
(714) 261-7800

Katena Products, Inc.
4 Stewart Court
Denville, NJ 07834
(201) 989-1600

Lab Safety Supply
P.O. Box 1368
Janesville, WI 53547-1368
(800) 356-0783

Lorvic Corporation
8810 Frost Avenue
St. Louis, MO 63134
(314) 524-7444

Mallinckrodt, Inc.
675 McDonnell Boulevard
P.O. Box 5840
St. Louis, MO 63134
(314) 895-2000

Markson Science, Inc.
10201 South 51st Street
Phoenix, AZ 85044
(800) 528-5114

Milex Products, Inc.
5915 Northwest Highway
Chicago, IL 60631
(312) 631-6484

Millipore Corporation
80 Ashby Road
Bedford, MA 07130
(800) 225-1380

Minnesota Valley Engineering, Inc.
407 Seventh Street, N.W.
New Prague, MN 56071
(612) 758-4400

Nalge Company
P.O. Box 20365
Rochester, NY 14602-0365
(716) 586-8800

National Instruments
12109 Technology Boulevard
Austin, TX 78727
(512) 250-9119

Motion Analysis Corporation
93 Strong Circle
Santa Rosa, CA 95401
(707) 579-6500

PEL-Freeze Biologicals
P.O. Box 68
Rogers, AR 72756
(800) 643-3426

Pharmacia LKB Biotechnology, Inc.
800 Centennial Avenue
P.O. Box 1327
Piscataway, NJ 08855
(201) 457-8000

Rainin Instrument Company, Inc.
Mack Road
Woburn, MA 01808-4628
(800) 472-4646

Scientific Manufacturing Industries
1399 65th Street
Emeryville, CA 94608

Sefi-Medical Instruments
P.O. Box 7295
Haifa 30170, Israel
04-2516J1 TLX: 46400 ext. 8796

Serono Diagnostics, Inc.
100 Longwater Circle
Norwell, MA 02061
(800) 345-3127

Sigma Chemical Company
P.O. Box 14508
St. Louis, MO 63178
(800) 325-3010

So-Low Environmental
Equipment Company, Inc.
10310 Spartan Drive
Cincinnati, OH 45215
(413) 772-9410

Southland Cryogenics, Inc.
2424 Lacy Lane
Carrollton, TX 75006
(214) 243-1311

Syva Company
P.O. Box 10058
Palo Alto, CA
(415) 493-2200

Tetko Company
420 Sawmill River Road
Elmsford, NY 10523
(914) 941-7767

Thomas Scientific
99 High Hill Road at I-295
P.O. Box 99
Swedesboro, NJ 08085
(609) 467-2000

T.S. Scientific
P.O. Box 198
Perkasie, PA 18944
(215) 257-4756

Victor Industries
810 North Main
Harrisonburg, VA 22801
(703) 434-4411

VITRO Dynamics, Inc.
P.O. Box 285
Rockaway, NJ 07866
(201) 625-1707

Whitehall Laboratories
685 Third Avenue
New York, NY 10017
(800) 223-2329 (Talkline) for information

Xytex Corporation
1100 Emmett Street
Augusta, GA 30904
(800) 241-9722

Zygotek Systems, Inc.
130 Maple Street, Suite 232
Springfield, MA 01103
(413) 732-8065

APPENDIX IV

SEMEN ANALYSIS

An integral part of the infertility evaluation of a couple is the examination of the male's semen, or what is commonly referred to as a sperm count. This term is somewhat inaccurate, as the semen analysis involves more than just counting the number of sperm. A semen analysis is an accurate measurement of the number of sperm, their motility, and their normality. The information gained from this examination is probably the single most important test in the evaluation of the male partner.

Patient Instructions for Collection of a Specimen

1. Refrain from any sexual activity including masturbation for 2-3 days.

2. The semen specimen should be collected by masturbation. Alternate methods may be discussed but are not recommended. Do not collect the specimen in a condom as these contain spermicidal agents which will alter the results of the analysis.

3. The specimen should be collected in a container provided by this office.

4. Bring the specimen to the laboratory within one hour after collection. Do not expose the specimen to extremes of temperature. If you are unable to deliver the specimen to the laboratory within one hour, a private room is available at the clinic for collection of the specimen.

5. Please complete the form below and hand it to the receptionist along with the specimen.

Name: _____ Spouse: _____ Date: _____

Address: _____

_____ Phone: (_____) _____

_____ Zip Code: _____

Dr. _____

1. What time was specimen collected? _____

2. Was any of the specimen lost or spilled during collection? *THIS IS VERY IMPORTANT!* Yes_____ No_____

3. I was abstinent (did not ejaculate) for _____ days before producing the present sample.

4. Comments: _____

_____

_____

_____

Prepared by B.A. Keel, 1989 (see chapter 3).

APPENDIX V

SEMEN ANALYSIS

Code #_____

Patient Name _____ Spouse _____

Date _____

Doctor _____

Abstained _____ days

☐ Sperm Mucus Panel ☐ Andrology Profile ☐ Wash and Rise IUI_____ IVF_____ SPA _____ ☐ Retrograde Ejaculation ☐ Other _____

	PARAMETER	OBSERVATION	NORMAL	POST TREATMENT
1.	Count	_____ x10^6/ml	20-200 x10^6/ml	_____ x10^6/ml
2.	Motility	_____ %	> 40%	_____ %
3.	Velocity	_____ um/sec	> 20um/sec	_____ um/sec
4.	Motile Density*	_____ x10^6/ml	> 8 x 10^6/ml	_____ x10^6/ml
5.	Motility Index**	_____ um/sec	> 8 um/sec	_____ um/sec
6.	Morphology	_____ % Normal	> 60% Normal	_____ % Normal
7.	Volume	_____ ml	1.5 - 5.5; mean 3.5	_____ ml
8.	Liquefaction	_____ min	10 - 30 min	_____ min
9.	Viscosity	_____	Normal to 1+	_____
10.	Agglutination	_____	Slight to absent	_____
11.	Mucus Penetration	_____ mm	> 30 mm	_____ mm

* % Motility x Total Density
** % Motility x Average Velocity

Oval (Norm.)	Abnormal Tail	Immature	No Head	Bent Head	Amor-phous	Small Head	Large Head	Two Head	Taper. Head

12. Comments_____
_____
_____
_____

_____   _____
Technologist   Andrologist

Prepared by B.A. Keel, 1989 (see chapter 3).

APPENDIX VI
The Diagnosis of Oocyte Maturation

1. Cellular Morphology
   a. Mature (preovulatory) oocyte
      — Round and even ooplasm, lightly colored, homogeneous in granularity
      — An expanded and radiant (sunburst) corona radiata
      — Cumulus cells which are present in a thin mucopolysaccharide mass (the expanded cumulus)
   b. Immature (unripened) oocyte
      — Centrally darkened and unevenly shaped ooplasm
      — A compact layer of cells surrounding the oocyte (the compact corona)
      — Either no cumulus mass present or a dense cumulus

2. Nuclear morphology
   a. Metaphase II— Cellular characteristics as noted above with mature oocytes; first polar body present in the perivitelline space
   b. Metaphase I — Cellular characteristics as noted above with either mature or immature oocytes; no first polar body, no germinal vesicle present
   c. Prophase I — Cellular characteristics as noted above for immature oocytes (typically); distinct germinal vesicle present

3. Insemination timetable
   MII: Inseminated 3—5 h after collection.
   MI: Inseminated 2—3 h after first polar body observed (oocytes examined each 3 h).
   PI: Inseminated 2—3 h after first polar body observed or at standard time of 29 h post collection.
   DEG: Not inseminated.
   FZ: Not inseminated.

Prepared by L. Veeck, 1989 (see Chapter 19).

APPENDIX VII A

CENTER FOR REPRODUCTIVE MEDICINE

UNIVERSITY OF KANSAS SCHOOL OF MEDICINE

IVF LABORATORY MEDIA PREPARATION SHEET

HAMS F-10

Date:_____

Prepared by:_____

9.8 g/L powdered Hams F-10   Lot #_____Co._____

0.075 g/L Benzyl Penicillin G   Lot #_____Co._____

0.050 g/L Streptomycin Sulfate   Lot #_____Co._____

0.2452 g/L Calcium Lactate L(+)   Lot #_____Co._____

1.680 g/L Sodium Bicarbonate   Lot #_____Co._____

0.5076 g/L $KHCO_3$ Lot #_____Co._____

qs to 100 ml

Osmolarity: 1st reading_____

        Adjusted reading_____

pH - unadjusted reading, no CO_2 equilibration_____

        Adjusted reading_____

MOUSE EMBRYO QUALITY CONTROL

                                    Mouse Run

                        I_____II_____III_____IV

% Blastocyst Development

May and Hanshew, Organization of the *In Vitro* Fertilization/Embryo Transfer Lab

APPENDIX VII B

CENTER FOR REPRODUCTIVE MEDICINE

UNIVERSITY OF KANSAS SCHOOL OF MEDICINE

IVF LABORATORY MEDIA PREPARATION SHEET

<u>DULBECCO'S PHOSPHATE BUFFERED SALINE (DPBS)</u>

Date:_____

Prepared by:_____

9.6 g/L powdered DPBS   Lot #_____Co._____

0.1 g/L CaCl$_2$ Lot #_____Co._____

0.075 g/L Benzyl Penicillin G   Lot #_____Co._____

0.075 g/L Streptomycin Sulfate   Lot #_____Co._____

qs to 1000 ml

Osmolarity: 1st reading_____

        Adjusted reading_____

pH - unadjusted reading, no CO$_2$ equilibration_____

40 u/ml Heparin_____

<u>MOUSE EMBRYO QUALITY CONTROL</u>

Mouse Run

I	II	III	IV

% Blastocyst Development

May and Hanshew, Organization of the *In Vitro* Fertilization/Embryo Transfer Lab

APPENDIX VII C

Date: _____

Order Number: _____

Contents of Order: _____

Date Mice Received: _____

Mouse Run Number: _____

Tech ID: _____

Mouse Number	Total Number Embryos	Oviduct	Cell Stage 1	Cell Stage 2
1		A		
		B		
2		A		
		B		
3		A		
		B		
4		A		
		B		
5		A		
		B		

Notes and Comments:

May and Hanshew, Organization of the *In Vitro* Fertilization/Embryo Transfer Lab

APPENDIX VII D

CENTER FOR REPRODUCTIVE MEDICINE
UNIVERSITY OF KANSAS SCHOOL OF MEDICINE
IVF Laboratory-Mouse Embryo Observation Form

Date:
Order Number:
Contents of Order:

Date Mice Received:
Mouse Run Number:
Tech I.D.:

Plate I.D.	Time/Day of Observation	Cell 1	Stage 2	3	4	5	6	8	Morula	Blastocyst	Degenerate	Hatched

May and Hanshew, Organization of the *In Vitro* Fertilization/Embryo Transfer Lab

APPENDIX VII E

CENTER FOR REPRODUCTIVE MEDICINE

UNIVERSITY OF KANSAS SCHOOL OF MEDICINE

IVF LABORATORY

Mouse Quality Assurance

Summary Sheet

Date:_____   Tech I.D.:_____

Order Number:_____

Contents of Order:_____

Date Mice Received:_____

Mouse Run Number:_____

_____

_____

Average Number Embryos/Mouse:_____

Average Number embryos developing to blastocyst:_____

Percent embryos developing to blastocyst:_____

Were any embryos cryopreserved?_____ (Y/N)

Number of embryos cryopreserved:_____

Number of embryos which survived cryopreservation:_____

Number of embryos developing to blastocyst following cryopreservation:_____

Percent of embryos developing to blastocyst following cryopreservation:_____

May and Hanshew, Organization of the *In Vitro* Fertilization/Embryo Transfer Lab

APPENDIX VII F

CENTER FOR REPRODUCTIVE MEDICINE

UNIVERSITY OF KANSAS SCHOOL OF MEDICINE

IVF - GIFT SEMENOLOGY DATA

Date_____

_____   _____
Wife's Last,   First Name   Husband's Last,   First Name

Semen Collection Time_____

Pre-Volume_____ ml_____

Pre-concentration_____ x 10^6/ml_____

Total Number _____ x 10^6_____

Pre-Motile_____ %_____

Pre-Progressive Motile_____ %_____

Motile Density (Motile sperm/ml)_____ x 10^6_____

Rise: Time in Incubator: In_____ Out_____

Comments:_____

_____

- -

Post-Concentration_____ /ml_____

Post-Motile_____ %_____

Post Progressive _____ %_____

Motile Density (motile sperm/ml)_____

Eggs Inseminated: Number_____

Insemination Volume (ul)_____

Number Sperm/Egg_____

Insemination Date_____Time:_____

Sperm Pre-Incubation Hours_____

May and Hanshew, Organization of the *In Vitro* Fertilization/Embryo Transfer Lab

APPENDIX VII G

CENTER FOR REPRODUCTIVE MEDICINE
UNIVERSITY OF KANSAS SCHOOL OF MEDICINE
IVF/ET LABORATORY
Oocyte Retrieval Record

Patient_____   Retrieval Date_____

FOLLICLE DATA:

Aspirate Tube #												
Ovary (L/R)												
Follicle #												
Tube Contents (Aspirate)												
Volume (ml)												
Color												
OOCYTE DATA:												
Oocyte #												
Granulosa Cells												
Mucus												
Cumulus												
Corona												
Oocyte Grade												
Incubation Time												
IVF/Transfer #												

Oocyte Classification Code:

1. Immature: Tight Corona and cumulus, no mucus
2. Intermediate: Slight to expanded cumulus; tight to moderate corona; mucus present
3. Mature: mucus; expanded cumulus; expanded, radiant corona; many granulosa cells
4. Post-Mature: Dark ooplasm; corona clumped and dark, granulosa cells clumped
5. Degenerate/Atreitic

Granulosa Cell Code: Aspirate Color Code: Aspirate Identification Code:

   N - None   Clr - Clear   1. Follicular Fluid
   F - Few   Stw - Straw Colored   2. Follicle Wash
   S - Some   Bld - Bloody   3. Apparatus Wash
   M - Many   4. Cul-de-sac
                                       5. Other (Blind Stick, etc.

May and Hanshew, Organization of the *In Vitro* Fertilization/Embryo Transfer Lab

APPENDIX VII H

CENTER FOR REPRODUCTIVE MEDICINE
UNIVERSITY OF KANSAS SCHOOL OF MEDICINE

IVF/ET LABORATORY

Oocyte/Embryo Observation Form

Patient_____   Retrieval Date:_____

OOCYTE/EMBRYO

Observation #1

Date					
Time					
Mucus					
Cumulus					
Corona					
Inseminate					
Degenerate					
Comments					
Drawing					
Photo					

Observation #2

Date					
Time					
Mucus					
Cumulus					
Corona					
Inseminate					
Fertilized					
Cleaved					
Comments					
Drawing					
Photo					

May and Hanshew, Organization of the *In Vitro* Fertilization/Embryo Transfer Lab

APPENDIX VII I

CENTER FOR REPRODUCTIVE MEDICINE

UNIVERSITY OF KANSAS SCHOOL OF MEDICINE

IVF LABORATORY
EMBRYO TRANSFER

Date: _____

Patient Name: _____

LABORATORY ONLY
_____

Insemination: Date: _____   Time: _____

Embryo Transfer:

                Removed From Culture: Time: _____

                             Transfer: Time: _____

                       Difference: Time: _____   Mins.

Amount Media Transferred: _____   Type Media: _____

Number Embryos Transferred: _____

Cell Stage: #1: _____ #2: _____ #3: _____ #4: _____ #5: _____

PHYSICIAN ONLY
_____

Patient Position: _____

Cervical Manipulation: Yes: _____ No: _____

                Method: _____

Catheter: Easy Passage: Yes: _____ No: _____

                Explain: _____

Leakage: Yes: _____ No: _____   Cramping: Yes: _____ No: _____

Bleeding: Yes: _____ No: _____   Comments: _____

Overall Estimate of Transfer (1-5): _____
        1= Easy   5= Failed

Initials of Transfer MD: _____   Tech ID: _____

May and Hanshew, Organization of the *In Vitro* Fertilization/Embryo Transfer Lab

APPENDIX VII J

CENTER FOR REPRODUCTIVE MEDICINE
UNIVERSITY OF KANSAS SCHOOL OF MEDICINE
IVF LABORATORY
Cryopreservation Media

Date: _____

Prepared By: _____

Dulbecco's PBS (DPBS)   Prepared On: _____

Human Serum Albumin   Lot Number: _____

Sucrose   Lot Number: _____

1,2 Propanediol (PDiol)   Lot Number: _____

Stock Solutions:

Solution 1: 11.0 ml PDiol + 6.85 gm Sucrose, q.s. to 100 ml with DPBS

Solution 2: 6.85 gm Sucrose, q.s. to 100 ml with DPBS

Solution 3: 11.0 ul PDiol, q.s. to 100 ml with DPBS

Filter Steralize Solutions 1-3

Working Solutions:

1. 1.5 M prop. diol/0.2 M sucrose/DPBS/0.3% HSA:
    45 ml solution 1 + 0.54 ml HSA.

2. 1.0 M prop. diol/0.2 M sucrose/DPBS/HSA:
    30 ml solution 1 + 15 ml solution 2 + 0.54 ml HSA.

3. 0.5 M prop. diol/0.2 M sucrose/DPBS/HSA:
    15 ml solution 1 + 30 ml solution 2 + 0.54 ml HSA.

4. 0.0 M prop. diol/0.2 M sucrose/DPBS/HSA:
    45 ml solution 2 + 0.54 ml HSA.

5. 1.5 M prop. diol/DPBS/HSA:
    45 ml solution 3 + 0.54 ml HSA.

6. 1.0 M prop. diol/DPBS/HSA:
    30 ml solution 3 + 15 ml DPBS + 0.54 ml HSA.

7. 0.5 M prop. diol/DPBS/HSA:
    15 ml solution 3 + 30 ml DPBS + 0.54 ml HSA.

8. 0.0 M prop. diol/DPBS/HSA:
    45 ml DPBS + 0.54 ml HSA

Percent mouse embryo survival: _____

Percent development to blastocyst: _____

May and Hanshew, Organization of the *In Vitro* Fertilization/Embryo Transfer Lab

APPENDIX VII K

CENTER FOR REPRODUCTIVE MEDICINE
UNIVERSITY OF KANSAS SCHOOL OF MEDICINE
IVF/ET LABORATORY
GIFT SUMMARY

Patient_____

Date_____

FOLLICLE # RETRIEVED OOCYTES	OOCYTE DISPOSITION	IVF INSEM.	HOURS IN CULTURE	DATE FROZEN	STAGE AT FREEZING	FREEZING DESIGNATION	THAW DATE	NUMBER BLASTOMERES VIABLE	SPECIAL TRM'T	COMMENTS

May and Hanshew, Organization of the *In Vitro* Fertilization/Embryo Transfer Lab

APPENDIX VII L

CENTER FOR REPRODUCTIVE MEDICINE
UNIVERSITY OF KANSAS SCHOOL OF MEDICINE
IVF LABORATORY
Frozen Embryo/Oocyte Log

Date Frozen	Patient Name	Dewar Number	Holder Number	Cane Number	Cane Color	Description of Straw	Number and Description Of Embryo	Number Transferred	Number Degenerate

May and Hanshew, Organization of the *In Vitro* Fertilization/Embryo Transfer Lab

APPENDIX VII M

CENTER FOR REPRODUCTIVE MEDICINE
UNIVERSITY OF KANSAS SCHOOL OF MEDICINE
IVF LABORATORY
Frozen/Thaw Embryo Transfer

Date: _____

Patient Name: _____

Insemination Date: _____ Time: _____

LABORATORY ONLY

Frozen/Thaw Information:

Removed From Liquid N2: Time: _____

Placed In Incubator: Time: _____

Stepwide Cryoprotectant Removal: Yes: _____ No: _____
If No, Comment:

Cell State: #1: _____ #2: _____ #3: _____ #4: _____ #5: _____
Appearance of Embryos:

Embryo Transfer:

Removed From Culture: Time: _____

            Transfer: Time: _____

          Difference: Time: _____ Mins.

Amount of Media Transferred: _____ ul   Type Media: _____

Number Embryos Transferred: _____

PHYSICIAN ONLY

Patient Position: _____ Cervical Manipulation: Yes: _____ No: _____

                                      Method: _____

Catheter: Easy Passage: Yes: _____ No: _____
Explain: _____

Leakage: Yes: _____ No: _____   Cramping: Yes: _____ No: _____

Bleeding: Yes: _____ No: _____   Comments: _____

Overall Eastimate of Transfer (1-5): _____ 1= Easy 5= Failed

Initials of Transfer MD: _____ Tech ID: _____

May and Hanshew, Organization of the *In Vitro* Fertilization/Embryo Transfer Lab

APPENDIX VII N

CENTER FOR REPRODUCTIVE MEDICINE

UNIVERSITY OF KANSAS SCHOOL OF MEDICINE

IVF LABORATORY
Temperature Log

Instrument: Year:

Serial Number:

Location:

Date	Degrees Centigrade	Tech ID	Date	Degrees Centigrade	Tech ID	Date	Degrees Centigrade	Tech ID

May and Hanshew, Organization of the *In Vitro* Fertilization/Embryo Transfer Lab

APPENDIX VII O

CENTER FOR REPRODUCTIVE MEDICINE

UNIVERSITY OF KANSAS SCHOOL OF MEDICINE

IVF LABORATORY
Incubator Quality Control

Serial Number: Year:
Location:

Date	Time	Degrees C 37° +/- 0.5	%CO$_2$ 5% +/- 0.5	Tech ID	Date	Time	Degrees C 37° +/1 0.5	% CO$_2$1 5% +/0 0.5	Tech ID

May and Hanshew, Organization of the *In Vitro* Fertilization/Embryo Transfer Lab

APPENDIX VII P

CENTER FOR REPRODUCTIVE MEDICINE

UNIVERSITY OF KANSAS SCHOOL OF MEDICINE

IVF LABORATORY
pH Meter Quality Control

Serial Number:
Location: Year:
7.0 Buffer Lot Number:
7.4 Buffer Lot Number:

Date	7.0 Buffer +/- 0.01	7.4 Buffer +/- 0.01	Tech ID	Date	7.0 Buffer +/- 0.01	7.4 Buffer +/- 0.01	Tech ID

May and Hanshew, Organization of the *In Vitro* Fertilization/Embryo Transfer Lab

APPENDIX VII Q

CENTER FOR REPRODUCTIVE MEDICINE

UNIVERSITY OF KANSAS SCHOOL OF MEDICINE

IVF LABORATORY
Osmometer Quality Control

Serial Number: 100 mOsm Lot Number: Year:
                                 290 mOsm Lot Number:
                            1000 mOsm Lot Number:

Date	100 mOsm Standard +/- 5	290 mOsm Standard +/- 5	1000 mOsm Standard +/- 5	Water Control 0-30	Tech ID

May and Hanshew, Organization of the *In Vitro* Fertilization/Embryo Transfer Lab

APPENDIX VII R

CENTER FOR REPRODUCTIVE MEDICINE

UNIVERSITY OF KANSAS SCHOOL OF MEDICINE

IVF Laboratory
Liquid N_2 Dewar

Quality Control   Year:

Date	Dewar ID	Liquid N_2 Level 33+/-5cm	Add Liquid N_2 Yes No	Tech ID	Date	Dewar ID	Liquid N_2 Level 33+/-5cm	Add Liquid N_2 Yes No	Tech ID

May and Hanshew, Organization of the *In Vitro* Fertilization/Embryo Transfer Lab

APPENDIX VII S

CENTER FOR REPRODUCTIVE MEDICINE

UNIVERSITY OF KANSAS SCHOOL OF MEDICINE

IVF LABORATORY
CO_2 Tank Record

Location:

Tank Started: Year:

Date	Tank Pressure	Regulator 5-10 psi	Tech ID	Date	Tank Pressure	Regulator 5-10 psi	Tech ID

May and Hanshew, Organization of the *In Vitro* Fertilization/Embryo Transfer Lab

APPENDIX VII T

CENTER FOR REPRODUCTIVE MEDICINE

UNIVERSITY OF KANSAS SCHOOL OF MEDICINE

IVF LABORATORY
Instrument Maintenance

Instrument:

Serial Number: Year:

Location:

Date	Maintenance Performed	Tech ID	Date	Maintenance Performed	Tech ID

May and Hanshew, Organization of the *In Vitro* Fertilization/Embryo Transfer Lab

APPENDIX VIII
Rules for Dating the Endometrium

1. Fundal specimen.
2. Capsule must be present for accurate evaluation. Dating should be made from stratum spongiosum until day 23, and then compacta and spongiosa are important.
3. Date to the most advanced portion or feature (unless only a few glands advanced, and then take the majority).
4. Do not depend on abnormal endometria for accurate dating; i.e., chronic endometritis, polyps, etc.
5. At least 50% of the glands must have subnuclear vacuoles to say that ovulation has occurred.
6. Date a 2-day span; e.g., 16-17 days, 19-20 days, etc.

16th day
Subnuclear vacuoles
Pseudostratification
Mitoses, glands and stroma

17th day
More or less orderly row of nuclei
Cytoplasm above nuclei and subnuclear vacuoles below
Gland and stromal mitoses
Very, very, very minimal secretion

18th day
Vacuoles above and below nuclei
Gland mitoses rare
Improved linear arrangement of nuclei
Stromal mitoses rare
Bubbles of secretion seen at luminal border

19th day
A few vacuoles remain in cell. Mainly active evacuation with intraluminal secretion
No gland or stromal mitoses
May look like day 16 but *NO* pseudostratification

20th day
Peak secretion with "ragged" luminal border
Vacuoles are rare — all subnuclear vacuoles gone; inspissation may be beginning

21st day
Abrupt onset of stromal edema
Gland secretion prominent (inspissated)
"Naked" stromal nuclei begin to appear

22nd day
Peak edema
Marked appearance of "naked" stromal nuclei; stromal cells small and dense filamentous cytoplasm
Active secretion, but subsiding
Rare stromal mitosis

23rd day
Prominent spiral arterioles
Periarteriolar cuffing with *enlargement of stromal cell nuclei and cytoplasm *(earliest predecidual change)
Stromal mitoses
Glands with secretory "exhaustion" — low columnar cells, luminal edges ragged

24th day
Definite predecidual cells around arterioles with early subepithelial changes
Greater stromal mitoses
Ragged cell borders; i.e., secretorily exhausted

25th day
Definite subcapsular predecidua
Inspissated secretion noted to begin
Early stromal infiltration with lymphocytes and occasional PMNs

26th day
Generalized decidual reaction—decidual islands in stroma
Polymorphonuclear leukocytic invasion (lymphocytes may accompany or precede)

27th day
Solid sheet of decidua
Marked leukocytic infiltrate polyps
Inspissated secretion with variable intracellular secretory activity

28th day
Focal necrosis and hemorrhage
Peak leukocytic infiltration polyps prominent
Cells may show secretory exhaustion or may show active secretion (VARIABLE)
Beginning stromal clumping and fragmentation of glands

Menstruating
Disruption of capsular layer
Stromal clumping
Glandular break-up and hemorrhage
Variable leukocytic infiltration
Edema
After 24 h, metaplastic alterations on surface

INDEX